AF680997

ANTITHROMBOTICS

Developments in Cardiovascular Medicine

VOLUME 126

The titles published in this series are listed at the end of this volume.

ANTITHROMBOTICS

Pathophysiological Rationale for Pharmacological Interventions

edited by

ARNOLD G. HERMAN

Professor of Pharmacology,
University of Antwerp (UIA),
Antwerp, Belgium

KLUWER ACADEMIC PUBLISHERS

DORDRECHT / BOSTON / LONDON

ISBN 0-7923-1413-1

QV
190
A633
1991

Published by Kluwer Academic Publishers,
P.O. Box 17, 3300 AA Dordrecht, The Netherlands.

Kluwer Academic Publishers incorporates
the publishing programmes of
D. Reidel, Martinus Nijhoff, Dr W. Junk and MTP Press.

Sold and distributed in the U.S.A. and Canada
by Kluwer Academic Publishers,
101 Philip Drive, Norwell, MA 02061, U.S.A.

In all other countries, sold and distributed
by Kluwer Academic Publishers Group,
P.O. Box 322, 3300 AH Dordrecht, The Netherlands.

Printed on acid-free paper

All Rights Reserved
© 1991 Kluwer Academic Publishers
No part of the material protected by this copyright notice may be reproduced or
utilized in any form or by any means, electronic or mechanical,
including photocopying, recording or by any information storage and
retrieval system, without written permission from the copyright owner.

Printed in the Netherlands

Contents

Preface vii

List of contributors ix

1. Platelet activation and aggregation: rationale for combining antithrombotic drugs
A.G. Herman 1

2. Role of nitric oxide in endothelial cell - platelet interactions
M.W. Radomski and S. Moncada 27

3. Platelets and megakaryocytes in vascular disease
J.F. Martin and P.M.W. Bath 49

4. Thrombosis in relation to atherosclerosis
N. Woolf 63

5. Pharmacological inhibition of the ADP-GP IIb/IIIa-fibrinogen pathway of platelet aggregation
J.-P. Cazenave, C. Gachet and F. Lanza 83

6. Calcium fluxes in platelets and endothelial cells, mechanisms and functional significance
T.J. Hallam 99

7. Inhibition of platelet function by cyclic nucleotides and cyclic nucleotide-dependent protein kinases
U. Walter, C. Nolte, J. Geiger, P. Schanzenbächer and K. Kochsiek 121

8. Pharmacological modification of platelet-derived cyclooxygenase product formation and its consequences for platelet-vessel wall interactions
K. Schrör 139

9. Antithrombotics and the lipoxygenase pathway
M.R. Buchanan and S.J. Brister 159

10. Pathological expressions of platelet-vessel wall interactions: implications of serotonin
F. De Clerck 181

11. The involvement of PAF in thrombotic events
C.P. Page, C.M. Herd and W. Paul 195

12. Prostaglandins and -analogs in the treatment of platelet-vessel wall interaction
H. Sinzinger 205

13. Adjuvant agents to enhance and sustain reperfusion with t-PA: studies in experimental dog models
H.K. Gold, T. Yasuda, I.K. Jang, L. Guerrero, J.T. Fallon, R.C. Leinbach and D. Collen 221

14. Effect of dietary marine lipids on (anti-)thrombotic mechanisms
G. Hornstra 233

Index 251

Preface

A number of exciting new developments have occurred during the last few years concerning the platelet-vessel wall interaction. Although they may be obvious and clear to the specialist in the field, for the clinician the area has become rather confusing. Time has come to review current knowledge on the pathophysiology of the platelet-vessel wall interaction and show how this knowledge can constitute the rationale for pharmacotherapeutic interventions.

A symposium was organized in Antwerp during which a number of outstanding speakers gave an overview of what is new on a particular topic and how this information can be translated to possible clinical applications.

The proceedings of the symposium are not only of interest to the practising physician, but contain enough new fundamental data to be of use for all those who are interested in the role of platelets in the etiopathogenes of cardiovascular diseases.

Arnold G. Herman
Antwerp, July 1991

List of Contributors

M.R. Buchanan
Department of Pathology
McMaster Clinic
Hamilton General Hospital
237 Barton Street East
HAMILTON, Ontario
Canada L8L 2X2

Co-author: S.J. Brister

J.-P. Cazenave
Regional Centre of Blood Transfusion
10, Rue Spielmann
F-67085 STRASBOURG Cedex
France

Co-authors: C. Gachet and F. Lanza

F. De Clerck
Department of Cardiovascular Pharmacology
Janssen Research Foundation
Turnhoutseweg 30
B-2340 BEERSE
Belgium

H.K. Gold
Cardiac Unit
Massachusetts General Hospital
Fruit Street
BOSTON, MA 02114
U.S.A.

Co-author: D. Collen

T.J. Hallam
Roche Products Ltd.
P.O. Box 8
WELWYN GARDEN CITY, Herts. AL7 3AY
U.K.

A.G. Herman
Department of Pharmaceutical Sciences
University Hospital
Universiteitsplein 1
B-2610 ANTWERP (Wilrijk)
Belgium

G. Hornstra
Department of Human Biology
University of Limburg
P.O. Box 616
6200 MD MAASTRICHT
The Netherlands

J.F. Martin
Department of Medicine
King's College School of Medicine and Dentistry
LONDON SE5 9PE
U.K.

Co-author: P.M.W. Bath

C.P. Page
Pharmacology Group
King's College
University of London
Manresa Road
LONDON SW3 6LX
U.K.

Co-authors: C.M. Herd and W. Paul

M.W. Radomski
The Wellcome Research Laboratories
Langley Court
South Eden Park Road
BECKENHAM, Kent BR3 3BS
U.K.

Co-author: S. Moncada

K. Schrör
Institute for Pharmacology
Heinrich-Heine-University Düsseldorf
Moorenstrasse 5
DW-4000 DÜSSELDORF 1
Germany

H. Sinzinger
Wilhelm Auerswald Atherosclerosis
Research Group (ASF) Vienna
Nadlergasse 1
A-1090 VIENNA
Austria

U. Walter
Clinical Research Unit
Medical University Clinic
Josef-Schneider-Strasse 2
DW-8700 WÜRZBURG
Germany

Co-authors: C. Nolte, J. Geiger, P.
Schanzenbächer and K. Kochsiek

N. Woolf
Department of Histopathology
University College and
Middlesex School of Medicine
Mortimer Street
LONDON W1P 7PN
U.K.

PLATELET ACTIVATION AND AGGREGATION : RATIONALE FOR COMBINING ANTITHROMBOTIC DRUGS

A.G. HERMAN

ABSTRACT

Exposure of the GPIIb/IIIa receptor, the final common pathway of aggregation, can be obtained via different mechanisms and by different stimuli. The synthesis of thromboxane A_2 can be blocked by aspirin and thromboxane synthase inhibitors, whereas its activity can be blocked by antagonists or by combined synthase inhibitors/antagonists. Agents that increase cAMP/cGMP prevent the exposure of the GPIIb/IIIa receptor and by also inhibiting the release reaction, are likely to have a broader spectrum of activity than pure GPIIb/IIIa receptor antagonists.

Combination of antithrombotic drugs has the possible advantage that different pathways of aggregation are affected, that the release of growth factors and/or procoagulants could be inhibited, that the presence of synergism will increase the efficacy and that other (mainly vascular) effects could be modulated. A multitude of in vitro and in vivo experimental data prove the superiority of such a combination and careful analysis of the clinical studies point also in that direction.

A. G. Herman (ed.), Antithrombotics, 1–26.
© 1991 *Kluwer Academic Publishers. Printed in the Netherlands.*

1. INTRODUCTION

Platelet activation is initiated by the interaction of various agonists with their respective receptor at the platelet surface. When activation finally results in the exposure and activation of the GPIIb/IIIa receptor, binding will occur with fibrinogen and platelet aggregation will ensue. Exposure of the GPIIb/IIIa, which is the final common pathway (Fig. 1) leading to aggregation, can however be obtained via different mechanisms and by different stimuli.

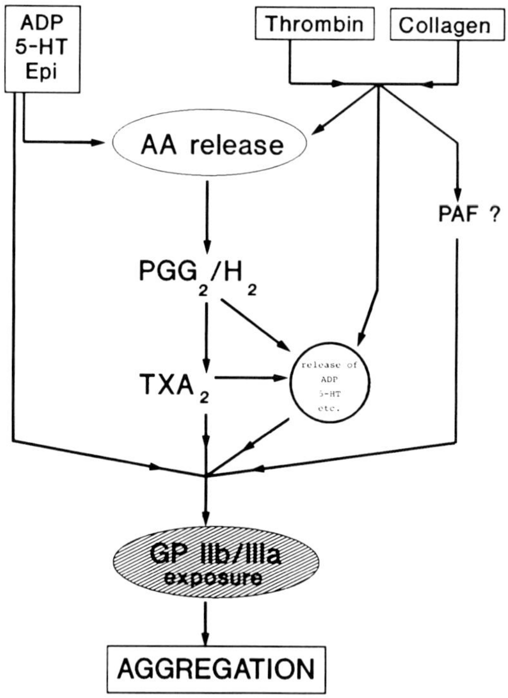

FIG. 1.

Different pathways of platelet activation lead to the exposure of the GPIIb/IIIa receptor which results in platelet aggregation after the binding of fibrinogen.
AA = arachidonic acid; PGG_2/H_2 = prostaglandin endoperoxides G_2 and H_2; 5-HT = 5-hydroxytryptamine; ADP = adenosine diphosphate; Epi = epinephrine.

Although most of the agonists can release arachidonic acid, which is subsequently metabolised to the potent pro-aggregating substance thromboxane A_2 (TXA_2), some of them can bypass this arachidonic acid pathway and activate the GPIIb/IIIa receptor either directly or indirectly via the release of adenosine diphosphate (ADP) and 5-hydroxytryptamine (5-HT, serotonin) from the dense granules, or via a third, still not fully determined pathway, which might involve the production of platelet-activating factor (PAF). From this it becomes clear that these agonists can still induce the exposure of the GPIIb/IIIa receptor, even when the arachidonic acid pathway is not longer fully operative. Furthermore, since no mediator is responsible for the aggregation, depending on the peculiarities of a given situation, all of them could be equally involved or one of them could play a more dominant role. It should also be realised that some of the mediators released from the platelet act synergistically (1), or can even potentiate each other (2), and by interfering with the production or activity of only one of the mediators, one often overlooks the possibility of the potentiating effect of the others.

Platelet aggregation should not only be looked upon as being implicated in the process of (acute) thrombosis with all its possible clinical consequences, but also as being involved in the processes of smooth muscle proliferation, migration and neo-intima formation as a result of the release of growth factors (a.o. platelet-derived growth factor and transforming growth factor ß) from the alpha-granules. The latter phenomenon could be important in the etiopathogenesis of e.g. atherosclerosis and, although blockade of the aggregation might indeed prevent the immediate occlusion of the vessel lumen, it does not obligatory implie the continuous blockade of the release of the platelet-derived vasoactive substances (such as TXA_2 and 5-HT) or platelet-derived growth factors.

2. ANTI-AGGREGATING AGENTS : MODE OF ACTION

Inhibition of aggregation can be obtained either by suppressing all pro-aggregating activity which is, or can be made available to the platelets, or by stimulating those factors which are normally present in the body and which have anti-aggregating activity.

2.1. INHIBITION OF PRO-AGGREGATING ACTIVITY

2.1.1. Antagonism of the pro-aggregating stimuli

The formation of thrombin can be prevented by heparin and the oral anticoagulants, whereas its platelet-aggregating activity can be inhibited by heparin, hirudin (an irreversible inhibitor) or argatroban, the latter being a synthetic competitive thrombin antagonist. Although these agents have been shown to prevent thrombosis in various animal models (3), their efficacy could be markedly increased by conjunction with antiplatelet agents and/or fibrinolytic agents (see Gold et al., this volume).

Although the receptor antagonists to ADP have not yet been tested clinically, a drug which specifically interferes with ADP induced aggregation, i.e. ticlopidine, has been shown in various clinical trials to interfere efficaciously with platelet aggregation (see Cazenave et al., this volume). Although its mode of action is not completely understood, it probably impairs the ADP signal transduction which might involve an inhibitory G-protein (4). Ketanserin, a selective 5-HT_2 antagonist, prevents the pro-aggregating as well as the vasoconstrictor activity of 5-HT and has been shown, either alone or in combination with other anti-aggregating substances, to exert some beneficial effects in animal models as well as in humans (see De Clerck, this volume).

A number of orally active PAF antagonists have been developed which selectively inhibit PAF induced platelet aggregation (5). Since they do not have a marked influence on bleeding time (6), it is suggested that PAF is not physiologically important in haemostasis (see Herd et al., this volume).

2.1.2. The arachidonic acid pathway

i) Cyclooxygenase inhibitors

Aspirin and aspirin-like drugs block the cyclooxygenase thereby preventing the formation of the prostaglandin endoperoxides G_2 (PGG_2) and H_2 (PGH_2) and TXA_2. Although aspirin, which blocks the cyclooxygenase irreversibly, is so far the most widely investigated anti-aggregating substance, its use carries a number of drawbacks. Since it blocks the cyclooxygenase not only in the platelets but also in the endothelial (and other) cells, it inherently diminishes also the synthesis of the endogenously produced anti-aggregating prostacyclin. Since a nearly complete inhibition of the TXA_2 biosynthesis is required to establish its full antiplatelet activity, reduction of the dosage administered is however limited and therefore only partly removes this possible drawback (7). Furthermore, since the prostacyclin production by the endothelial cells largely thrives on the prostaglandin endoperoxides provided by the platelets colliding with the endothelial cells, even a small dose of aspirin will, via its inhibitory effect on the platelet cyclooxygenase, decrease the prostacyclin production at the sites where it is mostly needed i.e. at places where there is an increased platelet-vessel wall interaction (8, 9). This possible interference with the biosynthesis of prostacyclin not only reduces the drug's own clinical efficacy, but also diminishes the anti-aggregating activity of other substances which require the continuous and uninhibited production of prostacyclin (10). Finally, aspirin blocks only one pathway of aggregation and its anti-aggregating activity is easily overcome by either increasing the dose of the aggregating stimulus (e.g. collagen, thrombin) or by adding a cofactor, even in subtreshold dosis, such as epinephrine or 5-HT (see Buchanan and Brister, this volume).

Furthermore, since platelets, which adhere to collagen are still able to release the content of their granules, even in the presence of aspirin, additional antagonists (e.g. 5-HT antagonists) may be required to further antagonise the pro-aggregating, vasoactive and smooth muscle proliferating effects of these mediators released (cfr. infra).

ii) Thromboxane synthase inhibitors

These substances not only inhibit the formation of the potent pro-aggregating TXA_2, but also redirect the metabolism of the prostaglandin endoperoxides towards the PGI_2 synthesis : the blood emerging from a skin wound contains higher levels of PGI_2 as compared to the circulating plasma levels and they are further increased after the administration of a thromboxane synthase inhibitor (11, 12, 13).

However, the clinical efficacy of these inhibitors has so far been rather disappointing mainly because inhibition of the thromboxane synthase results in the accumulation of the endoperoxides G_2/H_2. The latter, despite that part of it could be redirected to the endothelium for the PGI_2 synthesis, can also interact with the platelet and vascular smooth muscle TXA_2 receptor, thereby inducing platelet aggregation and vasoconstriction. The beneficial effects of the thromboxane synthesis inhibitor are apparently offset by the accumulation of the platelet precursor prostaglandin endoperoxides which have similar effects as TXA_2.

iii) Thromboxane receptor antagonists

The competitive thromboxane receptor antagonists prevent the interaction with its receptor of not only TXA_2 but also of its precursor i.e. the prostaglandin endoperoxides. Therefore, these substances should inhibit platelet aggregation more effectively than the thromboxane synthesis inhibitors but, because they are "competitive" antagonists, their anti-aggregating activity can easily be overcome by the generation and presence of high amounts of TXA_2 which will displace the antagonist from its receptor.

iv) Combined thromboxane synthase inhibitors and thromboxane antagonists

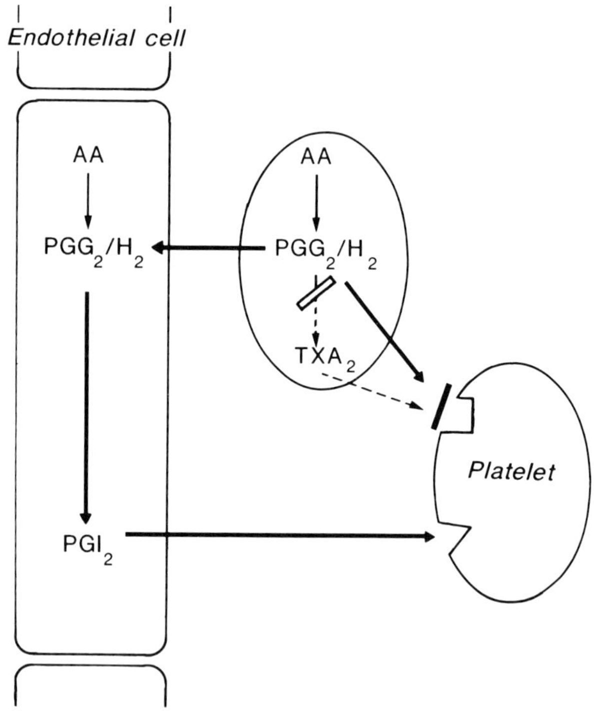

FIG. 2

Combinations of a thromboxane synthase inhibitor and a thromboxane antagonist. Inhibition of thromboxane synthase (▭) results in the accumulation of the endoperoxides G_2/H_2 which are redirected to the endothelium for the (increased) PGI_2 synthesis, but will also interact with the TXA_2 receptor. By incorporating TXA_2-antagonistic activity (▬) in one and the same molecule, the anti-aggregating activity of the thromboxane synthase inhibitor is no longer offset since the accumulated prostaglandin endoperoxides are no longer able to interact efficaciously with the (now blocked) receptor.

These drugs, which combine two activities i.e. they inhibit the thromboxane synthase and at the same time they antagonise the effects of TXA_2 and the prostaglandin endoperoxides G_2/H_2 at the receptor level, have the theoretical advantage that they should offset each others negative as pects (Fig. 2). As mentioned above, the effect of the thromboxane synthase inhibitor is blunted by the accumulation of the prostaglandin endoperoxides and their subsequent interaction with the TXA_2 receptor. By incorporating TXA_2-antagonistic activity in one and the same molecule, the anti-aggregating activity of the thromboxane synthase inhibitor is no longer offset since the accumulated prostaglandin endoperoxides are no longer able to interact efficaciously with the (now blocked) receptor. Furthermore, by inhibiting the formation of TXA_2, that part of the molecule which has TXA_2 antagonist activity now faces only small amounts of TXA_2 and is therefore in a much better position to antagonise the pro-aggregating effects of the (even accumulated) prostaglandin endoperoxides. These substances have been shown to reduce the formation of TXA_2, to increase the production of PGI_2 (14, 15) and to prolong bleeding time in healthy volunteers (16), to reduce elevated levels of platelet-derived ß-thromboglobulin in patients with atherosclerosis obliterans (17).

2.1.3. Agents that increase platelet cAMP/cGMP

The final common pathway i.e. exposure of the GPIIb/IIIa receptor, can be inhibited by agents which increase cyclic adenosine monophosphate (cAMP) and, most likely, also cyclic guanosine monophosphate (cGMP). As shown in Fig. 3 these agents obviously have a much broader spectrum of activity, not only since they will interfere with "all known" pathways of aggregation, but also with the release of substances from the dense (ADP, 5-HT) as well as from the alpha-granules (growth factors). The main endogenously produced stimuli for the platelet adenylate cyclase are most likely prostacyclin and, to a lesser extent PGD_2, whereas nitric oxide is a potent stimulator of the guanylate cyclase. In relation to the platelet-vessel wall interaction (Fig. 4), prostacyclin and nitric oxide are mainly derived from the endothelial cells, whereas the latter can also be made by the platelet under certain conditions (18, 19). Increasing the prostacyclin and/or nitric oxide production will lead to an increased stimulation of the adenylate and/or guanylate cyclase resulting in an increased intracellular concentration of cAMP and/or GMP which will result in the prevention or inhibition of platelet aggrega-

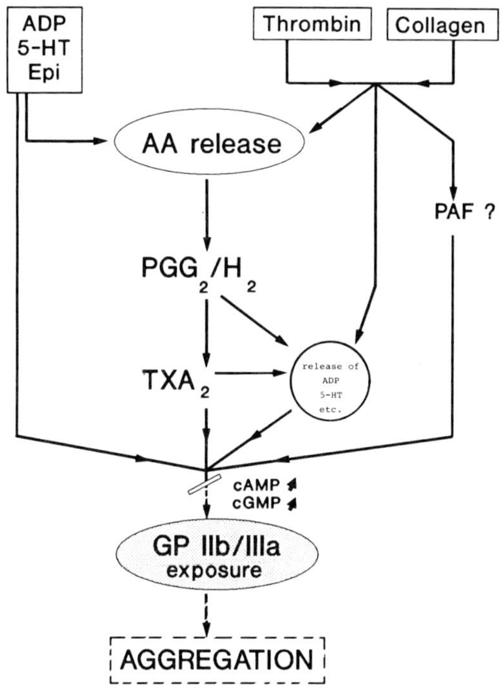

FIG. 3

Increase of cAMP and cGMP results in an inhibition (▭) of the exposure of GPIIb/IIIa, the final common pathway of aggregation. A much broader spectrum of activity can be expected, since they not only interfere with all known pathways of aggregation, but also with the release of substances from the dense (ADP, 5-HT) as well as from the alpha-granules (growth factors).

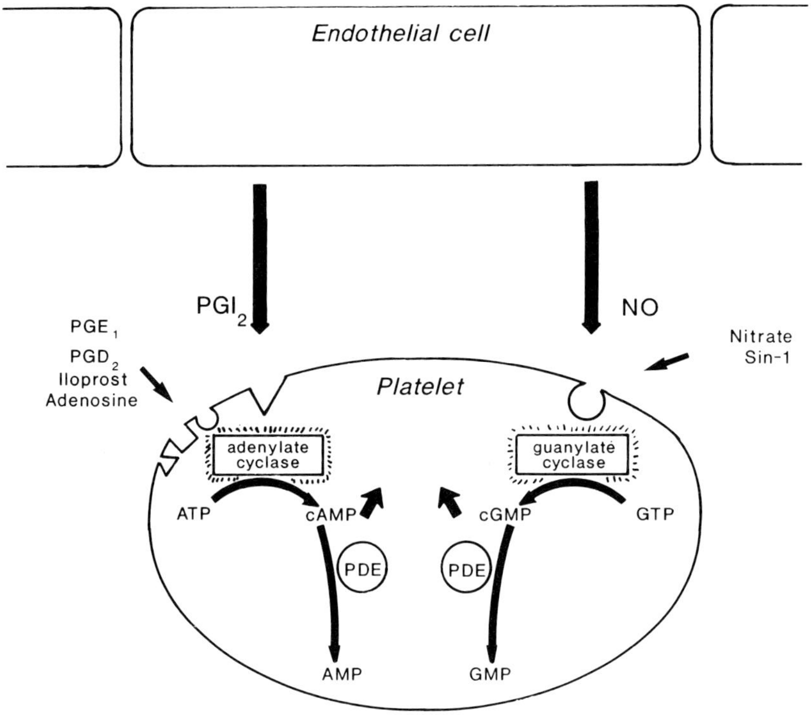

FIG. 4

Increased stimulation of the adenylate and guanylate cyclase will result in increased intracellular concentrations of cAMP and cGMP. This can be obtained by stimulating the production of PGI_2 or nitric oxide in the endothelial cell or by administration of prostaglandins E_1 or D_2, PGI_2-analogs such as iloprost or organic nitrates or SIN-1, the active metabolite of molsidomine.

gation (see Walter et al., this volume). Furthermore, since both cyclic nucleotides act synergistically, even subtreshold amounts of prostacyclin or nitric oxide are able to inhibit efficaciously platelet aggregation. Stimulation of the adenylate and/or guanylate cyclase is the mechanism of action whereby a number of substances such as prostaglandin E_1, iloprost, adenosine, organic nitrates and SIN-1, the active metabolite of molsidomine, exert their anti-aggregating activity.

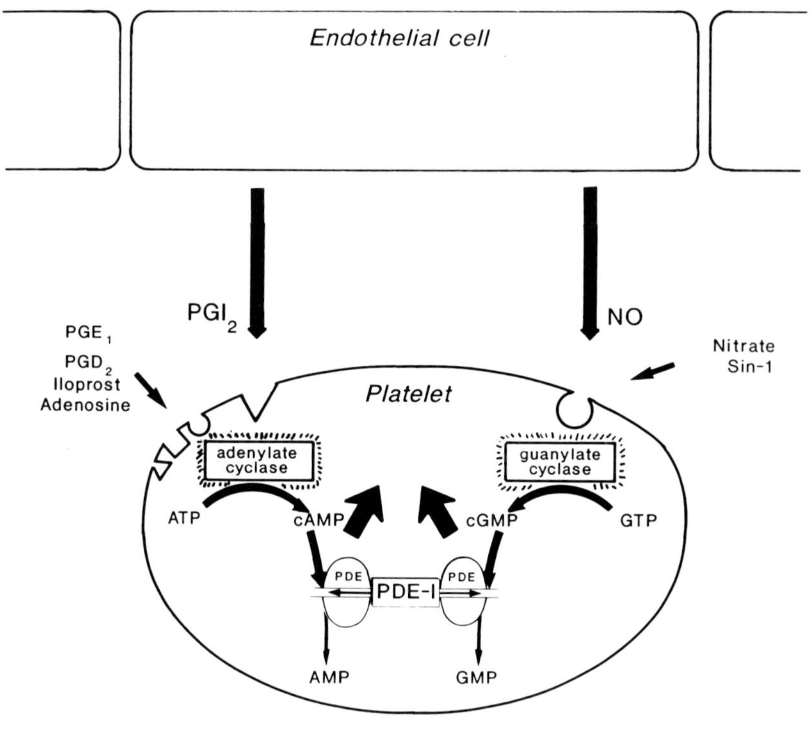

FIG. 5

The combined use of stimulators of the adenylate and/or guanylate cyclase with inhibitors of the phosphodiesterases (PDE-I) will lead to an important increase in the intracellular concentration of cAMP and/or cGMP in the platelet.

Increase of intracellular nucleotides can also be obtained by specific inhibitors of the cAMP- and/or cGMP specific phosphodiesterases (e.g. dipyridamole, zaprinast). The combined use of stimulators of the adenylate and/or guanylate cyclase with inhibitors of the phosphodiesterases will obviously lead to an important increase in the intracellular concentration of both nucleotides (Fig. 5). This is best illustrated by the experiments reported by Bult et al. (20) in which very low amounts of prostacyclin and nitric oxide, which at these concentrations are inactive even when used in combination, become effective as inhibitors of platelet aggregation in the presence of the cGMP-phosphodiesterase inhibitor dipyridamole (Fig. 6).

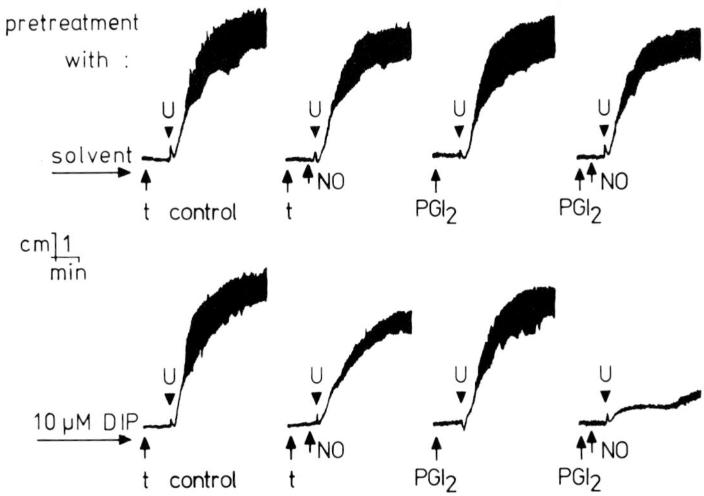

FIG. 6

Dipyridamole potentiates the anti-aggregating activity of nitric oxide (NO) and PGI_2. Subtreshold concentrations of PGI_2 (0.3 nM) and NO (3 μM), which are nearly inactive even used in combination (upper tracing) become effective as inhibitors of platelet aggregation in the presence of the cGMP-phosphodiesterase inhibitor dipyridamole (lower tracing). Aggregation in platelet-rich plasma was induced by 3 μM U-46619. (Adapted from information appearing in Thromb. Haemostașis, Bult et al., 1991, in press).

2.1.4. Inhibition of the fibrinogen binding to GPII/bIIIa

Blocking the GPIIb/IIIa receptor abolishes the binding of fibrinogen to the platelets which will result in inhibition of platelet aggregation. This can be obtained either by monoclonal antibodies, by GPIIb/IIIa related peptides, by fibrinogen-related peptides which contain the arginine-glycine-aspartic (RGD) sequence (21, 22, 23) and by RGD containing peptides present in some snake venoms (24, 25,

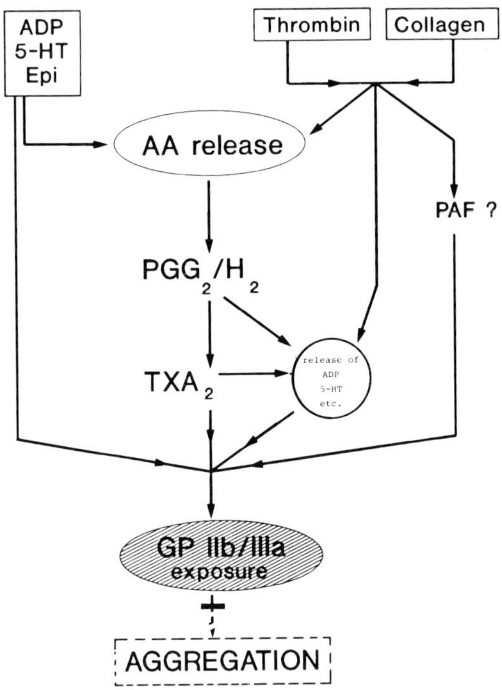

FIG. 7

Blockade of the GPIIb/IIIa receptor (▬) abolishes the binding of fibrinogen to the platelets which will lead to inhibition of platelet aggregation. Since, however, this inhibition is not the result of increased intracellular levels of cAMP and/or cGMP, the release reaction from the dense as well as from the alpha-granules can still occur, depending on the type or intensity of the pro-aggregating stimulus involved.

26). Since blocking the final common pathway of aggregation (Fig. 7) will result in a broader spectrum of anti-aggregating activity, as was also discussed for agents which prevent the exposure of GPIIb/IIIa by increasing the intracellular levels of cAMP and/or cGMP, there is however a distinct difference between both categories of drugs. Indeed, since blockade of the GPIIb/IIIa receptor and subsequent inhibition of the binding of fibrinogen, is not the result of increased levels of cAMP and/or cGMP, the release reaction from the dense as well as from the alpha-granules can still continue, whereby vasoactive substances (e.g. 5-HT) and growth factors can still be released, even in the absence of overt platelet aggregation. Furthermore, due to the lack of selectivity, these substances are likely to interfere with the normal haemostasis, as indicated by their increase of the bleeding time (27). The use of these substances might currently be limited to administration during acute episodes since, being peptides, oral administration is at present not feasible, their half-life is short and they are potentially immunogenic.

2.1.5. Other anti-aggregating drugs

Sulfinpyrazone, which is a competitive inhibitor of the platelet cyclooxygenase, inhibits platelet aggregation, but the exact mechanism of its antithrombotic effect is not well understood (28).

Penicillin G, cephalothin and related antibiotics inhibit aggregation probably by coating the platelet membrane (29) and a similar mechanism may explain the anti-platelet effects of dextran (30).

2.2. STIMULATION OF THE ENDOGENOUS ANTI-AGGREGATING ACTIVITY

A number of physiological stimuli and substances have been described which are able to augment the biosynthesis and/or activity of prostacyclin and/or nitric oxide (for review see ref. 31, 32). In relation to the phenomena of thrombosis and atherosclerosis, in which gross flow disturbances could be expected, it is interesting to note that flow-induced shear stress, acting upon the luminal endothelial surface as viscous drag, as well as pulsatile stretching of the endothelial cells are important stimuli for the release of prostacyclin (33) and nitric oxide (34, 35).

3. COMBINATION OF ANTITHROMBOTIC DRUGS

3.1. RATIONALE

The profile of an "ideal" antithrombotic drug is summarised in table 1.

TABLE 1

PROFILE OF AN "IDEAL" ANTITHROMBOTIC

- Interference with all pathways of aggregation
- No interference with normal haemostasis
  i.e. only active at the site of "thrombosis"
- No interference with normal coagulation
  i.e. no interference with fibrinolytic activity
- Selective interference with release of growth factors
  i.e. no interference with normal tissue repair
- No major side effects
- Easy way of administration
- Reasonable price
- "Clinical" efficacy

Since no such ideal antithrombotic is currently available, the nearest one can possibly get is eventually by the combination of drugs which have a different mechanism of action thereby increasing the spectrum of activity.
The possible advantages of combining antithrombotics are that :

a) **Different pathways of aggregation could be affected.** Since it is very unlikely that only one pro-aggregating stimulus will be involved, and since different mediators produce aggregation via different pathways, one can expect a higher chance to "hit" the whole process of aggregation by combining different drugs which affect the various pathways differently.
Affecting the final common pathway by inhibiting the

exposure of GPIIb/IIIa via an increase in intracellular cAMP/cGMP seems so far the best way of tackling the problem since this will also lead to an inhibition of the release reaction (cfr. supra).

b) **The release of growth factors and/or procoagulants could be affected.**
Platelets not only aggregate but contribute also to the process of coagulation by virtue of the exposure of their membrane and by releasing pro-coagulant factors from their alpha-granules. The latter contain also growth factors and by inhibiting the release reaction from these alpha-granules the process of fibrinolysis will be favoured (see Gold et al., this volume) and the proliferation of the vascular smooth muscle cells will be reduced which a.o. is involved in the etiopathogenesis of atherosclerosis.
In this context it is interesting to note that in a recently published article (36) on the follow-up of the United States Physician's Health Study, the continuous use of 325 mg of aspirin on alternate days was unable to reduce the incidence of angina pectoris, which might be an indication of the progression of atherosclerosis in which platelet-derived growth factors are likely to be involved and whose release was not affected by the continuous administration of aspirin.

c) **The presence of synergism will increase efficacy which can lead to a reduction of dosage and a decreased risk of side effects.**
This has repeatedly been shown in various in vitro and in vivo experimental conditions and is best illustrated in a recently reported animal experiment (Fig. 8) in which the combination of a thromboxane synthase inhibitor and a thromboxane antagonist resulted in an increased reduction of the mortality observed in mice after the intravenous injection of collagen (8). The outcome was dramatically ameliorated by a further association of a phosphodiesterase inhibitor and this amelioration was completely abolished by the addition of aspirin to the treatment. Indeed, since the beneficial effect of the combination of a thromboxane synthase inhibitor with a thromboxane antagonist is mainly due to the shift of the prostaglandin endoperoxide metabolism towards endothelially produced PGI_2, inhibition of the biosynthesis of the latter by aspirin will therefore completely annihilate the beneficial effect of this combination. This also illustrates how the <u>wrong choice</u> in a particular combination can

completely abolish the efficacy of either one of the drugs used or the synergistic activity of the combination.

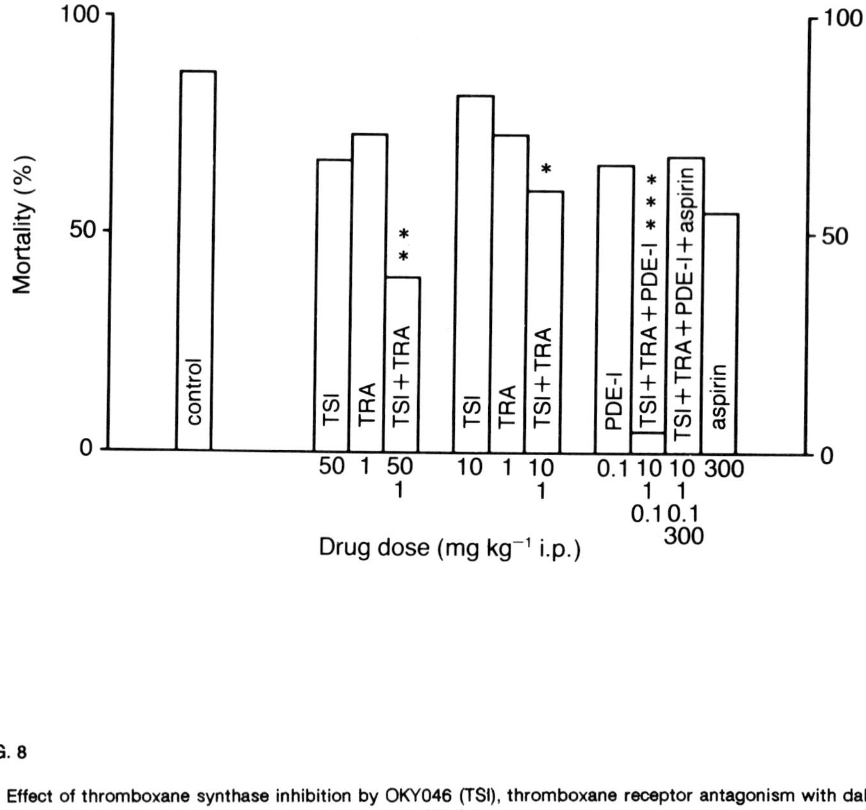

FIG. 8

Effect of thromboxane synthase inhibition by OKY046 (TSI), thromboxane receptor antagonism with daltroban (TRA), phosphodiesterase inhibition with enprofylline (PDE-I), and cyclooxygenase inhibition with aspirin alone or in various combinations, on the mortality due to lung platelet thrombo-embolism provoked in mice by the intravenous injection of collagen plus epinephrine. A synergism between OKY0456 and daltroban and between OKY046 plus daltroban and enprofylline is observed. Aspirin abolishes this synergism.

*, $p < 0.05$; **, $p < 0.01$; ***, $p < 0.0005$.

Adapted from information appearing in Trends Pharmacol. Sci., Gresele et al., 1991, 12, 160-163).

d) **Other (vascular) effects could be beneficial**
Some of the mediators released during platelet aggregation not only affect other platelets but have also profound vascular activity. This is the case for the prostaglandin endoperoxides, for TXA_2 and for 5-HT, and aspirin, which will only block the generation of the endoperoxides and TXA_2, has no influence on the pro-aggregating and vasoconstrictor activity of 5-HT. Very elegant experiments with human saphenous veins have recently been reported (37) in which it was shown that the contraction of human venous ring segments elicited by aggregating platelets could only partly be inhibited by pretreatment of the platelets with aspirin (Fig. 9).

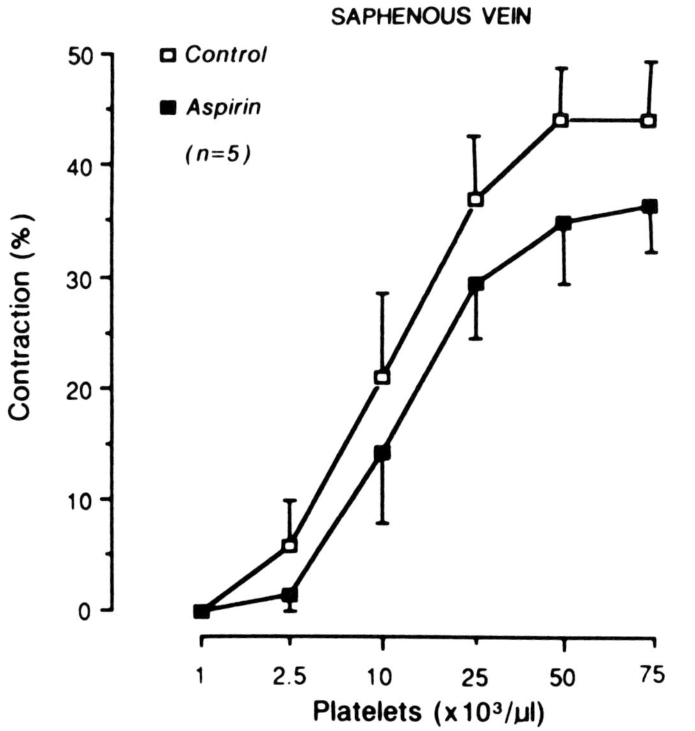

FIG. 9

Isolated rings of human saphenous vein without endothelium (□), which were suspended in organ chambers, contracted to aggregating platelets (1-75 x $10^3/\mu l$). Pretreatment of the platelets with aspirin (10 $\mu mol/l$) reduced, but did not abolish the platelet-induced contraction (■ ; $p < 0.05$).
(Adapted from information appearing in Lancet, Yang et al., 1991, 337, 939-943).

The combination of a thromboxane receptor antagonist and 5-HT_2 antagonist was, however, much more effective to inhibit the platelet induced vasoconstriction (Fig. 10).

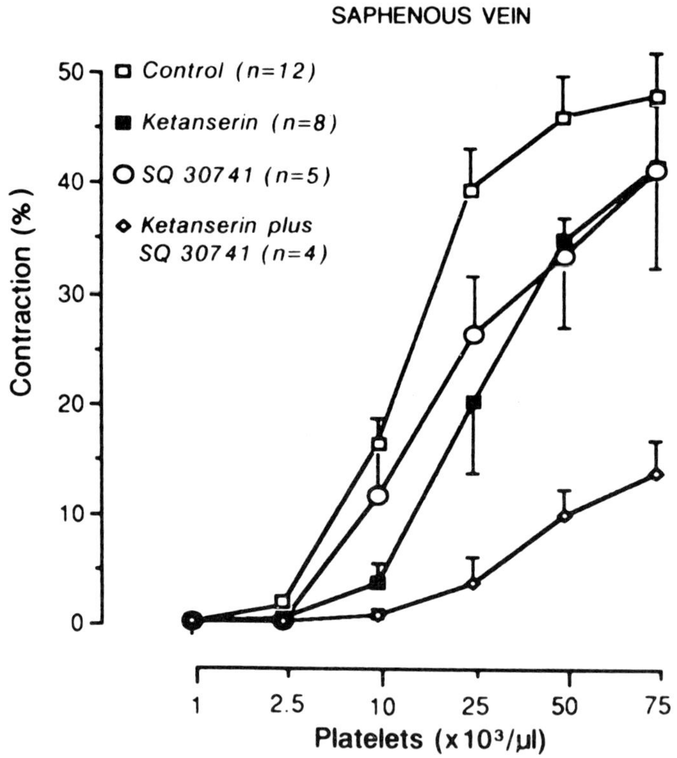

FIG. 10

Isolated rings of human saphenous vein without endothelium (□) which were suspended in organ chambers, contracted to aggregating platelets (1-75 x $10^3/\mu l$). The serotonergic antagonist ketanserin (■) and the thromboxane antagonist SQ39741 (O) reduced the platelet-induced aggregation ($p < 0.05$). This reduction was much more pronounced in the presence of both ketanserin and SQ30741 (◇).
(Adapted from information appearing in Lancet, Yang et al., 1991, 337; 939-943).

3.2. CLINICAL EFFICACY

In the last few years much of the debate about the clinical efficacy of the anti-aggregating and antithrombotic drugs has focused on the question whether aspirin alone is as affective as aspirin in combination with other substances.

By careful analysis of the studies in which these drugs were used for secundary prevention of myocardial infarction or stroke (see refs. 38, 39, 40, 41, 42) one had firstly to resort to the statistical technique of "meta-analysis" of the various studies in order to prove that aspirin could be effective and secondly, that aspirin alone was often only effective for the combined endpoints (myocardial infarction, stroke and vascular death) but not always for each item separately. Furthermore, even well know statisticians do not always agree amongst each other about the interpretation of the meta-analysis of these studies (see ref. 38, 41 and 43)!

One of the pitfalls present in the controversy about aspirin versus aspirin in combination is the still ongoing discussion about the correct dosage of aspirin which should be used in these combinations. As already published by Moncada and Korbut (10) the association of a high dose of aspirin can completely abolish the anti-aggregating activity of the phosphodiesterase inhibitor dipyridamole. The recently reported RISC study, in which 75 mg of aspirin per day reduced significantly the risk of myocardial infarction and death in patients with unstable angina or non-Q wave myocardial infarction, is an indication that lower doses of aspirin are active by itself and that the efficacy might be increased by combining this low dose with another anti-aggregating drug with different mode of action.

More attention should also be paid to the choice of the drugs used in a particular combination as has been illustrated by the experiments reported by Gresele et al. (Fig. 8). A third factor which should not be overlooked (and probably has been !) in these meta-analyses, is the concomitant use of other medications. Indeed, in the light of the more recent discoveries about the anti-aggregating activity of the nitrovasodilators and their efficacy after intravenous or oral administration in short-term mortality reduction in patients with acute myocardial infarction (42), one can imagine that the concomitant use of these substances could have favoured one or the other treatment schedule.

4.4. CONCLUSION

It is now generally accepted that anti-aggregating drugs are efficacious in the secondary prevention of myocardial infarction, stroke and a number of other cardiovascular disorders (Table 2).

TABLE 2

EFFICACY OF ASA VERSUS OTHER ANTITHROMBOTICS

	ASA	ASA and/or other*	Comments
Unstable angina	+	+	
Acute MI	+	+	
Secundary prevention MI	±	+	ASA only sign. meta-analysis
Primary prevention	±	NT (?)	
Stable angina	-	-	Useless
PTCA	+	+	+ Only for immediate reocclusion
Bypass surgery	+	+	+ Only for early graft occlusion
Prosthetic valves	-	+	
TIA + sec. prev. Stroke	±	+	ASA only sign. for combined endpoints by meta-analysis
Atherosclerosis obliterans	+	+	
Diabetic retinopathy	NT (?)	+	
Membranous glomerulo-nephritis	NT (?)	+	
Extracorporeal circulation	+		

* including anticoagulants NT (?) = not tested to our knowledge

(Based on ref. 40, 41, 42, 43, 44, 45)

The past and future of these substances can best be summarised by quoting the conclusion of the paper by Gresele et al. (4) "Although some initial success has been obtained with the clinical use of the currently available platelet-suppressive agents, there is still room for improvements in the clinical efficacy of antiplatelet therapy. The limited success of antiplatelet therapy may be due to the fact that only one of the multiple pathways leading to platelet activation is blocked by the available platelet inhibitors. The search for new and more effective approaches to platelet-suppressive therapy should consider the combined use of substances (or the use of drugs with combined actions) that interfere with several of the biochemical events involved in platelet activation.

Strategies aimed at increasing intraplatelet cAMP levels may be particularly effective, because an increase in this second messenger would suppress the range of biochemical events leading to platelet activation".

REFERENCES

1. RADOMSKI, M.W., PALMER, R.M.J. and MONCADA, S. (1987) 'The anti-aggregating properties of vascular endothelium : interactions between prostacyclin and nitric oxide', Br. J. Pharmac. 91, 639-646.

2. BAUMGARTNER, H.R. and BORN, G.V.R. (1960) 'Effects of 5-hydroxytryptamine on platelet aggregation', Nature 218, 137-141.

3. HERAS, M., CHESEBRO, J.H., PENNY, W.J., BAILEY, K.R., BADIMON, L. and FUSTER, V. (1989) 'Effects of thrombin inhibition on the development of acute platelet thrombus deposition during angioplasty in pigs', Circulation 79, 657-665.

4. GACHET, C., CAZENAVE, J.-P., OHLMANN, P., BOULOUX, C., DEFREYN, G., DRIOT, F. and MAFFRAND, J.-P. (1990) 'The thienopyridine ticlopidine selectively prevents the inhibitory effects of ADP but not of adrenaline on cAMP levels raised by stimulation of the adenylate cyclase of human platelets by PGE_1', Biochem. Pharmacol. 40, 2683-2687.

5. BRAQUET, P., TOUQUI, L., SHEN, T.Y. and VARGAFTIG, B.R. (1987) 'Perspectives in platelet activating factor research', Pharmacol. Rev. 39, 97-145.

6. ADAMUS, W.S., HUER, H., MEADE, C.J., FREY, G. and BRECHT, H.M. (1988) 'Inhibitory effect of oral WEB 2086, a novel selective PAF-acether antagonist, on ex vivo platelet aggregation', Eur. J. Clin. Pharmacol. 35, 237-240.

7. REILLY, I.A.G. and FITZGERALD, G.A. (1987) 'Inhibition of thromboxane formation in vivo and ex vivo : implications for therapy with platelet inhibitory drugs', Blood 69, 180-186.

8. GRESELE, P., DECKMYN, H., NENCI, G.G. and VERMYLEN, J. (1991) 'Thromboxane synthase inhibitors, thromboxane receptor antagonists and dual blockers in thrombotic disorders', Trends Pharmacol. Sci. 12, 160-163.

9. KYRLE, P.A., EICHLER, H.G., JÄGER, U. and LECHNER, K. (1987) 'Inhibition of prostacyclin and thromboxane A_2 generation by low-dose aspirin at the site of plug formation', Circulation 75, 1025-1029.

10. MONCADA, S. and KORBUT, R. (1978) 'Dipyridamole and other phosphodiesterase inhibitors act as antithrombotic agents by potentiating endogenous prostacyclin', Lancet, i, 1286-1289.

11. DECKMYN, H., VAN HOUTTE, E., VERSTRAETE, M. and VERMYLEN, J. (1983) 'Manipulation of the local thromboxane and prostacyclin balance in vivo by the antithrombotic compounds dazoxiben, acetylsalicylic acid and nafazatrom', Biochem. Pharmacol. 32, 2757-2762.

12. GRESELE, P., ARNOUT, J., DECKMYN, H., HUYBRECHTS, E., PIETERS, G. and VERMYLEN, J. (1987) 'Role of proaggregatory and anti-aggregatory prostaglandins in hemostasis', J. Clin. Invest. 80, 1435-1445.

13. NOWAK, J. and FITZGERALD, G.A. (1989) 'Redirection of prostaglandin endoperoxide metabolism at the platelet-vascular interface in man', J. Clin. Invest. 83, 380-385.

14. GRESELE, P., DECKMYN, H., ARNOUT, J., NENCI, G.G. and VERMYLEN, J. (1989) 'Characterization of N, N'-bis (3-picolyl)-4(methoxy-isophtalamide (Picotamide) as a dual thromboxane synthase inhibitor/thromboxane A_2 receptor antagonist in human platelets', Thromb. Haemostasis 61, 479-484.

15. DE CLERCK, F., BEETENS, J., DE CHAFFOY DE COURCELLES, D., FREYNE, E. and JANSSEN, P.A.J. (1989) 'R68070 : thromboxane synthase inhibition and thromboxane A_2/-prostaglandin endoperoxide receptor blockade combined in one molecule - I, Biochemical profile in vitro', Thromb. Haemostasis 61, 35-42.

16. HOET, B., FALCON, C., DE REYS, S., ARNOUT, J., DECKMYN, H. and VERMYLEN, J. (1990) 'R68070, a combined thromboxane-endoperoxide receptor antagonist and thromboxane synthase inhibitor, inhibits human platelet activation in vitro and in vivo : comparison with aspirin', Blood 75, 646-653.

17. HOET, B., ARNHOUT, J., VAN GEET, C., DECKMYN, H., VERHAEGHE, R. and VERMYLEN, J. (1990) 'Ridogrel, a combined thromboxane synthase inhibitor and receptor blocker, decreases elevated plasma ß-thromboglobulin levels in patients with documented peripheral arterial disease', Thromb. Haemostasis 64, 87-90.

18. RADOMSKI, M.W., PALMER, R.M.J. and MONCADA, S. (1990) 'Characterization of the L-arginine : nitric oxide pathway in human platelets', Br. J. Pharmac. 101, 325-328.

19. RADOMSKI, M.W., PALMER, R.M.J. and MONCADA, S. (1990) 'An L-arginine/nitric oxide pathway present in human platelets regulates aggregation', Proc. Natl. Acad. Sci. USA. 87, 5193-5197.

20. BULT, H., FRET, H.R.L., JORDAENS, F.H. and HERMAN, A.G. (1991) 'Dipyridamole potentiates platelet inhibition by nitric oxide', Thromb. Haemostasis, in press.

21. COLLER, B.S. (1985) 'A new murine monoclonal antibody reports an activation-dependent change in the confirmation and/or microenvironment of the platelet glycoprotein IIb/IIIa complex', J. Clin. Invest. 76, 101-108.

22. PLOW, E.F., PIERSCHBACHER, M.D., RUOSLAHTI, E., MARGUERIE, G.A. and GINSBERG, M.H. (1985) 'The effect of Arg-Gly-Asp-containing peptides on fibrinogen and von Willebrand factor binding to platelets', Proc. Natl. Acad. Sci. USA. 82, 8057-8061.

23. HAVERSTICK, D.M., COWAN, J.F., YAMADA, K.M. and SANTORO, S.A. (1985) 'Inhibition of platelet adhesion to fibronectin, fibrinogen and von Willebrand factor substrates by a synthetic tetrapeptide derived from the cell-binding domain of fibronectin', Blood 66, 946-952.

24. HUANG, T-F., HOLT, J.C., LUKASIEWICZ, H. and NIEWIAROWSKI, S. (1987) 'Trigramin : a low molecular weight peptide inhibiting fibrinogen interaction with platelet receptors expressed on glycoprotein IIb-IIIa complex', J. Biol. Chem. 262, 16157-16163.

25. GAN, Z-R., GOULD, R.J., JACOBS, J.W., FRIEDMAN, P.A. and POLOKOFF, M.A. (1988) 'Echistatin : a potent platelet aggregation inhibitor from the venom of the viper, Echis carinatus', J. Biol. Chem. 263, 19827-19832.

26. DENNIS, M.S., HENZEL, W.J. PITTI, R.M., LIPARI, M.T., NAPIER, M.A., DEISHER, T.A., BUNTING, S. and LAZARUS, R.A. (1990) 'Platelet glycoprotein IIb-IIIa protein antagonists from snake venoms. Evidence for a family of platelet-aggregation inhibitors', Proc. Natl. Acad. Sci. USA. 87, 2471-2475.

27. COLLER, B.S., FOLTS, J.D., SMITH, S.R. and SCUDDER, L.E. (1987) 'Abolition of in vivo platelet thrombus formation with monoclonal antibodies to the platelet GPIIb/IIIa receptor : correlation with platelet aggregation and bleeding time', Thromb. Haemostasis 58, 244.

28. HANSON, S.R., HARKER, L.A. and BJORNSSON, T.D. (1985) 'Effect of platelet-modifying drugs on arterial thromboembolism in baboons : aspirin potentiates the antithrombotic actions of dipyridamole and sulfinpyrazone by mechanism(s) independent of platelet cyclooxygenase inhibition' J. Clin. Invest. 75, 1591-1599.

29. CAZENAVE, J-P., PACKHAM, M.A., GUCCIONE, M.A. and MUSTARD, J.F. (1973) 'Effects of penicillin G on platelet aggregation, release and adherence to collagen' Proc. Soc. Exp. Biol. Med. 142, 159-166.

30. HARKER, L.A. and FUSTER, V. (1986) 'Pharmacology of platelet inhibitors', J. Am. Coll. Cardiol. 8 (suppl. B), 21B-32B.

31. MONCADA, S. (1982) 'Biological importance of prostacyclin', Br. J. Pharmac. 76, 3-31.

32. MONCADA, S., PALMER, R.M.J. and HIGGS, E.A. (1991) 'Nitric oxide : physiology, pathophysiology and pharmacology', Pharmacol. Rev., in press.

33. QUADT, J.F.A., VOSS, R. and TEN HOOR, F. (1982) 'Prostacyclin production of the isolated pulsatingly perfused rat aorta', J. Pharmacol. Method 7, 263-270.

34. POHL, U., HOLTZ, J., BUSSE, R. and BASSENGE, E. (1986) 'Crucial role of the endothelium in the vasodilator response to increased flow in vivo', Hypertension 8, 37-44.

35. POHL, U., HERLAN, K., HUANG, A. and BASSENGE, E. (1990) 'EDRF-mediated, shear-induced dilation opposes myogenic vasocontriction', Am. J. Physiol., in press.

36. MANSON, J.E., GROBBEE, D.E., STAMPFER, M.J., TAYLOR, J.O., GOLDHABER, S.Z., GAZIANO, M., RIDKER, P.M., BURING, J.E. and HENNEKENS, C.H. (1990) 'Aspirin in the primary prevention of angina pectoris in a randomized trial of United States Physicians', Am. J. Med. 89, 772-776.

37. YANG, Z., STULZ, P., VON SEGESSER, L., BAUER, E., TURINA, M. and LUSCHER, T.F. (1991) 'Different interactions of platelets with arterial and venous coronary bypass vessels', Lancet 337, 939-943.

38. ANTIPLATELET TRIALISTS' COLLABORATION (1988) 'Secondary prevention of vascular disease by prolonged antiplatelet treatment', Br. Med. J. 296, 320-331.

39. STEIN, B., FUSTER, V., ISRAEL, D.H., COHEN, M., BADIMON, L., BADIMON, J.J. and CHESEBRO, J.H. (1989) 'Platelet inhibitor agents in cardiovascular disease an update', J. Am. Coll. Cardiol. 14, 813-836.

40. VERSTRAETE, M. (1990) 'Les anti-aggrégants en 1990', La Revue de Med. Int. 11, 209-215.

41. SZE, P.C., REITMAN, D., PINCUS, M.M., SACKS, H.S. and CHALMERS, T.C. (1988) 'Antiplatelet agents in the secondary prevention of stroke', Stroke 19, 436-442.

42. YUSUF, S., SLEIGHT, P., HELD, P. and McMAHON, S. (1990) 'Routine medical management of acute myocardial infarction. Lessons from overvieuws of recent randomized controlled trials', Circulation 82 (suppl II), II117-II134.

43. REITMAN, D., SACKS, H.S., CHALMERS, T.C., SZE, P. and PINCUS, M.D. (1988) 'Letter to the Editor', Stroke 19, 1447-1448.

ROLE OF NITRIC OXIDE IN ENDOTHELIAL CELL - PLATELET INTERACTIONS

M.W. RADOMSKI and S. MONCADA

ABSTRACT. Nitric oxide (NO) is synthesized by constitutive and inducible NO synthases. The formation of NO by the constitutive enzyme and subsequent stimulation of the soluble guanylate cyclase in the vascular system is part of the control mechanisms which regulate haemostasis and counteract thrombosis. An impaired production of NO may result in platelet activation and thrombosis. In contrast, a prolonged activation of constitutive and/or the expression of inducible NO synthases may provide amounts of NO capable of inhibiting platelet function and inducing bleeding diathesis. Finally, the pharmacological administration of drugs which generate NO or compounds which modulate the activity of NO synthases may prove to be of therapeutic value for restoration of the haemostatic balance.

1. Introduction

The vascular endothelium is a dynamic structure which regulates the function of the vascular wall and blood - borne elements by releasing soluble mediators with high biological activity.

The discovery of prostacyclin (PGI_2) in 1976 [1] and the appreciation of its potent platelet - inhibitory properties focused research attention on defining the role of this eicosanoid in the regulation of platelet haemostasis. The following 15 years have witnessed a great deal of research dedicated to understanding the physiological role of this substance, its changes in pathophysiology and its therapeutic potential [2-5].

In 1980, Furchgott and Zawadzki [6] demonstrated that the vascular relaxation induced by acetylcholine was dependent on the presence of the endothelium and provided evidence that this effect was mediated by a labile humoral factor which they after named endothelium- derived relaxing factor (EDRF). This discovery sparked an intensive research effort aimed at identifying the biological role and the chemical structure of EDRF [7]. The first demonstration that EDRF was nitric oxide gas (NO) came from the experiments by Moncada and colleagues who showed that the biological actions and pharmacological reactivity of EDRF and NO on the vascular strips and on platelets are indistinguishable . Moreover, endothelial cells released NO in quantities sufficient to account for the vasodilator and platelet inhibitory effects of EDRF [8-16].

The purpose of this article is to comment on the biological importance of NO as a regulatory mediator which controls platelet

A. G. Herman (ed.), Antithrombotics, 27–48.
© 1991 *Kluwer Academic Publishers. Printed in the Netherlands.*

haemostasis and prevents thrombosis. We will also review the pharmacological implications of the inhibitory activity of NO on platelets.

2. Biosynthesis of nitric oxide

Both endothelial cells and platelets have the capacity to synthesize NO. The amino acid L- arginine (L- Arg) is the precursor for the synthesis of this mediator . The enzyme responsible for this reaction in both structures is a Ca^{2+}- and NADPH - dependent N^G-,C^G-dioxygenase which uses a guanidino nitrogen atom of L -Arg and incorporates molecular oxygen to form NO and L -citrulline [17-19].

Studies with inhibitors of NO synthase indicate that vascular endothelium constantly generates NO. This led to the suggestion that this mediator can be considered as the endogenous nitrovasodilator [20]. The physiological stimuli for the generation of NO are not yet fully understood but pulsatile flow and shear stress seem to be two of the major determinants [21-23]. In contrast to endothelial cells, platelets do not constantly generate NO and in the resting platelets the synthesis of NO is not detectable . However, NO synthase becomes activated during platelet aggregation [18,24]. Mechanisms which transduce the message carried by physiological stimuli to trigger the synthesis of NO have not been fully elucidated; however, since constitutive platelet/endothelial NO synthase is strictly Ca^{2+} -dependent (in a very narrow range of Ca^{2+} concentrations from 0.1 to 1.0 µM), it is likely that this divalent cation controls the activation of NO synthase _in vivo_ [17,18,24]. An increase in $[Ca^{2+}{}_i]$ in the endothelium may result from the stimulation of stretch-activated cation- selective channels which are permeable for Ca^{2+} [25,26] whereas the same process in platelets is likely to be a consequence of platelet activation by different aggregating agents [27].

3. Nitric oxide transduction mechanism- guanylate cyclase system

Nitric oxide has a high binding affinity for haem iron and therefore it reacts with haemoproteins including soluble guanylate cyclase (SGC). This binding results in the conversion of guanosine 5'-triphosphate to guanosine 3',5'- monophosphate (cyclic GMP) which stimulates cyclic GMP - dependent protein kinase. The subsequent biochemical effects triggered by this nucleotide in platelets may result in: inhibition of phosphorylation of myosin light chains and of protein kinase C , stimulation of phosphorylation of the beta-subunit of glycoprotein I, and modulation of phospholipase A_2- and C- mediated responses [28-35]. Stimulation of NO release in cultured endothelium results in activation of SGC activity and elevation of cyclic GMP levels in the endothelium itself [36-38]. Cyclic GMP causes inhibition of inositol 1,4,5- triphosphate formation, probably by a G protein - mediated mechanism [39].

Intracellular Ca^{2+} is the main target for cyclic GMP - controlled platelet responses and an increase in SGC activity results in a reduction of $[Ca^{2+}{}_i]$ in platelets [29,32,33,40]. Receptor - mediated Ca^{2+} influx and mobilization are regulated by cyclic GMP in platelets. It appears that this nucleotide inhibits Ca^{2+} influx more potently than Ca^{2+} mobilization [40].

The concentrations of cyclic GMP are not only controlled by the synthesizing enzyme (SGC) but also by degrading enzymes (cyclic nucleotide phosphodiesterases, PDE). The separation of PDE from human platelets yields three activities [41]. The first enzyme is relatively specific for cyclic GMP. The second has low affinity for both cyclic AMP and GMP; however, low levels of cyclic GMP stimulate the rate of hydrolysis of cyclic AMP by this enzyme [42]. The third enzyme is relatively specific for cyclic AMP and its activity is inhibited by low levels of cyclic GMP [43]. Thus, NO - mediated increases in cyclic GMP can also significantly affect cyclic AMP levels and modulate platelet function. In bovine and porcine aortic endothelial cells both cyclic GMP - stimulated PDE and cyclic AMP-stimulated PDE have been identified [44,45]. It has been suggested that the levels of cyclic GMP in endothelium are regulated by the former enzyme [45].

4. Biological effects of nitric oxide

In endothelium, accumulation of cyclic GMP may down- regulate the release of NO from these cells [39]. The autocrine down- regulating role of NO synthase in platelets has recently been described [18,24]. The stimulation of platelets by aggregating agents results in activation of NO synthase, most likely via a Ca^{2+}- and L -Arg-dependent mechanism. The resultant NO activates the SGC and increases cyclic GMP, whose actions down- regulate aggregation [18,24,46] (Fig.1). Nitric oxide synthase - cyclic GMP is not the only system capable of down- regulating platelet aggregation. Murray et al. [47] have recently shown that platelet activation is linked to sensitization of adenylate cyclase and increased formation of cyclic AMP.

Cultured and fresh endothelial cells when stimulated with bradykinin release NO in quantities sufficient to inhibit platelet adhesion [12,13,48]. Moreover, isolated coronary and pulmonary vasculature release NO which inhibits platelet adhesion under constant flow conditions [49-52].

Platelet aggregation _in vitro_ induced by a variety of agonists is inhibited by NO released from fresh or cultured endothelial cells [9,10,53-60]. This NO also causes disaggregation of platelet aggregates [10]. Moreover, stimulation of NO release _in vivo_ by cholinergic stimuli, or by substance P, results in inhibition of platelet aggregation induced by ADP, or collagen [61-63]. Thus, a concerted action of endothelial and platelet NO synthases may regulate platelet activation causing inhibition of adhesion and aggregation, down- regulation of aggregation and induction of disaggregation (Fig.1).

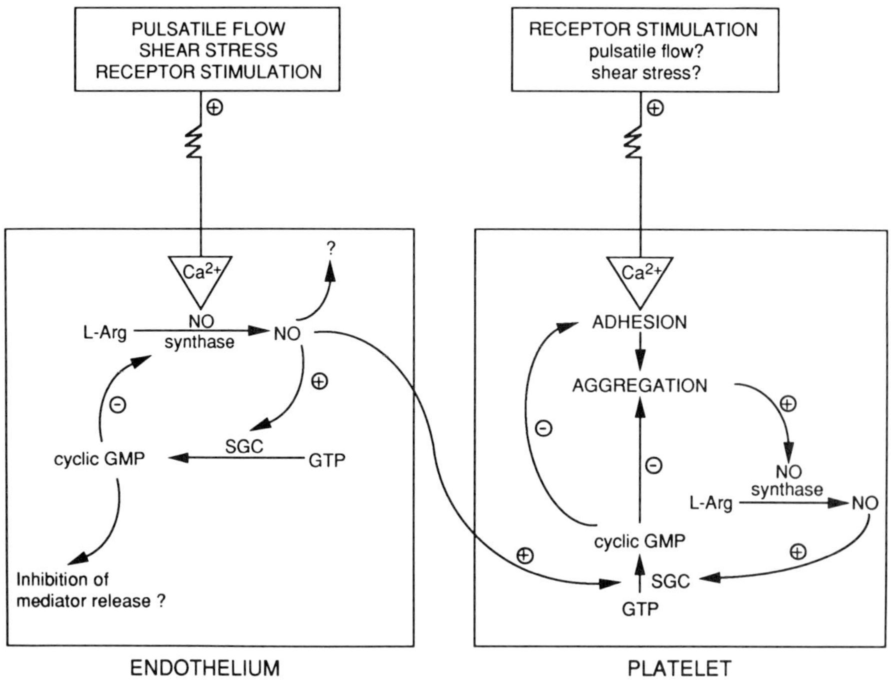

Fig.1. Regulation of endothelium- platelet interactions by NO synthase. (+) denotes activation , (-) denotes inhibition.

5. Synergistic model of regulation of platelet aggregation

Platelets and endothelial cells produce and /or secrete agents which directly inhibit platelet aggregation. In addition to NO, the inhibitory activity of PGI_2, prostaglandin D_2 (PGD_2) , tissue plasminogen activator (TPA) and adenosine triphosphate (ATP) have been described [1,64-67]. Under basal conditions in vivo the synthesis and release of a single inhibitor is unlikely to account for regulation of platelet aggregation. Indeed, the amounts of PGI_2 present in human plasma are too low to affect platelet function on their own [68]. Nitric oxide and prostacyclin synergize with each other as inhibitors of platelet aggregation and inducers of disaggregation [10,56]. Synergistic inhibition of platelet aggregation has been also reported in the interactions of NO with PGD_2 and of PGI_2 with TPA [69,70]. Thus, it is likely that platelet aggregation *in vivo* is down-regulated by synergistic interactions between inhibitors which may counterbalance the activating action of synergistically acting proaggregating agents [71-77].

6. Platelet pathology and synthesis of nitric oxide

Atherosclerosis is the most important cause of thrombotic disease. The capacity of the endothelium to synthesize NO is reduced both in experimental animals [78-83] and human coronary atherosclerosis [84-86]. Moreover, NO has been found to inhibit mitogen release from stimulated human platelets [87]. Mitogens such as platelet -derived growth factor released from injured or stimulated platelets may be responsible for the production of atherosclerotic proliferative lesions which underlie arterial constriction, thrombosis and plaque formation [88,89]. Thus, impaired NO production could be one of precipitating or perpetuating factors of atherosclerosis.

Decreased formation of NO can lead directly to thrombosis. Laser - induced endothelial damage *in vivo*, which inhibits EDRF release, results in platelet aggregation [90]. More effective release of EDRF may be responsible for the better patency of human arterial coronary than venous bypass grafts [91]. Inhibition of NO synthesis in the rabbit by N^G-nitro- L- arginine methyl ester (L-NAME) potentiates the pulmonary accumulation of and prolongs the disaggregation of ^{111}Indium -labelled platelets induced by submaximal doses of ADP, PAF and thrombin [92]. Moreover, in experimental coronary stenosis in rabbits a massive spreading and formation of aggregates on the surface of damaged endothelium were detected only when animals were pretreated with L-NMMA [93]. These data indicate that the failure of the haemostatic system to produce NO may have serious thrombotic repercussions.

Experimental and clinical studies have demonstrated that lipopolysaccharides of the outer membrane of gram - negative bacteriae (LPS, endotoxins) are responsible for the development of clinical manifestations of septicaemia and endotoxin shock . Severe hypotension and disturbances in the haemostatic- thrombotic balance are among the major clinical symptoms . Classically, bleeding diathesis in septicaemia has been ascribed to disseminated intravascular coagulation with consumption coagulopathy, fibrinolysis and/or thrombocytopenia [94-98]. There is, however, evidence that bleeding diathesis in sepsis may occur without endotoxin - induced coagulopathy or thrombocytopenia [99-102]. We have recently found that the stimulation of fresh and cultured endothelial cells by LPS and interferon -γ results in the expression of an inducible NO synthase. This enzyme is Ca^{2+}- independent, its expression is inhibited by glucocorticoids, and it produces large amounts of NO which are sufficient to inhibit platelet aggregation [103,104] (Fig. 2) . Thus, bleeding complications that accompany endotoxaemia may result from the expression of an inducible NO synthase which leads to the inhibition of platelet function. The haemostatic defect seems to occur also in uraemia which is characterized by an accumulation of metabolites of the urea cycle, a prolonged bleeding time and decreased platelet adhesion and aggregation [105,106] . Remuzzi and colleagues have shown that the prolonged bleeding time in uraemic rats can be normalized by systemic administration of L-NMMA [106]. All these observations suggest that an excessive formation of NO resulting from immunological or non- immunological stimulation of NO -synthase may disturb the haemostatic balance and favour bleeding diathesis.

7. Pharmacology of nitric oxide and related compounds

7.1. Pharmacology of nitric oxide formation and action

Under physiological conditions, there is little effect of L -Arg administered acutely on the formation of NO by the intact endothelium and by resting platelets [17,18,24]. This may be due to a high plasma and intracellular content of L- Arg which may down- regulate both transport and activation of NO synthase as well as to the presence of arginase, an enzyme which redirects L- Arg towards metabolites of the urea cycle [107-111]. However, transport of L -Arg into cultured endothelial cells which have previously been depleted of this amino acid is up- regulated and, under these circumstances, L- Arg causes the formation of NO [17,112]. In addition, NO synthase is activated during platelet aggregation [18,24]. The activated enzyme converts L -Arg to NO leading to the inhibition of platelet aggregation [18,24,113,114] (Fig.3).
L- arginine can also augment the formation of NO by vessels of cholesterol- fed rabbits [115]. Thus, it is likely that NO synthase is activated during the course of vascular disorders and therefore an acute or chronic administration of L- Arg may have pharmacological significance.
D - arginine and L -homoarginine showed no or little substrate activity [17,18]. N^G-monomethyl-L-arginine (L-NMMA), L-NAME and N-iminomethyl-L-arginine (L-NIO) have been shown to be potent and selective inhibitors of NO synthases in platelets and in the vessel wall . Administration of inhibitors of NO synthase causes a disruption of the NO -mediated transduction mechanism which in the cardiovascular system is detected as vasoconstriction and platelet activation [18,24,92,93,116-120] (Fig.3). In humans, short- lasting administration of L-NMMA into the brachial artery and into the veins on the back of the hand at doses at least 100- fold below those likely to have a systemic effect resulted in severe arterial and venous

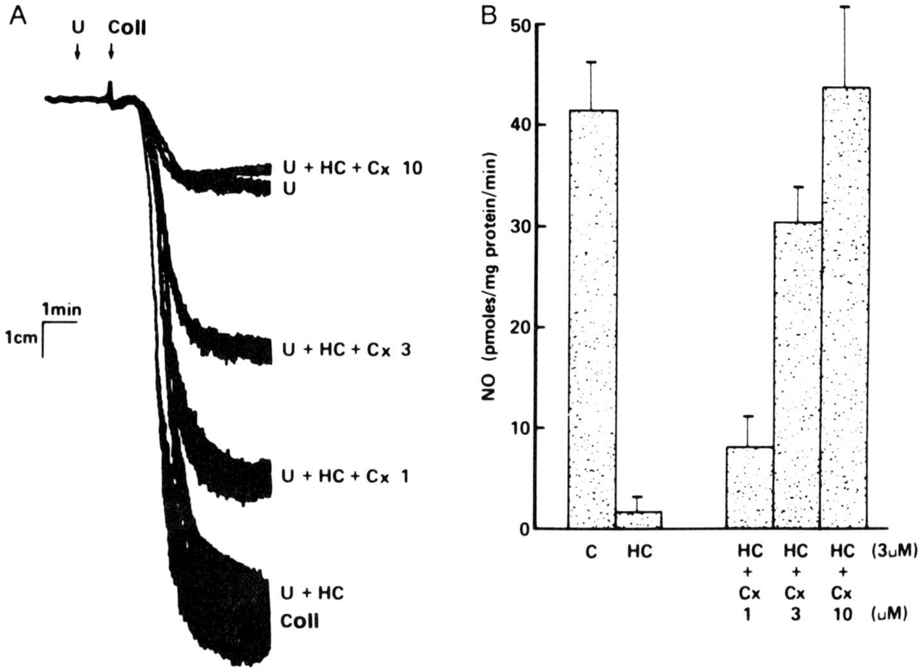

Fig.2. Nitric oxide synthesized by inducible NO synthase (B) inhibits platelet aggregation (A). The enzyme was expressed in cultured porcine endothelial cells by endotoxin and interferon-γ(103). The induction resulted in synthesis of NO (C) which caused inhibition of platelet aggregation (U) induced by collagen (4 µg/ml, Coll). This induction was inhibited by hydrocortisone (3 µM, HC), an effect prevented in a concentration-dependent manner by cortexolone (Cx), a partial agonist on the glucocorticoid receptor. From (103) with permission.

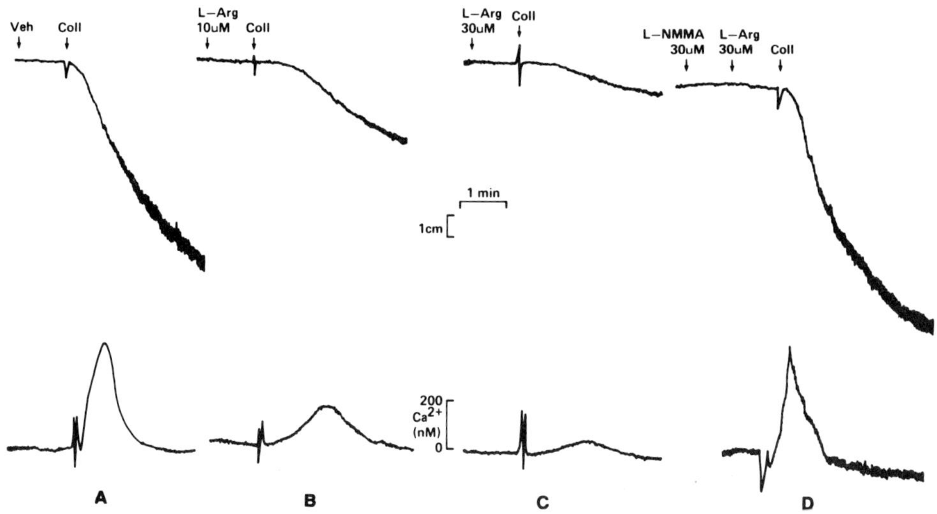

Fig.3. Pharmacological effects of L-Arg and L-NMMA on aggregation of human washed platelets. Platelets were isolated from blood using prostacyclin (159), labelled with aequorin (160) and aggregation (upper panel) and $[Ca^{2+}{}_i]$ (lower panel) were monitored in a Chronolog platelet ionized calcium aggregometer. Collagen (1 µg/ml) - induced platelet aggregation resulted in a maximal increase in light transmission and $[Ca^{2+}{}_i]$ (A). These effects were inhibited by L- Arg (10 and 30 µM) (B and C). The inhibitory effect of L- Arg (30 µM) was prevented by L-NMMA (D).

constriction [121,122]. Therefore , caution should be exercised when considering long- lasting administration of NO synthase inhibitors aimed at achieving systemic haemostatic effects . However, a limited administration of these compounds may prove of value for stimulation of local haemostasis.

The chemical half-life of released NO is very short since it is inactivated within few seconds . Several studies have shown that superoxide anions (O_2^-), which are often generated together with NO, largely contribute to the inactivation of this mediator [5,7-12,54,58,123,124]. Superoxide anion dismutase (SOD), a scavenger of O_2^-, significantly prolongs and unmasks the antiaggregating and disaggregating activity of subthreshold amounts of NO [9,10,58]. The clinical platelet inhibitory potential of SOD remains to be investigated.

Since the initial demonstration of its interaction with EDRF [125], oxyhaemoglobin (Hb) has become one of the most widely used agents for inhibition of biological effects of NO. Low concentrations of free Hb (0.1-10 μM) are needed for inactivation of NO generated in vitro in amounts which inhibit platelet aggregation [9-12,49-52]. However, when contained within red blood cells the concentration of Hb required for inactivation of the platelet inhibitory effect of NO is 40 to 50 times higher [60]. In addition, the vasodilator action of NO released by acetylcholine is not modified by infusion of homologous Hb into human volunteers [126]. These data, in conjunction with the important rheological observation that in the blood erythrocytes stream to the centre and platelets to the endothelial side of the vessel [127], suggest that Hb does not interact readily with NO in vivo. However, even in physiological conditions, some erythrocytes are inevitably lysed and free Hb may be present in plasma in those areas of the vasculature where shear stress is high [128]. Therefore, it is interesting that Hb does not reverse the inhibitory effect of L-Arg on platelet aggregation in vitro suggesting that this haemoprotein does not normally penetrate the platelet membrane efficiently [18]. In contrast, when platelet aggregation is induced in vivo with a resultant increase in cell permeability and lysis, endogenous or pharmacologically administered Hb may gain easier access to NO - generating cells and inactivate the platelet inhibitory effect of NO [63].

7.2. Pharmacology of nitrovasodilators

Nitrovasodilators are generally accepted as basic medication in almost all patients with angina pectoris unless there are clear contraindications [129]. These drugs are believed to exert their antianginal effect by direct dilatation of the coronary vasculature or by decreasing oxygen demand secondary to a reduction in cardiac work [130]. There is, however, increasing evidence that platelet activation plays an important role in the pathogenesis of ischaemic heart disorder [131] . Recognition of the potent antiplatelet properties of endogenous NO raises the possibility that the antianginal effect of nitrovasodilators may also depend on inhibition of platelet activation. Pharmacological evidence indicates that the pharmacodynamical effects of nitrovasodilators are due to the release of NO [132]. Nitrovasodilators can be classified according to their ability to liberate NO in vitro [133]. The first group comprises compounds that release NO spontaneously without the need for any other cofactor. This group includes sodium nitroprusside (SNP), S-nitroso-N-acetylpenicillamine (SNAP) and SIN-1, the active metabolite of molsidomine. The second group consists of agents such as glyceryl trinitrate (GTN) and other organic nitrates which liberate NO in the presence of an additional thiol compound . When arranged according to their ability to liberate NO spontaneously in vitro the following order of potency is obtained: SIN-1>SNAP>SNP>>GTN [134]. The platelet inhibitory effects of nitrovasodilators in vitro correlate well with their ability to liberate NO spontaneously and to stimulate SGC . The relatively low efficacy of GTN and other organic nitrates in stimulating platelet SGC and inhibiting aggregation in vitro may be due to the limited capacity of platelets to liberate NO from nitrovasodilators [135]. This view is supported by the observation that N-acetylcysteine, a reduced thiol known to enhance the release of NO from GTN in vitro [133], greatly potentiates the intraplatelet increase in cyclic GMP and the inhibition of platelet aggregation caused by GTN [136].

The platelet inhibitory effectiveness of molsidomine and SIN-1 in vivo is well documented. Experimental thrombosis of the coronary and mesenteric artery, as well as venous thrombosis of the jugular vein and mesenteric venules, are effectively inhibited by molsidomine or SIN-1 [137-140]. In addition, inhibition of platelet aggregation was observed after oral administration of molsidomine to healthy volunteers or following intravenous infusion of SIN-1 in patients suffering from myocardial infarction [141]. The data on the platelet inhibitory effect of GTN in vivo are less clear. In normal pigs [142], the deposition of ^{111}In- labelled platelets on arterial segments following injury using balloon angioplasty is inhibited by i.v. infusion of GTN when arterial injury is deep (extending through the internal elastic lamina) rather than mild (deendothelialization only). In contrast, transdermal or sublingual administration of GTN to healthy volunteers did not result in inhibition of platelet aggregation ex vivo or prolongation of bleeding time respectively [143,144]. However, i.v. administration of this nitrate for 24h to patients suffering from acute myocardial infarction significantly inhibited platelet adhesion and aggregation to fibrillar collagen [145]. Thus, the platelet inhibitory effect of GTN may depend not only on the route of administration of this drug but also on the extent of vascular injury. Deep vascular injury and exposition of smooth muscle cells to flowing blood may enhance the platelet inhibitory action of GTN, an effect already reported in vitro [146].

8. Inhibition of platelet aggregation by cyclic nucleotides- a case for a synergistic approach

Combinations of pharmacological agents are often used clinically for the therapeutic advantages they may provide over single agents. The pharmacological rationale behind the use of synergistic combinations is to enhance the effectiveness of and to limit the side effects of their constituents, which on their own must be administered at a higher dose than when used in combination. Organic nitrates such as GTN, isosorbide mononitrates and isosorbide dinitrate, and other NO generators such as SNP and SIN-1, synergize with PGI_2 to inhibit platelet aggregation *in vitro* [147-150]. This effect is reciprocal and is dependent on the release of NO, since the same interaction is observed between NO gas and PGI_2 . In addition NO and PGI_2 synergize with each other as inducers of platelet disaggregation [10]. This synergy is also observed when nitrovasodilators are combined with stable prostacyclin analogues such as iloprost and RS93427 [151-153] or with the anitiaggregatory prostaglandin E_1 and TPA [154]. More importantly, this prostaglandin and isosorbide dinitrate synergize in reducing deposition and increasing survival time of ^{111}In - labelled platelets in patients with peripheral vascular disease [155]. Synergistic platelet inhibitory interactions have also been reported between NO , PGI_2 and agents which inhibit breakdown of their respective target cyclic nucleotide (i.e. PDE inhibitors) or between NO and SOD which prolongs the half-life of this mediator [9-12]. Thus, evidence has accumulated in support of the hypothesis that synergistic use of drugs which interfere with the action and metabolism of cyclic nucleotides in platelets offers an interesting strategy for the development of more effective antiplatelet drugs [156,157].

9. Concluding remarks

Nitric oxide synthesized by the enzyme NO synthase is part of a multifactorial, synergistic, down - regulating system which controls platelet haemostasis. The constituents of this system are produced not only by the endothelium but also by the platelets themselves. Thus, the discoveries of endothelium - dependent relaxation and of NO synthase have opened a new chapter in our knowledge on the homeostasis of the vascular wall. Several important questions remain to be answered. Determination of the structure and of mRNA for the constitutive and inducible NO synthases will advance our understanding of the mechanisms which regulate the activities of these enzymes. The role (detrimental or beneficial) of an inducible NO synthase in atherosclerosis and vascular thrombotic disease remains to be investigated. Much is still to be learned about the antithrombotic pharmacology of nitrovasodilators and a clinical commitment should be sought to substantiate this knowledge. Pharmacological synthesis of a new (preferably platelet- selective) generation of nitrovasodilators capable of long- lasting, spontaneous NO release poses an interesting challenge for the pharmaceutical industry. The cytoprotective properties of NO also require further attention [158]. Finally, as with all biomedical discoveries, knowledge gained should be applied to the prevention of disease states, and studies should be undertaken to investigate the effects of dietary supplementation with L- arginine for the prophylaxis of atherosclerosis, its ischaemic and thrombotic complications and of other manifestations of thromboembolic disease.

ACKNOWLEDGEMENTS:
We thank Mrs. Annie Higgs for help in preparation of the manuscript.

REFERENCES:

1. Moncada, S., Gryglewski, R.J., Bunting, S., Vane, J.R. (1976) An enzyme isolated from arteries transforms prostaglandin endoperoxides to an unstable substance that inhibits platelet aggregation. Nature 263,663-665.
2. Moncada, S., Vane, J.R. (1979) Pharmacology and endogenous roles of prostaglandin endoperoxides, thromboxane A_2 and prostacyclin. Pharmacol.Rev.30,293-331.
3. Moncada, S. (1982) Biological importance of prostacyclin Br.J.Pharmacol.76,3-31.
4. Vane, J.R. (1982) Prostacyclin: a hormone with a therapeutic potential. The Sir Henry Dale Lecture for 1981. J.Endocrinol.95,3P-43P.
5. Moncada,S., Palmer, R.M.J., Higgs, E.A. (1990) Platelet- vessel wall interactions: Eicosanoids and EDRF in: Atherosclerosis Reviews vol.21, eds. A. Leaf, P.C. Weber, Raven Press, New York, pp.71-77.
6. Furchgott, R.F., Zawadzki, J.V. (1980) The obligatory role of endothelial cells in the relaxation of arterial smooth muscle by acetylcholine. Nature 288,373-376.
7. Moncada, S., Palmer, R.M.J, Higgs, E.A. Nitric oxide: physiology, pathophysiology and pharmacology. Pharmacol. Rev., 1991 submitted.
8. Palmer, R.M.J., Ferrige, A.G., Moncada, S. (1987) Nitric oxide accounts for the biological activity of endothelium - derived relaxing factor. Nature 327,524-526.
9. Hutchinson, P.J.A., Palmer, R.M.J., Moncada, S. (1987) Comparative pharmacology of EDRF and nitric oxide on vascular strips. Eur. J. Pharmacol. 141,445-451.
10. Radomski, M.W., Palmer, R.M.J., Moncada, S. (1987) Comparative pharmacology of endothelium - derived relaxing factor, nitric oxide and prostacyclin in platelets. Br. J. Pharmacol. 92,181-187.
11. Radomski, M.W., Palmer, R.M.J., Moncada S. (1987) The anti - aggregating properties of vascular endothelium: interactions between prostacyclin and nitric oxide. Br.J.Pharmacol. 92,639-646.
12. Radomski, M.W, Palmer, R.M.J., Moncada, S. (1987) Endogenous

nitric oxide inhibits human platelet adhesion to vascular endothelium. Lancet ii,1057-1058.
13. Radomski, M.W., Palmer, R.M.J., Moncada, S. (1987) The role of nitric oxide and cGMP in platelet adhesion to vascular endothelium. Biochem. Biophys. Res. Commun. 148,1482-1489.
14. Ignarro, L.J, Buga, G.M., Wood, K.S., Byrns, R.E., Chaudhuri, G. (1987) Endothelium- derived relaxing factor produced and released from artery and vein is nitric oxide. Proc. Natl. Acad. Sci. USA 84,9265-9269.
15. Khan, M.T., Furchgott, R.F. (1987) Additional evidence that endothelium - derived relaxing factor is nitric oxide in: Pharmacology M.J. Rand, and C. Roper (eds.). Elsevier Amsterdam, pp.341-344.
16. Kelm, M., Feelisch, M., Spahr, R., Piper, H.M., Noack, E., Schrader, J. (1988) Quantitative and kinetic characterization of nitric oxide and EDRF released from cultured endothelial cells. Biochem. Biophys. Res. Commun. 154,236-244.
17. Palmer, R.M.J., Ashton, D.S., Moncada, S. (1988) Vascular endothelial cells synthesize nitric oxide from L -arginine. Nature 333,664-666.
18. Radomski, M.W., Palmer, R.M.J., Moncada, S. (1990) An L-arginine/nitric oxide pathway present in human platelets regulates aggregation. Proc. Natl. Acad. Sci. USA 87,5193-5197.
19. Leone, A.M., Palmer, R.M.J., Knowles, R.G., Francis, P.L., Ashton, D.S., Moncada, S. Constitutive and inducible nitric oxide synthases are L -arginine N^G-,C^G- dioxygenases. J. Biol. Chem., 1991 submitted.
20. Moncada, S., Palmer, R.M.J.,Higgs, E.A. (1988) The discovery of nitric oxide as the endogenous nitrovasodilator. Hypertension 12,365-372.
21. Pohl, U., Busse, R., Kuon, E., Bassenge, E. (1986) Pulsatile perfusion stimulates the release of endothelial autacoids. J. Appl. Cardiol. 1,215-235.
22. Rubanyi, G.M., Romero, J.C., Vanhoutte, P.M. (1986) Flow- induced release of endothelium - derived relaxing factor. Am. J. Physiol. 250,H1145-H1149.
23. Drexler, H., Zeiher, A.M., Wollschlager, H., Meinertz, T., Just, H., Bonzel, T. (1989) Flow- dependent coronary artery dilatation in humans. Circulation 80,466-474.
24. Radomski, M.W., Palmer, R.M.J., Moncada, S. (1990) Characterization of the L -arginine: nitric oxide pathway in human platelets. Br. J. Pharmacol. 101,325-328.
25. Lansman, J.B., Hallam, T.J., Rink, T.J. (1987) Single stretch-activated ion channels in vascular endothelial cells as mechanotransducers ? Nature 325,811-813.
26. Ohno, M., Ochiai, M., Taguchi, J., Hara, K., Akatsuka, N., Kurokawa, K. (1990) Stretch may enhance the release of endothelium-derived relaxing factor in rabbit aorta. Biochem. Biophys. Res. Commun. 173,1038-1042
27. Siess, W. (1989) Molecular mechanisms of platelet activation. Physiol. Rev. 69,58-178.

28. Waldmann, R., Bauer, S., Gobel, C., Hofmann, F., Jakobs, K.H., Walter, U. (1986) Demonstration of cGMP- dependent protein kinase and cGMP- dependent phosphorylation in cell- free extracts of platelets. Eur J. Biochem. 158,203-210.

29. Nakashima, S., Tohmatsu, T., Hattori, H., Okano, Y., Nozawa, Y. (1986) Inhibitory action of cyclic GMP on secretion, polyphosphoinositide hydrolysis and calcium mobilization in thrombin-stimulated human platelets. Biochem. Biophys. Res. Commun. 135,1099-1104.

30. Waldmann, R., Nieberding, M., Walter, U. (1987) Vasodilator-stimulated protein phosphorylation in platelets is mediated by cAMP - and cGMP - dependent protein kinases. Eur. J. Biochem. 167,441-448.

31. Waldmann, R., Walter U. (1989) Cyclic nucleotide elevating vasodilators inhibit platelet aggregation at an early step of the activation cascade. Eur. J. Pharmacol. 159,317-320.

32. Walter U. Physiological role of cGMP and cGMP - dependent protein kinase in the cardiovascular system. (1989) Rev. Physiol. Biochem. Pharmacol. 113,41-88.

33. Matsuoka, I., Nakahata, N., Nakanish, H. (1989) Inhibitory effect of 8-bromo cyclic GMP on an extracellular Ca^{2+}- dependent arachidonic acid liberation in collagen - stimulated rabbit platelets. Biochem. Pharmacol. 38,1841-1847.

34. Sane, D.C., Bielawska, A., Greenberg, C.S., Hannun, Y.A. (1989) Cyclic GMP analogs inhibit thrombin- induced arachidonic acid release in human platelets. Biochem. Biophys. Res. Commun. 165,708-714.

35. Ignarro, L.J. (1989) Heme- dependent activation of soluble guanylate cyclase by nitric oxide: regulation of enzyme activity by porphyrins and metalloporphyrins. Sem. Hematol. 26,63-76.

36. Martin, W., White, D.G., Henderson, A.H. (1988) Endothelium - derived relaxing factor and atriopeptin II elevate cyclic GMP levels in pig aortic endothelial cells. Br. J. Pharmacol. 93,229-239.

37. Doni, M.G., Whittle, B.J.R., Palmer, R.M.J., Moncada, S. (1988) Actions of nitric oxide on the release of prostacyclin from bovine endothelial cells in culture. Eur. J. Pharmacol. 151,19-25.

38. Boulanger, C., Schini, V.B., Moncada, S., Vanhoutte, P.M. (1990) Stimulation of cyclic GMP production in cultured endothelial cells of the pig by bradykinin, adenosine diphosphate, calcium ionophore A23187 and nitric oxide. Br. J. Pharmacol. 101,152-156.

39. Lang, D., Lewis, M.J. (1991) Inhibition of inositol 1,4,5-triphosphate formation by cyclic GMP in cultured aortic endothelial cells of the pig. Br. J. Pharmacol. 102,277-281.

40. Morgan, R.O., Newby, A.C. (1989) Nitroprusside differentially inhibits ADP - stimulated calcium influx and mobilization in human platelets. Biochem. J. 258,447-454.

41. Hidaka, H., Asano, T. (1976) Human blood platelet 3':5'- cyclic nucleotide phosphodiesterase. Biochim. Biophys. Acta 429,485-497.

42. Grant, P.G., Mannarino, A.F., Colman, R.W. (1990) Purification and characterization of a cyclic GMP- stimulated cyclic nucleotide phosphodiesterase from the cytosol of human platelets. Thromb. Res.

59,105-119.
43. Grant, P.G., Colman, R.W. (1984) Purification and characterization of a human platelet cyclic nucleotide phosphodiesterase. Biochemistry 23,1801-1807.
44. Lugnier, C., Schini, V. (1988) Characterization of cyclic nucleotide phosphodiesterases in cultured bovine aortic endothelial cells. Br. J. Pharmacol. 94,406P.
45. Souness, J.E., Diocee, B.K., Martin, W., Moodie, S.A. (1990) Pig aortic endothelial -cell cyclic nucleotide phosphodiesterases. Use of phosphodiesterase inhibitors to evaluate their roles in regulating cyclic nucleotide levels in intact cells. Biochem. J. 266,127-132.
46. Radomski, M.W., Palmer, R.M.J., Moncada, S. (1991) Modulation of platelet aggregation by an arginine: nitric oxide pathway. TIPS, 12,87-88.
47. Murray, R., Shipp, E., FitzGerald, G.A. (1990) Prostaglandin endoperoxide/thromboxane A_2 receptor desensitization. Cross- talk with adenylate cyclase in human platelets. J. Biol. Chem. 265,21670-21675.
48. Sneddon, J.M., Vane, J.R. (1988) Endothelium- derived relaxing factor reduces platelet adhesion to bovine endothelial cells. Proc. Natl. Acad. Sci. USA 85,2800-2804.
49. Venturini, C.M., Del Vecchio, P.J., Kaplan, J.E. (1989) Thrombin induced platelet adhesion to endothelium is modified by endothelial derived relaxing factor (EDRF). Biochem. Biophys. Res. Commun. 159,349-354.
50. Venturini, C.M., Minnear, F.L., Del Vecchio, P.J., Fenton II, J.W., Kaplan, J.E. (1990) Thrombin - induced platelet adhesion to endothelial cells in culture and under flow conditions: Role of endothelium - derived relaxing factor and prostacyclin. In: Endothelium - derived relaxing factors G.M. Rubanyi, and P.M. Vanhoutte (eds.) S. Karger, Basel , pp.315-324.
51. Pohl, U., Busse, R. (1989) EDRF increases cyclic GMP in platelets during passage through the coronary vascular bed. Circ. Res. 65,1798-1803.
52. Wiesmuller, G., Bernards, W., Klaus, W., Rosen, R. (1989) Role of endothelium on platelet adhesion and aggregation in isolated rabbit hearts. Naunyn Schmmiedeberg's Arch. Pharmacol. 340S:R58.
53. Azuma, H., Ishikawa, M., Sekizaki, S. (1986) Endothelium - dependent inhibition of platelet aggregation. Br. J. Pharmacol. 88,411-415.
54. Furlong, B., Henderson, A.H., Lewis, M.J., Smith, J.A. (1987) Endothelium - derived relaxing factor inhibits in vitro platelet aggregation. Br. J. Pharmacol. 90,687-692.
55. Busse, R., Luckhoff, A., Bassenge, E. (1987) Endothelium- derived relaxant factor inhibits platelet activation. Naunyn Schmiedeberg's Arch. Pharmacol. 336,566-571.
56. Macdonald, P.S., Read, M.A., Dusting, G.J. (1988) Synergistic inhibition of platelet aggregation by endothelium- derived relaxing factor and prostacyclin. Thromb. Res. 49,437-449.
57. Hawkins, D.J., Meyrik, B.O., Murray, J.J. (1988) Activation of guanylate cyclase and inhibition of platelet aggregation by

endothelium- derived relaxing factor released from cultured cells. Biochim. Biophys. Acta 969,289-296.
58. Bult, H., Fret, H.R.L., van den Bossche, R.M, Herman, A.G.(1988) Platelet inhibition by endothelium - derived relaxing factor from the rabbit perfused aorta. Br. J. Pharmacol. 95,1308-1314.
59. Alheid, U., Reichwehr, I., Forstermann, U. (1989) Human endothelial cells inhibit platelet aggregation by separately stimulating platelet cyclic AMP and cyclic GMP. Eur. J. Pharmacol. 164,103-110.
60. Houston, D.S., Robinson, P., Gerrard, J.M. (1990) Inhibition of intravascular platelet aggregation by endothelium - derived relaxing factor: reversal by red blood cells. Blood 76,953-958.
61. Bhardwaj, R., Page, C.P., May, G.R., Moore, P.K. (1988) Endothelium -derived relaxing factor inhibits platelet aggregation in human whole blood in vitro and in the rat in vivo. Eur. J. Pharmacol. 157,83-91.
62. Hogan, J.C., Lewis, M.J., Henderson, A.H. (1988) In vivo EDRF activity influences platelet function. Br. J. Pharmacol. 94,1020-1022.
63. Humphries, R.G., Tomlinson, W., O'Connor, S.E., Leff, P. (1990) Inhibition of collagen- and ADP - induced platelet aggregation by substance P in vivo: Involvement of endothelium- derived relaxing factor. J. Cardiovasc. Pharmacol. 16,292-297.
64. Whittle, B.J.R., Moncada, S., Vane, J.R. (1978) Comparison of prostacyclin (PGI_2), prostaglandin E_1 and D_2 on platelet agregation in different species. Prostaglandins 16,373-388.
65. Loscalzo, J., Vaughan, D.E. (1987) Tissue plasminogen activator promotes platelet disaggregation in plasma. J. Clin. Invest. 79,1749-1755.
66. Terres, W., Umnus, S., Mathey, D.G., Bleifeld, W. (1990) Effects of streptokinase, urokinase, and recombinant tissue plasminogen activator on platelet aggregability and stability of platelet aggregates. Cardiovasc.Res. 24,471-477.
67. Soslau, G., Parker, J. (1989) Modulation of platelet function by extracellular adenosine triphosphate. Blood 74,984-993.
68. Blair, I.A., Barrow, S.E., Waddell, K.A., Lewis, P.J., Dollery, C.T. (1982). Prostacyclin is not a circulating hormone in man. Prostaglandins 23,579-589.
69. Radomski, M.W. (1989) Vascular endothelium in haemostasis and thrombosis. Role of prostacyclin and EDRF. Acta Physiol. Pol. 40,S97-S109 (in Polish).
70. Schafer, A.I., Zavoico, G.B., Loscalzo, J., Mass, A.K. (1987) Synergistic inhibition of platelet activation by plasmin and prostaglandin I_2. Blood 69,1504-1507.
71. Grant, J.A., Scrutton, M.C. (1980) Positive interaction between agonists in the aggregation response of human blood platelets: Interaction between ADP, adrenaline and vasopressin. Br. J. Haematol. 44,109-125.
72. Kaibuchi, K., Takai, Y., Sawamura, M., Hoshijima, M., Fujikura, T., Nishizuka, Y. (1983) Synergistic functions of protein phosphorylation and calcium mobilization in platelet activation. J.

Biol. Chem. 258,6701-6704.
73. Ardlie, N.G, Cameron, H.A, Garrett, J. (1984) Platelet activation by disease. Thromb. Res. 36,315-322.
74. Ardlie, N.G., Bell, L.K., McGuiness, J.A. (1987) Synergistic potentiation by epinephrine of collagen or thrombin- induced calcium mobilization in human platelets. Thromb. Res. 46,519-526.
75. Ware, J.A., Smith, M., Salzman, E.W. (1987) Synergism of platelet - aggregating agents. Role of elevation of cytoplasmic calcium. J. Clin. Invest. 80,267-271.
76. Gazzaniga, P.P., Di Macco, G., La Mancusa, R., Oddi, A., Pappalardo, G., Pulcinelli, F.M., Reggio, D. (1988) In vitro enhancement of human platelet aggregation by somatostatin. Experientia 44,892-894.
77. Siess, W., Lapetina, E.G. (1989) Platelet aggregation induced by alpha$_2$- adrenoceptor and protein kinase C activation. Biochem. J. 263,377-385.
78. Verbeuren, T.J., Jordaens, F.H., Zonnekeyn, L.L, Van Hove, C.E., Coene, M.C., Herman, A.G. (1986) Effect of hypercholesterolemia on vascular reactivity in the rabbit. I. Endothelium - dependent and endothelium - independent contractions and relaxations in isolated arteries of control and hypercholesterolemic rabbits. Circ. Res. 58,552-564.
79. Sreeharan, N., Jayakody, R.L., Senaratne, M.P.J., Thomson, A.B.R., Kappagoda, C.T. (1986) Endothelium - dependent relaxation and experimental atherosclerosis in rabbits. Can. J. Physiol. Pharmacol. 64,1451-1453.
80. Shimokawa, H., Tomoike, H., Nabeyama, S., Yamamoto, H., Araki, H., Nakamura, M. (1983) Coronary artery spasm induced in atherosclerotic miniature swine. Science 221,560-561.
81. Shimokawa, H., Vanhoutte, P.M. (1989) Hypercholesterolemia causes generalized impairment of endothelium - dependent relaxation to aggregating platelets in porcine arteries. J. Am. Coll. Cardiol. 13,1402-1408.
82. Jayakody, L., Kappagoda, T., Senaratne, M.P.J., Thomson, A.B.R. (1988) Impairment of endothelium - dependent relaxation : an early marker for atherosclerosis in the rabbit. Br. J. Pharmacol. 94,335-346.
83. Sellke, F.W., Armstrong, M.L., Harrison, D.G. (1990) Endothelium - dependent vascular relaxation is abnormal in the coronary microcirculation of the atherosclerotic primates. Circulation 81,1586-1593.
84. Bossaller, C., Habib, G.B., Yamamoto, H., Williams, C., Wells, S., Henry, P.D. (1987) Impaired muscarinic endothelium- dependent relaxation and cyclic guanosine 5'- monophosphate formation in atherosclerotic human coronary artery and rabbit aorta. J. Clin. Invest. 79,170-174.
85. Forstermann, U., Mugge, A., Alheid, U., Haverich, A., Frolich, J. (1988) Selective attenuation of endothelium- mediated vasodilation in atherosclerotic human coronary arteries. Circ. Res. 62,185-190.
86. Chester, A.H., O'Neil, G.S., Moncada, S., Tadjkarimi, S., Yacoub,

M.H. (1990) Low basal and stimulated release of nitric oxide in atherosclerotic epicardial coronary arteries. Lancet 336,897-900.
87. Barrett, M.L., Willis, A.L., Vane, J.R. (1989) Inhibition of platelet - derived mitogen release by nitric oxide (EDRF). Agents and Actions 27,488-491.
88. Ross, R., Glomset, J.A. (1976) The pathogenesis of atherosclerosis (First of two parts). New Engl. J. Med. 295,369-377.
89. Ross, R., Glomset, J.A. (1976) The pathogenesis of atherosclerosis (Second of two parts). New Engl. J. Med. 295,420-425.
90. Rosenblum, W.I., Nelson, G.H., Povlishock, J.T. (1987) Laser - induced endothelial damage inhibits endothelium- dependent relaxation in the cerebral microcirculation of the mouse. Circ. Res. 60,169-176.
91. Luscher, T.F., Yang, Z., Diederich, D., Buhler, F.R. (1989) Endothelium- derived vasoactive substances: Potential role in hypertension, atherosclerosis, and vascular occlusion. J. Cardiovasc. Pharmacol. 14,S63-S69.
92. May, G.R., Crook, P., Moore, P.K., Page, C.P. (1991) The role of nitric oxide as an endogenous regulator of platelet and neutrophil activation within the pulmonary circulation of the rabbit. Br. J. Pharmacol. 102,759-763.
93. Cedro Ceremuzynska, K., Lembowicz, K., Pytel, B. N^G-monomethyl-L-arginine increases platelet deposition on damaged endothelium in vivo. A scanning electron microscopy study, in preparation.
94. Corrigan Jr, J.J., Ray, W., May, N. (1968) Changes in the blood coagulation system associated with septicemia. New. Engl. J. Med. 279,851-856.
95. Van Deventer, S.J.H., Buller, H.R., Ten Cate, J.W., Sturk, A., Pauw, W. (1988) Endotoxaemia: an early prediction of septicaemia in febrile patients. Lancet ii,605-609.
96. Suffredini, A.F., Fromm, R.E., Parker, M.M., Brenner, M., Kovacs, J. A., Wesley, R.A., Parrillo, J.E. (1989) The cardiovascular response of normal humans to the administration of endotoxin. New. Engl. J. Med. 321,280-287.
97. Suffredini, A.F., Harpel, P.C., Parillo, J.E. (1989) Promotion and subsequent inhibition of plasminogen activation after administration of intravenous endotoxin to normal subjects. New Engl. J. Med. 320,1165-1172.
98. Deventer, S.J.H., Buller, H.R., ten Cate, J.W., Aarden, L.A., Hack, C.E., Sturk, A. (1990) Experimental endotoxemia in humans: analysis of cytokine release and coagulation, fibrinolytic, and complement pathways. Blood 76,2520-2526.
99. Bhargava, M., Kumari, S., Bhargava, S.K. (1978) Impairment of platelet function in neonatal septicaemia. Indian J. Med. Res. 68,964-969.
100. Anaya- Galindo, R., Poucel, S., Ponton, Y.G.L. (1980) Thrombocytopathy possibly due to sepsis. A new clinical entity. Rev. Invest. (Mex.) 32,391-399.
101. Saba, H.I., Saba, S.R., Morelli, G., Harmann, R.C. (1984) Endotoxin - mediated inhibition of human platelet aggregation. Thromb. Res. 34,19-33.

102. Davis, R.B., Johnson, M.F. (1986) Effects of bacterial endotoxin and platelet activating factor (PAF) on human platelet aggregation in native whole blood. Thromb. Res. 44,565-573.
103. Radomski, M.W., Palmer, R.M.J, Moncada, S. (1990) Glucocorticoids inhibit the expression of an inducible, but not the constitutive, nitric oxide synthase in vascular endothelial cells. Proc. Natl. Acad. Sci. USA 87,10043-10047.
104. Rees, D.D., Cellek, S., Palmer, R.M.J., Moncada, S. (1990) Dexamethasone prevents the induction by endotoxin of a nitric oxide synthase and the associated effects on vascular tone: an insight into endotoxin shock. Biochem. Biophys. Res. Commun. 173,541-547.
105. Remuzzi, G.(1988) Bleeding in renal failure. Lancet ii,1205-1208.
106. Remuzzi, G., Perico, N., Zoja, C., Corna, D., Macconi, D., Vigano G. (1990) Role of endothelium - derived nitric oxide in the bleeding tendency of uremia. J. Clin. Invest. 86,1768-1771.
107. Barbul, A. (1986) Arginine: biochemistry, physiology, and therapeutic implications. J. Parenteral Enteral Nutr. 10,227-238.
108. Glass, R.E., Goode, A.W., Houghton, B.J., Rowell, L.W. (1986) Plasma arginine in cancer of the gastrointestinal tract: effect of surgical treatment. Gut 27,844-848.
109. Van Haeften, T.W., Konings, C.H. (1989) Arginine pharmacokinetics in humans assessed with an enzymatic assay adapted to a centrifugal analyzer. Clin. Chem. 35,1024-1026.
110. Konings, C.H. (1980) A kinetic procedure for the estimation of arginine in serum using arginine kinase. Clin. Chim. Acta 176,185-194.
111. Villaneuva, V.R., Giret, M. (1980) Human platelet arginase. Mol. Cel. Biochem. 33,97-100.
112. Baydoun, A.R., Emery, P.W., Pearson, J.D., Mann, G.E. (1990) Substrate- dependent regulation of intracellular amino acid concentrations in cultured bovine aortic endothelial cells. Biochem. Biophys. Res. Commun. 173,940-948.
113. Caren, R., Corbo, L. (1973) Response of plasma lipids and platelet aggregation to intravenous arginine. Proc. Soc. Exp. Biol. Med. 143,1067-1071.
114. Houston, D.S., Gerrard, J.M., McCrea, J., Glover, S., Butler, A.M. (1983).The influence of amines on various platelet responses. Biochim. Biophys. Acta 734,267-273.
115. Girerd, X.J., Hirsch, A.T., Cooke, J.P., Dzau, V.J., Creager, M.A. (1990) L -arginine augments endothelium- dependent vasodilatation in cholesterol- fed rabbits. Circulation Res. 67,1301-1308.
116. Rees, D.D., Palmer, R.M.J., Hodson, H.F., Moncada, S. (1989) A specific inhibitor of nitric oxide formation from L- arginine attenuates endothelium - dependent relaxation. Br. J. Pharmacol. 96,418-424
117. Palmer, R.M.J., Rees, D.D., Ashton, D.S., Moncada, S. (1988) L-arginine is the physiological precursor for the formation of nitric oxide in endothelium- dependent relaxation. Biochem. Biophys. Res. Commun. 153,1251-1256.
118. Moncada, S., Palmer, R.M.J. (1990) The L- arginine pathway in the

vessel wall. In: Nitric oxide from l- arginine. A bioregulatory system. S. Moncada, E.A. Higgs (eds.) Elsevier Science Publishers B.V.(Biomedical Division), pp.19-33.
119. Rees, D.D., Schulz, R., Hodson, H.F., Palmer, R.M.J., Moncada, S. (1990) Identification of some novel inhibitors of the vascular nitric oxide synthase in vivo and in vitro. In: Nitric oxide from L - arginine. A bioregulatory system. S. Moncada , E.A. Higgs (eds.) Elsevier Science Publishers B.V. (Biomedical Division) , pp.485-487.
120. Rees, D.D., Palmer, R.M.J., Moncada, S. (1989) Role of endothelium - derived nitric oxide in the regulation of blood pressure. Proc. Natl. Acad. Sci. USA 86,3375-3378.
121. Vallance, P., Collier, J., Moncada, S. (1989) Effect of endothelium - derived nitric oxide on peripheral arteriolar tone in man. Lancet ii,997-1000.
122. Vallance, P., Collier, J., Moncada, S. (1989) Nitric oxide synthesised from L -arginine mediates endothelium- dependent dilatation in human veins in vivo. Cardiovasc. Res. 23,1053-1057.
123. Gryglewski, R.J., Palmer, R.M.J., Moncada, S. (1986) Superoxide anion is involved in the breakdown of endothelium - derived vascular relaxing factor. Nature 320,454-456.
124. Rubanyi, G.M., Vanhoutte, P.M. (1986) Superoxide anions and hyperoxia inactivate endothelium- derived relaxing factor. Am. J. Physiol. 250,H822-H827.
125. Martin, W., Villani, G.M., Jothianandan, D,. Furchgott, R.F. (1985) Selective blockade of endothelium - dependent and glyceryl trinitrate- induced relaxation by hemoglobin and by methylene blue in the rabbit aorta. J. Pharmacol. Exp. Ther. 232,708-716.
126. Vallance, P., Benjamin, N., Collier, J. (1988) Erythropoietin, haemoglobin, and hypertensive crisis. Lancet ii,1107.
127. Born G.V.R. (1980) Haemodynamic and biochemical interactions in intravascular platelet aggregation. In : Blood cells and vessel walls:functional interactions, Ciba Foundation Symposium 71 , Elsevier Amsterdam, pp.61-77.
128. Radomski, M.W., Gryglewski, R.J. (1989) Physiological role of megakaryocyte - platelet axis in vascular haemostasis. In: Cell: ultrastrucuture and function vol 4, J. Kawiak , Z. Osuchowska , A. Przelecka (eds.) Panstwowe Wydawnictwo Naukowe Warszawa , pp.111-148, in Polish.
129. Jansen, W., Prenze, R., Kumper, H., Tauchert, M. (1990) Interval treatment of coronary artery disease with sustained- release isosorbide -5- mononitrate. Am. J. Cardiol. 65,16J-22J.
130. Needleman, P., Corr, P.B., Johnson Jr, E.M. (1985) Drugs used for the treatment of angina: organic nitrates, calcium channel blockers, and beta- adrenergic antagonists. In: The pharmacological basis of therapeutics, A. Goodman Gilman , L.S. Goodman , T.W. Rall T, F. Murad (eds.), Macmillan Publishing Company New York , pp. 806-826.
131. Fuster, V., Badimon, L., Badimon, J., Adams, P.C., Turitto, V., Chesebro, J.H. (1987) Drugs interfering with platelet functions: mechanisms and clinical relevance. In: Thrombosis and Haemostasis 1987 M. Verstraete , J. Vermylen , R. Lijnen , J. Arnout (eds.) Leuven

University Press , pp. 349-418.
132. Feelisch, M., Noack, E.A. (1987) Correlation between nitric oxide formation during degradation of organic nitrates and activation of guanylate cyclase. Eur. J. Pharmacol. 139,19-30.
133. Feelisch, M., Noack, E. (1987) Nitric oxide (NO) formation from nitrovasodilators occurs independently of hemoglobin or non-heme iron. Eur. J. Pharmacol. 142,465-469.
134. Feelisch, M. Experimentelle Untersuchungen zum intrazellularen Wirkungsmechanismus der Nitrovasodilatatoren und der endothelabhangigen Gefassregulation. Beweis fur Bildung von Stickoxid (NO) als gemeinsamem, intermediarem Wirkungsvermittler. Ph.d thesis, Dusseldorf 1988; in German.
135. Gerzer, R., Karrenbrock, B., Siess, W, Heim, J.M. (1988) Direct comparison of the effects of nitroprusside, SIN 1, and various nitrates on platelet aggregation and soluble guanylate cyclase activity. Thromb. Res. 52,11-21.
136. Loscalzo, J. (1985) N- acetylcysteine potentiates inhibition of platelet aggregation by nitroglycerin. J. Clin. Invest. 76,703-708.
137. Basista, M., Grodzinska, L., Swies, J. (1985) The influence of molsidomine and its active metabolite SIN-1 on fibrinolysis and platelet aggregation. Thromb. Haemost. 54,746-749.
138. Bredin, H.K., Weichert, W. (1987) Inhibition of platelet thrombus formation in rat mesenteric vessels by molsidomine and SIN-1. Path. Biol. 35,223-225 (in French).
139. Just, M., Martorana, P.A., Nitz, R.E. (1987) Inhibition of platelet function in animals by molsidomine. Path. Biol. 35,226-228 (in French).
140. Reden, J. (1990) Molsidomine. Blood Vessels 27,282-294.
141. Wautier, J.L., Weill, D., Kadeva, H., Maclouf, J., Soria, C. (1989) Modulation of platelet function by SIN-1A, a metabolite of molsidomine. J. Cardiovasc. Pharmacol. 14,S111-S114.
142. Lam, J.Y.T., Chesebro, J.H., Fuster, V. (1988) Platelets, vasoconstriction, and nitroglycerin during arterial wall injury. A new antithrombotic role for an old drug. Circulation 78,712-716.
143. Hogan, J.C., Lewis, M.J., Henderson, A.H. (1989) Glyceryl trinitrate and platelet aggregation: effects of N- acetyl-cysteine. Br. J. Clin. Pharmacol. 27,617-619.
144. Ritter, J.M., Benjamin, N., Doktor, H.S., Barrow, S.E., Mant, T.G. K., Schey, S., Stewart- Long, P. (1990) Effects of selective thromboxane antagonist (GR32191B) and of glyceryl trinitrate on bleeding time in man. Br. J. Clin. Phamacol. 29,431-436.
145. Gebalska, J. (1990) Platelet adhesion and aggregation in relation to clinical course of acute myocardial infarction. M.D. thesis, Warsaw (in Polish).
146 Benjamin, N., Dutton, J.N., Ritter, J.M. (1991) Inhibition of platelet aggregation bv vascular smooth muscle cells and glyceryl trinitrate- evidence for generation of NO. Br. J. Pharmacol., 102,847-850.
147. Forster, W. (1980) Significance of prostaglandins and thromboxane A_2 for the mode of action of cardiovascular drugs. In: Advances in

prostaglandin and thromboxane research vol.7 B. Samuelsson , P.W. Ramwell, R. Paoletti (eds.) Raven Press New York , pp. 609-618.
148. Levin, R.L., Weksler, B.B., Jaffe, E.A. (1982) The interaction of sodium nitroprusside with human endothelial cells and platelets: nitroprusside and prostacyclin synergistically inhibit platelet function. Circulation 66,1299-1307.
149. De Caterina, R., Giannessi, D., Bernini, W., Mazzone, A. (1988) Organic nitrates: Antiplatelet effects of organic nitrates. Thromb. Haemost. 59,207-211.
150. Bult, H., Fret, H.R.L., Herman, A.G. (1989) Interaction between SIN-1 and prostacyclin in inhibiting platelet aggregation. J. Cardiovasc. Pharmacol. 14,S120-S123.
151. Willis, A.L., Smith, D.L., Loveday, M., Fulks, J., Lee, C.H., Hedley, L., Van Antwerp, D. (1989) Selective anti- platelet aggregation synergism between a prostacyclin- mimetic RS93427 and the nitrodilators sodium nitroprusside and glyceryl trinitrate. Br. J. Pharmacol. 98,1296-1302.
152. Gryglewski, R.J., Korbut, R., Trabka- Janik, E., Zembowicz, A., Trybulec, M. (1989) Interaction between NO donors and iloprost in human vascular smooth muscle, platelets and leukocytes. J. Cardiovasc. Pharmacol. 14,S124-S128.
153. Lidbury, P.S., Antunes, E., de Nucci, G., Vane, J.R. (1989) Interactions of iloprost and sodium nitroprusside on vascular smooth muscle and platelet aggregation. Br. J. Pharmacol. 98,1275-1280.
154. Stamler, J.S., Vaughan, D.E., Loscalzo, J. (1989) Synergistic disaggregation of platelets by tissue- type plasminogen activator, prostaglandin E_1, and nitroglycerin. Circ. Res. 65,796-804.
155. Sinzinger, H., Fitscha, P., O'Grady, J., Rauscha, F., Rogatti, W., Vane, J.R. (1990) Synergistic effect of prostaglandin E_1 and isosorbide dinitrate in peripheral vascular disease. Lancet 335,627-628.
156. Moncada, S., Radomski, M.W., Palmer, R.M.J. (1988) Endothelium - derived relaxing factor. Identification as nitric oxide and role in the control of vascular tone and platelet function. Biochem. Pharmacol. 19,2495-2501.
157. Radomski, M.W., Esplugues, J.V. (1988) Regulatory properties of vascular endothelium: Focus on prostacyclin and endothelium - derived relaxing factor. Meth. and Find. Exptl. Clin. Pharmacol. 10,537-541.
158. Radomski, M.W., Palmer, R.M.J., Read, N.G., Moncada, S. (1988) Isolation and washing of human platelets with nitric oxide. Thromb. Res. 50,537-546.
159. Radomski, M., Moncada, S. (1983). An improved method for washing of platelets with prostacyclin. Thromb.Res. 30,383-389.
160. Yamaguchi, A., Suzuki, H., Tanoue, K., Yamazaki, H. (1986). Simple method of aequorin loading into platelets using dimethyl sulfoxide. Thromb.Res. 44,165-174.

PLATELETS AND MEGAKARYOCYTES IN VASCULAR DISEASE

J. F. MARTIN

P. M. W. BATH

ABSTRACT. Platelets are actively involved during atherogenesis and coronary thrombosis. Platelets are formed from bone marrow megakaryocytes and changes in their function result from alterations in megakaryocytes. Atherosclerosis, its risk factors such as hypercholesterolaemia, and its complications including myocardial infarction, are associated with a prethrombotic state consisting of large megakaryocytes containing increased amounts of DNA, and large hyperreactive platelets. The cause for these changes in thrombogenesis require further study; such knowledge will aid the formulation of pharmacological agents capable of modulating the process.

1. Introduction

Current opinion on the sequence of events during acute myocardial infarction (AMI), unstable angina (UA) and sudden cardiac death suggests that the initial event, in many cases, involves rupture or ulceration of an atherosclerotic plaque (Falk (1983), Davies and Thomas (1984), Falk (1985)). This results in exposure of thrombogenic components of the vessel wall intercellular matrix, including collagen, to platelets and other blood elements. Platelets aggregate and adhere to the vessel wall leading to the development of mural thrombus and subsequently complete thrombosis and obstruction of the coronary artery (DeWood et al. (1980)). Parts of the thrombus may then break off leading to peripheral embolisation (Falk (1985)). Platelet activation results in

A. G. Herman (ed.), Antithrombotics, 49–62.
© 1991 *Kluwer Academic Publishers. Printed in the Netherlands.*

the release of potent mediators of platelet aggregation and vasoconstriction, for example serotonin and thromboxane A_2, which lead to coronary artery spasm.

The sequence of events occurring during atherogenesis is less clear but monocyte adhesion to endothelium and migration into the vessel wall constitute early events (Ross (1986)). Monocytes subsequently take up altered LDL becoming foam cells. Smooth muscle cells migrate through the vessel wall and proliferate (Ross (1986)). Alteration in endothelial cell function may constitute the initial event in atherosclerosis and results in the increased movement of cells and factors into the vessel wall. The role of platelets during atherogenesis is unclear but they are an important source of smooth muscle cell mitogens, including platelet-derived growth factor (Ross et al. (1974)).

This Chapter discusses the role of platelets and their precursor cell, the bone marrow megakaryocyte, in vascular disease, including coronary artery thrombosis, arteriosclerosis, and its risk factors. To appreciate platelet and MK pathology in vascular disease it is necessary first to understand their physiology.

2. Platelet Physiology

Thrombogenesis is unique in mammalian biology since MKs, the bone marrow cells which produce platelets, are, by their nature, polyploid. Hence, MK DNA content (or ploidy) is greater than the normal 2N diploid state. Endomitosis results in repeated doubling of DNA such that MK ploidy varies between 4N and 128N with a normal modal value of 16N. The cytoplasm from one MK can produce between 1000 and 2000 platelets (Trowbridge et al. (1984)).

Platelets contain no nucleus or DNA but appear to contain some messenger RNA although it is unclear what function this serves. Hence, they are unlikely to be able to synthesise significant amounts of protein although they can take up some substances from the circulation, for example fibrinogen (Harrison et al. (1989)) and serotonin. The principle determinants of platelet content are proteins manufactured within the MK, for example von Willebrand factor (Cramer et al. (1988,1989)). Such proteins are coded for by MK genetic message; messenger RNA for platelet-derived growth factor is present in MKs (Gladwin et al. (1990)). Other substances may be taken up by MKs from their bone marrow environment (Harrison et al. (1989)). Similarly, platelet physical parameters, such as volume (Thompson et al. (1983)) and density (Martin and Penington (1983)), are also determined by the MK during thrombopoiesis.

MKs, platelets and their haemostatic function are closely linked such that they can be thought of as a single system, in other words, a megakaryocyte-platelet-haemostatic axis (MPHA). Alterations in function or physical characteristics at one level of the axis are generally associated with changes at other levels. The MPHA parameters most studied to date include MK size and ploidy, platelet count, size and density, and bleeding time, an in vivo test of platelet function (Harker and Slichter (1972)).

In the steady state, MK size and ploidy are positively correlated with each other (Levine et al. (1982)). Platelet count and mean platelet volume (MPV) are inversely related (Giles (1981), Bessman et al. (1980), Levin and Bessman (1983)) resulting in a near-constant platelet mass (the product of the count and volume). Platelet count appears to be principally determined by MK size and ploidy. In contrast, platelet size is dependent on the manner in which MK cytoplasm breaks up during platelet formation, In general, platelet density correlates with platelet volume (Martin et al. (1983)). Bleeding time (BT) correlates with platelet mass (Scheklik et al. (1986), Milner and Martin (1985)) and inversely with MK size and ploidy (Kristensen et al. (1988)). Men have larger MKs than women while their BT is shorter (Kristensen et al. (1988)).

Large platelets are functionally more reactive; in particular they produce more thromboxane A_2 per unit volume of platelet cytoplasm and are associated with a shortened BT (Martin et al. (1983), Jakubawski et al. (1983)). Large platelets contain more dense granules, aggregate preferentially and more rapidly after ADP and collagen challenge, and release more serotonin and β-thromboglobulin (Haver and Gear (1981), Thompson et al. (1982, 1983)).

2.1. ACUTE CHANGE IN THE MEGAKARYOCYTE-PLATELET-HAEMOSTATIC AXIS

The response of the MPHA to acute platelet destruction induced with the intravenous administration of anti-platelet serum (APS) includes the production of larger platelets (Martin et al. (1982,1983)) followed by an increase in MK ploidy, typically from a normal modal value of 16N to 32N or 64N (Odell et al. (1976), Martin et al. (1982,1983)). Although alterations in MK ploidy and size have not been studied in man, platelet size increases following cardiopulmonary bypass, a situation analogous to APS experiments since profound platelet loss occurs acutely during surgery (Martin et al. (1987)). Conversely, platelet hypertransfusion leads to a reduction in platelet size (Odell et al. (1967)) and MK ploidy (Penington and Olsen (1970)).

Experimental thrombocytosis can also be induced with low dose vincristine, a cytotoxic agent. The platelet count increased over 5 days and followed the change in MK modal ploidy from 16N to 32N (Harris and Penington (1984)). No changes in MPV were observed.

2.2. CHRONIC CHANGE IN THE MEGAKARYOCYTE-PLATELET-HAEMOSTATIC AXIS

Chronic alterations in the MPHA may also be induced in animals experimentally. Rats made chronically hypoxic increase their MPV slowly over 36 days as the platelet count falls (Metcalfe et al. (1984)); the MK modal ploidy increased from 16N to 32N over the same period.

Chronic destruction of platelets occurs if daily injections of APS are administered; rat MK ploidy and MPV increased (Martin et al. (1982)). Similarly, human immune thrombocytopenic purpura, a condition characterised by the subacute or chronic destruction of platelets is associated with an increase in MK and platelet size (Harker (1970), Branehog et al. (1975)).

2.3. A CONTROL MECHANISM FOR THE MEGAKARYOCYTE-HAEMOSTATIC AXIS

Interpretation of these results suggests the following feedback mechanism operates to regulate thrombopoiesis. Increased platelet destruction (as occurs following the acute administration of APS) leads to the production of large platelets. When increased platelet production occurs alone (for example after vincristine administration) MPV remains constant or falls while MK ploidy increases. With concurrent platelet destruction and production (as occurs during chronic hypoxia or APS administration) both MPV and MK ploidy increase. Hence, it has been postulated that platelet volume, and MK ploidy (and thus platelet count) are under separate and independent hormonal control (Martin (1989)).

3. The Megakaryocyte-Platelet-Haemostatic Axis during Atherogenesis

3.1. MEGAKARYOCYTES

Acute animal hypercholesterolaemia is associated with an increase in MK ploidy and size in parallel with the development of atheroma (Martin et al. (1985), Schick and Schick (1985)) suggesting that MKs may, in some way, influence or cause atherogenesis. This hypothesis is considerably supported by the observation that administration of APS in the presence of hypercholesterolaemia not only results in a further increase in MK size and ploidy but also in an acceleration in the rate of atherogenesis (Kristensen et al. (1990)).

MK ploidy has been compared in subjects with significant coronary artery atherosclerotic disease (necessitating surgical bypass grafting) and a control group with minimal or no coronary disease but requiring cardiac valvular surgery. The patients with coronary atherosclerosis had a higher MK ploidy (Bath et al. (1991)) again suggesting that alterations in MKs may be a risk factor for atherogenesis.

3.2. PLATELETS

Central to the "response-to-injury" hypothesis for the development of atherosclerosis was the interaction between platelets and de-endothelialised vessel wall (Ross and Glomset (1976)). Experimental removal of endothelium can be accomplished physically using a balloon-catheter or chemically using agents toxic to endothelial cells such as homocystine. Either way, platelets immediately adhere to the disrupted vessel wall and atherosclerotic-like lesions subsequently develop.

If endothelial injury is undertaken in the presence of anti-platelet drugs such as dipyridamole, or in the absence of platelets following the administration of APS, then the development of atherosclerotic-like lesions can be prevented. Although these experiments support the central role of platelets during experimental atherogenesis, they were dependent on the absence of functioning endothelium. In reality, the physical loss of endothelium occurs late during atherogenesis therefore down-rating the immediate importance of platelets in human atherosclerosis.

4. The Megakaryocyte-Platelet-Haemostatic Axis during Acute Coronary Syndromes

4.1. MEGAKARYOCYTES

The study of MKs during the early phase of AMI is difficult for ethical reasons. However, when bone marrow biopsy was carried out at in patients 18 days post-AMI it was found that the MKs were larger than those from patients with chest pain but without AMI (Trowbridge et al. (1984)). Evidence that these changes preceded AMI was obtained from a parallel study investigating male subjects who died from autopsy-proven sudden cardiac death and age-matched male controls suffering traumatic death but with no evidence of vascular disease; MKs were larger in the sudden cardiac death group and of similar size to those with myocardial AMI in the first study (Trowbridge et al. (1984)).

4.2. PLATELETS

4.2.1. *Physical parameters*. Statements relating to platelet count and MPV in AMI are complicated by the observation that two populations of patient may exist: those with a low count and increased volume (probably the majority), and those with normal count and volume (Trowbridge and Martin (1987)).

The platelet count may be either low in patients suffering from AMI (Cameron et al. (1983), Kishk et al. (1985)) or normal (Dalal et al. (1982), Kristensen et al. (1990)). The platelet count falls for several days post-AMI (Cameron et al. (1983)) while the magnitude of fall is related to the size of the infarct. There is evidence that platelet survival time is shortened following AMI suggesting that platelet consumption is increased during this time.

MPV is increased in patients with AMI when compared to healthy sex-matched controls (Martin et al. (1983)), male age-matched controls (Cameron et al. (1983)) and patients with non-coronary chest pain (Kishk et al. (1985), Erne et al. (1988)). In addition to an increase in MPV, the entire platelet volume distribution curve is shifted to the right (Trowbridge and Martin (1987), Erne et al. (1988)). Platelet mass is unchanged following AMI (Milner and Martin (1985)) suggesting that changes in platelet count and volume are broadly equivalent in magnitude but opposite in direction. Platelet density, a correlate of MPV, is also increased in AMI relative to healthy sex-matched controls (Martin et al. (1983)).

The changes in platelets and MKs associated with AMI can be explained by platelet consumption, leading to an increase in MPV, and a reactive increase in platelet production resulting from larger and higher ploidy MKs. An alternative possibility is that the high platelet volume is secondary to the selective consumption of small platelets (Sewell 1984) although this suggestion flies in the face of large platelets being more reactive than small ones.

The tendency to form platelet aggregates has been measured in AMI and may either be increased (Lowe et al. (1979), Fuchs et al. (1987)) or unchanged (Dalal et al. (1982)).

4.2.2. *Platelet function in vitro*. Several studies have recorded increased plasma concentrations of the platelet product, thromboxane B_2 (a stable metabolite of the vasoconstricting eicosanoid, thromboxane A_2) in AMI (de Boer et al. (1982), Walinsky et al. (1984), Nidorf et al. (1989)). These studies are difficult to interpret since plasma thromboxane A_2 concentrations are normally low and phlebotomy almost invariably results in some platelet activation with the concomitant release of platelet thromboxane A_2 into the plasma. Better estimations of plasma thromboxane A_2 can be made by analysing the urinary metabolite, 2,3-dinor-thromboxane B_2, or the plasma liver metabolite, 11-dehydro-thromboxane B_2 (Catella et al. (1986)); in both cases the concentrations are increased post myocardial AMI (Vesterquist et al. (1985), Fitzgerald et al. (1986), Henriksson et al. (1986)). Increased synthesis of thromboxane A_2 in the early phase of AMI can be inhibited by aspirin.

Serum thromboxane B_2 levels are also elevated in AMI. It is important to appreciate that plasma and serum levels of thromboxane A_2 measure different aspects of platelet function; plasma levels reflect the degree of platelet activation at that moment in time while serum levels reflect the overall potential for platelet activation. From the above data, it would seem that both platelet activation and the potential for activation are increased in AMI.

Other in vitro platelet function tests have been studied in patients with AMI; platelet products such as platelet factor 4 and β-thromboglobulin are elevated (Dana et al. (1976), Cortellaro et al. (1981), de Boer et al. (1982)). Platelet function undergoes diurnal variation such that platelets are more sensitive to aggregation induced by adenosine diphosphate or adrenaline during the morning at a time when most infarctions occur (Tofler et al. (1987)).

4.2.3. *Platelet function in vivo*. The principle measure of in vivo platelet function is the cutaneous BT. BT is shortened at the time of AMI (Cortellaro et al. (1981), Milner and Martin (1985), Kristensen et al. (1990)) but returns towards normal by 2 years post AMI (Kristensen 1988). A shortened BT in patients who had suffered from AMI 3 months to 5 years prior to study has also been reported (O'Brien et al. (1973)). Since the BT measurement is easy to perform and its shortening in AMI is not dependent on the length of time since the onset of chest pain (Milner and Martin (1985), Kristensen et al. (1990)), measurement of the BT may be useful in the initial diagnosis of AMI prior to the elevation of cardiac enzymes in those patients with non-diagnostic ECG's (Bath et al. (1991)).

Using aspirin as a probe for cyclooxygenase activity it has been found that the shortened BT in AMI lengthens significantly more after aspirin than in control patients with non-coronary chest pain (Kristensen et al. (1990)); however, the post-aspirin BT remains shorter relative to the control group and correlates with increased plasma adrenaline concentrations. This data suggests that the shortened BT in myocardial AMI is determined by at least two components: one related to increased adrenaline levels and the other to increased platelet cyclooxygenase activity.

4.3. UNSTABLE ANGINA

The vast majority of platelet research in patients suffering from acute coronary artery syndromes relates to AMI and sudden cardiac death. No work has been published on MK parameters in UA although many of the "control" group in the AMI study discussed above (Trowbridge et al. (1984)) probably had UA in which case MKs are significantly smaller in UA than in AMI.

Again, no formal studies have been performed on platelet volume in UA although the platelet count is similar to controls in one study (Kristensen et al. (1990)). Circulating platelet aggregates have been reported to be increased in UA (Fuchs et al. (1987)).

Conflicting evidence exists with respect to in vitro platelet function although methodological differences again may explain this. Plasma thromboxane B_2 concentrations and the urinary excretion of 2,3-dinor-thromboxane B_2 are raised in patients with UA while the latter may be higher than in patients with AMI (Fitzgerald et al. (1986)). Plasma concentrations of thromboxane B_2 have also been reported to be normal in patients with UA (Nidorf et al. (1988)). Altered platelet arachidonic acid metabolism, leading to increased thromboxane synthesis, has been found in subjects with UA as compared with angina and controls (Serneri et al. (1987)).

Platelet function in vivo, measured as the BT, was not significantly different in UA compared with control non-cardiac chest pain patients, and was significantly longer than in patients with AMI (Kristensen et al. (1990)).

4.4. THE MEGAKARYOCYTE-PLATELET-HAEMOSTATIC AXIS PRIOR TO ACUTE VASCULAR EVENTS

All the above studies reporting altered MK and platelet parameters in acute coronary syndromes involved measurements during or after the event. Hence, it is impossible to determine whether these changes occurred before the acute event, and therefore might be contributory in terms of determining the timing and severity of the event, or are a result of coronary thrombosis.

However, certain evidence is in favour of changes in the MPHA occurring prior to acute vascular events. Firstly, MKs are larger in victims of sudden cardiac death compared with those suffering from fatal trauma and therefore have to have changed prior to the event (Trowbridge et al. (1984)). Secondly, the shortened BT in myocardial AMI is not related to the time of measurement, unlike for cardiac enzyme and electrocardiographic changes (Milner and Martin (1985), Kristensen et al. (1990)). Lastly, thromboxane B_2 production remains raised (Nidorf et al. (1989)) and the BT shortened (O'Brien et al. (1973)) for several months post-AMI.

At least four hypotheses have been put forward to explain why MKs, and therefore platelets, may be altered prior to coronary thrombosis. Firstly, MKs may be congenitally different; secondly, a viral or other environmental factor may transform bone marrow MKs; thirdly, an alteration may occur in the control system regulating the MPHA, and lastly, a period of increased platelet destruction or consumption may precede AMI. To date, no evidence has been published which suggests if any of these hypotheses are correct.

4.5. PLATELETS AND SURVIVAL PROGNOSIS FOLLOWING ACUTE MYOCARDIAL INFARCTION

Several reports have suggested that platelet parameters measured post-AMI may predict survival. In a study involving 26 patients with AMI, Heptinstall and collegues found that death following AMI was associated with an increased platelet-release reaction (Heptinstall et al. (1980)).

Spontaneous platelet aggregation (SPA) was determined in 149 survivors of AMI at 3 months and the subjects followed-up for 5 years. Those subjects whose platelets underwent SPA within 10 minutes (SPA-positive group) had a relative risk of death of 5.4 times that for those subjects whose platelets did not aggregate within 20 minutes (SPA-negative group) (Trip et al. (1990)); 14.9% of the SPA-negative group suffered a cardiac event (cardiac death or recurrent non-fatal AMI) as opposed to 46.2% of the SPA-positive group.

Burr and collegues have studied 1716 patients 6 months post-AMI and found that the age-adjusted MPV was significantly elevated in those patients who suffered a further cardiac ischaemic event or who died (Martin et al. (1991)). The elevation in MPV was independent of other risk factors for ischaemic heart disease including subject social class, smoking status, blood pressure, white cell count, plasma fibrinogen and serum lipid concentrations.

5. Therapeutic manipulation of the Megakaryocyte-Platelet-Haemostatic Axis

Anti-platelet agents such as aspirin, sulphinpyrazone and eicosapentanoic acid (present in fish oil) have all been shown to prevent recurrent vascular events such as AMI and stroke. These agents all have an effect on platelet function including inhibition of platelet aggregation and prolongation of BT. However, it is unclear whether they have any influence on MKs or platelet physical parameters such as MPV. Analysis of MPV in the "diet and reinfarction trial" (DART) did not reveal any effect of fish oil on platelet size in spite of the observations that dietary fish supplementation was effective in the secondary prevention of AMI (Burr et al. (1990)) while a raised MPV was associated with subsequent death (Martin et al. (1991)). Similarly, fish oil had no effect on MPV, platelet count or MK ploidy (or in the development of atherosclerosis) in a study involving its administration to hypercholesterolaemic rabbits (Kristensen et al. (1988)).

The development and study of drugs which alter MK ploidy, gene expression, and platelet size is now required. Such agents might be superior to aspirin in vascular prevention since they would target the pathological basis of thrombotic disease, namely the prethrombotic state.

6. Acknowledgements

JFM is British Heart Foundation Professor of Cardiovascular Science, King's College School of Medicine and Dentistry, London, UK.

7. References

Bath PMW, Gladwin A-M, Carden N, Martin JF. (1991) 'Patients with atherosclerosis on coronary angiography have increased megakaryocyte DNA content compared to those with normal coronary arteries', Thromb Haemostas, Abstract In press.

Bath PMW, Kristensen SD, Martin JF, Milner PC. (1991) 'Bleeding time and diagnosis of acute myocardial infarction', Haemostasis 44, Letter In press.

Bessmann JD, Williams LJ, Gilmer PR. (1980) 'The inverse relation of platelet size and count in normal subjects, and an artifact of other particles', Am J Clin Path 76, 289-93.

Branehog I, Kutti J, Ridell B, Swolin B, Weinfeld A. (1975) 'The relation of thrombokinetics to bone marrow megakaryocytes in idiopathic thrombocytopenic purpura (ITP)', Blood 45, 551-62.

Burr ML, Fehily AM, Gilbert JF, Rogers S, Holliday RM, Sweetnam PM, Elwood PC, Deadman NM. (1989) 'Effect of changes in fat, fish, and fibre intakes on death and myocardial infarction: diet and reinfarction trial (DART)' Lancet ii 757-61.

Cameron HA, Phillips R, Ibbotson RM, Carson PHM. (1983) 'Platelet size in myocardial infarction', Br Med J 287, 449-51.

Catella F, Healy D, Lawson JA, FitzGerald GA. (1986) '11-dehydrothromboxane B2: a quantitative index of thromboxane A2 formation in the human circulation', Proc Natl Acad Sci 83, 5861-5.

Cortellaro M, Boschetti C, Fassio G, Baroni L, Polli EE. (1981) 'Haemostatic function changes in a trial on the secondary prevention of myocardial infarction with sulphinpyrazone', Acta Haematol 65, 193-204.

Cramer EM, Breton-Gorius J, Beesley JE, Martin JF. (1988) 'Ultrastructural demonstration of tubular inclusions coinciding with von Willebrand factor in pig megakaryocytes', Blood 71, 1533-8.

Cramer EM, Debili N, Martin JF, Gladwin A-M, Breton-Gorius J, Harrison P, Savidge GF, Vainchenker W. (1989) 'Uncoordinated expression of fibrinogen compared with thrombospondin and von Willebrand factor in maturing human megakaryocytes', Blood 73, 1123-9.

Dalal JJ, Penny WJ, Saunders KC, Sheridan DJ, Bloom AL, Henderson AH. (1982) 'Platelet counts and aggregates in coronary artery disease', Europ Heart J 3, 107-113.

Dana B, Ellman L, Carvalho A, Daggett WM, Hutter AM. (1976) 'Plasma heparin neutralising activity in coronary artery disease', Am J Cardiol 38, 9-11.

Davies MJ, Thomas A. (1984) 'Thrombosis and acute coronary-artery lesions in sudden cardiac ischemic death', New Engl J Med 310, 1137-40.

de Boer AC, Turpie AGG, Butt RW, Johnston RV, Genton E. (1982) 'Platelet release and thromboxane synthesis in symptomatic coronary artery disease', Circulation 66, 327-33.

DeWood MA, Spores J, Notske R, Mouser LT, Burroughs R, Golden MS, Lang HT, (1980) 'Prevalence of total coronary occlusion during the early hours of transmural myocardial infarction', New Engl J Med 303, 897-902.

Erne P, Wardle J, Sanders K, Lewis SM, Maseri A. (1988) 'Mean platelet volume and size distribution and their sensitivity to agonists in patients with coronary artery disease and congestive heart failure', Thromb Haemostas 59, 259-63.

Falk E. (1985) 'Unstable angina with fatal outcome: dynamic coronary thrombosis leading to infarction and/or sudden death. Autopsy evidence of recurrent mural thrombosis with peripheral embolization culminating in total vascular occlusion', Circulation 71, 699-708.

Falk E. (1983) 'Plaque rupture with severe pre-existing stenosis precipitating coronary thrombosis. Characteristics of coronary atherosclerotic plaques underlying fatal occlusive thrombi', Br Heart J 50, 127-34.

Fitzgerald DJ, Roy L, Catella F, FitzGerald GA. (1986) 'Platelet activation in unstable coronary disease', N Engl J Med 315, 983-9.

Fuchs J, Weinberger I, Rotenberg Z, Joshua H, Almozlino A, Agmon J. (1987) 'Circulating aggregated platelets in coronary artery disease', Am J Cardiol 60, 534-7.

Giles C. (1981) 'The platelet count and mean platelet volume', Br J Haematol 48, 31-7.

Gladwin AM, Carrier MJ, Beesley JE, Lelchuk R, Martin JF. (1990) 'Identification of mRNA for PDGF B-chain in human megakaryocytes isolated using a novel immunomagnetic separation method' Br J Haematol In press.

Harker LA, Slichter SJ. (1972) 'The bleeding time as a screening test for evaluation of platelet function', New Engl J Med 287, 155-9.

Harker LA. (1970) 'Thrombokinetics in idiopathic thrombocytopenic purpura', Br J Haematol 19, 95-104.
Harris RA, Penington DG. (1984) 'The effects of low-dose vincristine on megakaryocyte colony-forming cells and megakaryocyte ploidy', Br J Haematol 57, 37-48.
Harrison P, Wilbourn B, Debili N, Vainchenker W, Breton-Gorius J, Lawrie AS, Masse J-M, Savidge GF, Cramer EM. (1989) 'Uptake of plasma fibrinogen into the alpha granules of human megakaryocytes and platelets', J Clin Invest 84, 1320-4.
Haver VM, Gear ARL. (1981) 'Functional fractionation of platelets' J Lab Clin Med 97, 187.
Henriksson P, Wennmalm A, Edhag O, Vesterqvist O, Green K. (1986) 'In vivo production of prostacyclin and thromboxane in patients with acute myocardial infarction', Br Heart J 55, 543-8.
Heptinstall S, Mulley GP, Taylor PM, Mitchell JRA. (1980) 'Platelet-release reaction in myocardial infarction', Br Med J i, 80-1.
Jakubowski JA, Thompson CB, Vaillancourt R, Valeri CR, Deykin D. (1983) 'Arachidonic acid metabolism by platelets of differing size', Br J Haematol 53, 503.
Kishk YT, Trowbridge EA, Martin JF. (1985) 'Platelet volume subpopulations in acute myocardial infarction: an investigation of their homogeneity for smoking, infarct size and site', Clin Sci 68, 419-25.
Kristensen SD, Bath PMW, Martin JF. (1990) 'Differences in bleeding time, aspirin sensitivity and adrenaline between acute myocardial infarction and unstable angina', Cardiovasc Res 24, 19-23.
Kristensen SD, Bath PMW, Martin JF. (1988) 'The bleeding time is inversely related to megakaryocyte nuclear DNA content and size in man', Thromb Haemostas 59, 357-9.
Kristensen SD, Milner PC, Martin JF. (1988) 'Bleeding time and platelet volume in acute myocardial infarction - a 2 year follow up study', Thromb Haemostas 59, 353-6.
Kristensen SD, Roberts KM, Kishk YT, Martin JF. (1990) 'Accelerated atherogenesis occurs following platelet destruction and increases in megakaryocyte size and DNA content', Eur J Clin Invest 20, 239-47.
Kristensen SD, Roberts KM, Lawry J, Martin JF. (1988) 'The effect of fish oil on atherogenesis and thrombopoiesis in rabbits on high cholesterol diet', Artery 15, 250-8.
Levin J, Bessmann JD. (1983) 'The inverse relation between platelet volume and platelet number', J Lab Clin Med 101, 295-307.
Levine RF, Hazzard KC, Lamberg JD. (1982) 'The significance of megakaryocyte size', Blood 60, 1122-31.
Lowe GDO, Reavey MM, Johnston RV, Forbes CD, Prentice CRM. (1979) 'Increased platelet aggregates in vascular and non-vascular illness: correlation with plasma fibrinogen and effect of Ancrod' Thromb Res 14, 377-386.

Martin JF, Bath PMW, Burr ML. (1991) 'Increased platelet volume following myocardial infarction is associated with death and second infarction in a study of 1716 men', Throm Haemostas, Abstract In press.

Martin JF, Daniel TD, Trowbridge EA. (1987) 'Acute and chronic changes in platelet volume and count after cardiopulmonary bypass induced thrombocytopenia in man', Throm Haemostas 57, 55-58.

Martin JF, Penington DG. (1983) 'The relationship between the age and density of circulating 51-Cr labelled platelets in the sub-human primate', Thromb Res 30, 157-64.

Martin JF, Plumb J, Kilbey RS, Kishk YT. (1983) 'Changes in volume and density of platelets in myocardial infarction', Br Med J 287, 456-9.

Martin JF, Slater DN, Kishk YT, Trowbridge EA. (1985) 'Platelet and megakaryocyte changes in cholesterol-induced experimental atherosclerosis', Arteriosclerosis 5, 604-12.

Martin JF, Trowbridge EA, Salmon G, Plumb J. (1983) 'The biological significance of platelet volume: its relationship to bleeding time, platelet thromboxane B2 production and megakaryocyte nuclear DNA concentration', Thromb Res 32, 443-60.

Martin JF, Trowbridge EA, Salmon GL, Slater DN. (1982) 'The relationship between platelet and megakaryocyte volumes', Thromb Res 28, 447-59.

Martin JF. (1989) 'The relationship between megakaryocyte ploidy and platelet volume', Blood Cells 15, 108-117.

Metcalfe BC, Warren CW, Slater DN, et al. (1984) 'Changes in platelets and megakaryocytes in stimulated high altitude', Clin Sci 6, 76.

Milner PC, Martin JF. (1985) 'Shortened bleeding time in acute myocardial infarction and its relation to platelet mass', Br Med J 290, 1767-70.

Nidorf SM, Sturm M, Strophair J, Kendrew PJ, Taylor RR. (1989) 'Whole blood aggregation, thromboxane release and the lyso derivative of platelet activating factor in myocardial infarction and unstable angina', Cardiovasc Res 23, 273-8.

O'Brien JR, Etherington M, Jamieson S, Klaber MR. (1973) 'Stressed template bleeding-time and other platelet-function tests in myocardial infarction', Lancet i, 694-6.

Odell TT, Jackson CW, Reiter RS. (1967) 'Depression of the megakaryocyte-platelet system in rats by transfusion of platelets', Acta Haemat 38, 34-42.

Odell TT, Murphy JR, Jackson CW. (1976) 'Stimulation of megakaryocytopoiesis by acute thrombocytopenia in rats', Blood 48, 765-75.

Penington DG, Olsen TE. (1970) 'Megakaryocyte in states of altered platelet production: cell numbers, size and DNA content', Br J Haematol 18, 447-63.

Ross R, Glomset JA. (1976) 'The pathogenesis of atherosclerosis (i)', N Engl J Med 295, 369-77.
Ross R, Glomset J, Kariya B, Harker L. (1974) 'A platelet-dependent serum factor that stimulates the proliferation of arterial smooth muscle cells in vitro', Proc Natl Acad Sci 71, 1207-10.
Ross R. (1986) 'The pathogenesis of atherosclerosis - an update', N Engl J Med 314, 488-500.
Schick BP, Schick PK. (1985) 'The effect of hypercholesterolemia on guinea pig platelets, erythrocytes and megakaryocytes', Biochim Biophys Acta 833, 291-302.
Serneri GGN, Abbate R, Panetta A, Pinto S, Favilla S, Prisco D, Gensini GF. (1987) 'Altered intraplatelet arachidonic acid metabolism during the acute state of unstable angina', Thromb Res 46, 303-16.
Sewell R, Ibbotson RM, Phillips R, Carson P. (1984) 'High mean platelet volume after myocardial infarction: is it due to consumption of small platelets?', Br Med J 289, 1576-8.
Szczeklik A, Milner PC, Birch J, Watkins J, Martin JF. (1986) 'Prolonged bleeding time, reduced platelet aggregation, altered PAF-Acether sensitivity and increased platelet mass are a trait of asthma and hay fever', Thromb Haemostas 56, 283-7.
Thompson CB, Eaton KA, Princiotta SM, Rushin CA, Valeri CR. (1982) 'Size dependent platelet subpopulations: relationship of platelet volume to ultrastructure, enzymatic activity, and function', Br J Haematol 50, 509-19.
Thompson CB, Love DG, Quinn PG, Valeri CR. (1983) 'Platelet size does not correlate with platelet age', Blood 62, 487-94.
Tofler GH, Brezinski D, Schafer AI, Czeisler CA, Rutherford JD, Willich SN, Gleason RE, Williams GH, Muller JE. (1987) 'Concurrent morning increase in platelet aggregability and the risk of myocardial infarction and sudden cardiac death', New Engl J Med 316, 1514-8.
Trip MD, Cats VM, van Capelle FJL, Vreeken J. (1990) 'Platelet hyperreactivity and prognosis in survivors of myocardial infarction', N Engl J Med 322, 1549-54.
Trowbridge EA, Martin JF. (1987) 'The platelet volume distribution: a signature of the prethrombotic state in coronary heart disease?', Thromb Haemostas 58, 714-717.
Trowbridge EA, Slater DN, Kishk YT, Woodcock BW, Martin JF. (1984) 'Platelet production in myocardial infarction and sudden cardiac death', Thromb Haemostas 52, 167-71.
Vesterqvist O, Edhag O, Green K, Henriksson P. (1985) 'In vivo production of thromboxane in acute human myocardial infarction: a preliminary study', Thromb Res 37, 459-64.
Walinsky P, Smith JB, Lefer AM, Lebenthal M, Urban P, Greenspon A, Goldberg S. (1984) 'Thromboxane A2 in acute myocardial infarction', Am Heart J 108, 868-72.

THROMBOSIS IN RELATION TO ATHEROSCLEROSIS

N WOOLF

ABSTRACT

This communication discusses the role of thrombosis in relation to plaque growth and in the pathogenesis of acute ischaemic syndromes.

The presence of thrombosis on an arterial surface leads to a swift and striking proliferation of intimal smooth muscle cells and an increase in the extracellular matrix proteins which these cells produce. Smooth muscle proliferation is almost certainly mediated by binding of component growth factors such as PDGF to the muscle cells, and the events that follow such binding and the effects on the PDGF system of hypercholesterolaemia are discussed.

Thrombi occurring in relation to the pre–existing plaques vary from those which are only recognisable ultramicroscopically to those which are visible either on angiography or naked–eye examination of post–mortem samples.

Angiographically identifiable thrombi are found in a very high proportion of cases of acute myocardial ischaemia, and the morphological characteristics of any coronary artery plaques which are likely to lead to such thrombosis are briefly described.

A. Thrombosis in Ischaemic Heart Disease

In clinical terms coronary artery atherosclerosis may manifest itself in a number of different forms. These include:

1. STABLE ANGINA
2. UNSTABLE ANGINA
3. ACUTE MYOCARDIAL NECROSIS (INFARCTION)
4. SUDDEN DEATH
    a. with a history of previous infarction and NO prodromal chest pain.
    b. with NO history of previous infarction and with prodromal chest pain.

A. G. Herman (ed.), Antithrombotics, 63–81.
© 1991 *Kluwer Academic Publishers. Printed in the Netherlands.*

The angiographic correlate of stable angina is the presence of one or more segments of significant stenosis in the coronary artery tree (i.e. a reduction of lumenal cross sectional area by 75% or more). The appearance here is of a Type I stenosis i.e. one with a smooth lumenal outline and no undercutting of the margins of the stenosis. The histological correlate of a Type I stenosis is either a concentric or eccentric plaque with a well formed connective tissue cap and a relatively small basal atheromatous pool.

The other syndromes listed , in contrast to stable angina, are acute in onset , unexpected in their timing and constitute life–threatening hazards. In the histological sense what distinguishes them from stable angina in many instances, is the **acute development of thrombosis** , such thrombosis being related ,in virtually all cases, to **plaque injury**. An exception is the re–entrant tachycardia which can cause sudden death in patients with healed infarcts (1). The circumstances in the vessel wall under which acute thrombosis may occur are outlined in a later section of this paper.

Thrombosis, however, may play a part in the natural history of atherosclerosis , outwith it's now acknowledged role in the pathogenesis of acute ischaemic syndromes, its major contribution in this connection being to plaque growth (2).

B. Effect of Thrombosis on the Underlying Artery Wall: Factors Influencing Plaque Growth.

Plaque growth is mediated by proliferation of smooth muscle cells within the arterial intima and by the synthesis and secretion of connective tissue matrix proteins by these same smooth muscle cells (3). Smooth muscle cell proliferation is brought about by a growth–factor triggered switch in the phenotype of the smooth muscle cell from a "resting" or purely contractile phenotype to an actively proliferating and synthesizing one. This is a fundamental process in atherogenesis, and, indeed, in any form of vascular intimal thickening, irrespective of the presence or absence of thrombus.There is no doubt , however , that the interaction between the elements of a thrombus and a locally denuded artery wall greatly accelerates this connective tissue response and a similar sequence of events is seen in the pulmonary circulation as a result of the impaction of small pulmonary emboli. Endothelial denudation of one kind or another would seem to be the most likely antecedent for such thrombus–driven hyperplasia.

The speed and degree of intimal smooth muscle cell response to the presence of thrombus can be striking.

For example experimental denudation of the aortic intima of a full grown pig by rubbing with a small gauze swab , produces within three weeks, an intima ,at the site of injury, 10–12 times as thick as before (4). This rapid thickening is accompanied by an enormous increase in the cell population of the neo–intima formed at the site of injury as compared with normal intima. In the early stages of the reaction, it is not possible to determine, on morphological grounds, with any accuracy the lineage of these proliferating cells since they show no features of differentiation. Within 12 – 14 days of injury, however, some morphological features appear which indicate that these cells are differentiating into smooth muscle, and within three weeks, the light microscopic features are clearly those of muscle.

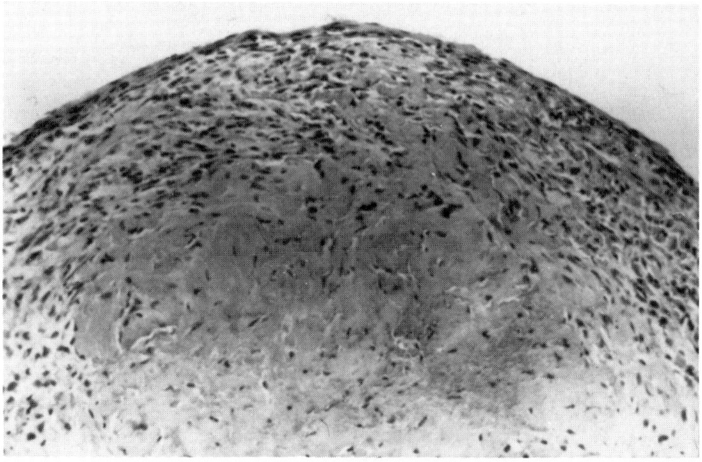

FIG.1. Section of pig aorta 10 days after intimal abrasion. There is an intimal elevation, the centre of which is occupied by darkly staining , rather structureless material which represents he remains of mural thrombus which has been incorporated into the underlying vessel wall. Above and around this is a an abundant cell population which, on transmission electron microscopy shows some of the differentiation features of smooth muscle. Note the new vascular channels appearing within the thrombus.

Haematoxylin and Eosin x 200

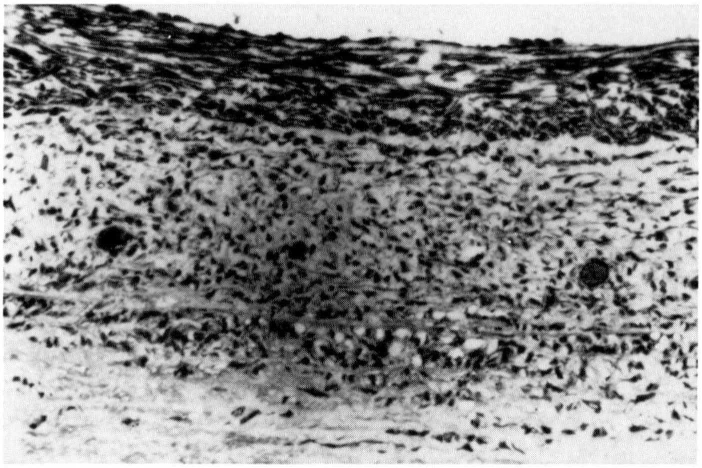

FIG. 2. Section of pig aorta 18 days after intimal abrasion. The intima is now thickened and shows the presence of a large cell population which has now assumed a more ordered pattern than is seen in the previous figure. New smooth muscle cells are arranged, in the superficial part of the neo–intima, in layers which lie parallel to the intimal surface. In the deeper parts of the neo–intima, the cells have a more haphazard arrangement and are surrounded by abundant new extra–cellular matrix.

Lendrum picro–Mallory x 300

THE MECHANISM OF INTIMAL HYPERPLASIA FOLLOWING THROMBUS FORMATION

Such myo–intimal hyperplasia appears to be dependent on the presence of components of thrombus rather than on endothelial injury as such, since intimal denudation in the presence of very low platelet counts is not followed by this striking hyperplastic response. The platelet can cause a smooth muscle cell proliferative reaction as a result of the release of platelet derived growth factor (PDGF) and , possibly, epidermal growth factor (EGF) which bind to receptors on the smooth muscle cell, from its alpha storage granules. Platelet–derived growth factor is what is described as a **competence** growth factor which exerts a mitogenic effect on cells which are out of cycle and, like fibroblast growth factor is also **chemotactic** for connective tissue cells (5,6). PDGF is a two chain protein which has an A and a B chain. Interestingly, the two chains are coded for on separate chromosomes, the A chain being coded for on chromosome 7 and the B chain on chromosome 22. The B chain of PDGF shows 87% homology with the gene product of the transforming oncogene of the simian sarcoma virus (

v–sis) and, more importantly with that of the cellular proto–oncogene c–sis, and this suggests a central role for PDGF in cell growth and proliferation (7,8).

Epidermal growth factor is a **progression** type of growth factor in that it can only exert a mitogenic effect on cells which are in cycle and its role in the post–thrombotic smooth muscle cell response is not yet established . It is possible also, that the fibrin component of the thrombus may also stimulate intimal hyperplasia since fibrin–D–dimer and fibrin degradation products have been shown to stimulate the production of DNA (9).

Binding of PDGF to its receptor serves as a molecular switch for the activation of a number of intra–cellular pathways. The phosphatidylinositol pathway is activated, there is an increase in both the intra–cellular calcium concentration and the cell pH and, within a few minutes, (in ex–vivo situations at least), transcription of the **c–fos** proto–oncogene commences, this being followed by activation of **c–myc** and actin transcription. In addition to its mitogenic effect on arterial smooth muscle cells, PDGF has a number of other effects on the cells to which it binds. These include increases in endocytosis, cholesterol synthesis and expression of the LDL–receptor (3).

Hypercholesterolaemia, a major risk factor in atherogenesis , affects the PDGF system in a number of ways. It causes **up–regulation** of:–

expression of the PDGF B chain receptor

synthesis of the PDGF B chain

transcription of the **c–fms** gene which codes for the macrophage– colony stimulating factor receptor

production of interleukin–1–B

production of transforming growth factor beta.

PDGF is also the molecular mechanism through which **transforming growth factor beta** and **interleukin–1** exert their growth promoting effects on cells since binding of these signals to their appropriate receptors is followed by activation of the genes coding for PDGF and increased synthesis of this growth factor.

C. Types of Thrombus Occurring in Relation to Atherosclerosis Plaques

Thrombi occurring in relation to plaques vary considerably in size. They may be :–

i. **ultramicroscopic** , being visible only on scanning electron microscopy

ii. **microscopic** , being visible on light microscopy in either conventionally prepared and stained sections or in immuno–histochemical preparations

iii. **visible either on angiography or on naked eye examination** of segments of coronary artery removed at necropsy

(i) MORPHOLOGY OF THE ENDOTHELIAL SURFACE OVER ATHEROSCLEROTIC PLAQUES: ULTRA-MICROSCOPIC THROMBI

It is a truism but an important one that human artery material can be studied by the pathologist at one moment only in relation to the natural history of atherosclerosis, and then under somewhat restricting circumstances. We are forced to rely therefore on animal models of atherogenesis for information as to the **sequence** of changes taking place at the blood/vessel wall interface during lesion development. In hyperlipidaemic models endothelial denudation does not occur as a pre–lesional event (10,11), and it seems intrinsically unlikely that lesions in such animals are initiated by thrombus formation. The first morphologically identifiable change in relation to the arterial endothelium in hyperlipidaemic animals is adhesion of monocytes to an intact endothelial surface, this being followed by migration of the monocytes into the sub–endothelial tissues (12). Scanning electron microscopy of the lesions which result from this process show focal intimal elevations under intact endothelium , the elevations consisting of masses of lipid–laden macrophages (13) which can be identified with ease in transmission electron micrographs. Some little time later, (usually 3–4 months after the initiation of the hyperlipidaemic state), defects appear in the overlying endothelium , revealing aggregated masses of lipid–filled macrophages. In some, but by no means all, of these defects platelet adhesion can be seen to have occurred (14).

Until recently it has been difficult, for a number of technical reasons, to acquire human arterial samples which are suitable for surface ultra–structural study. Samples of artery removed at surgery, in our experience, often show an unacceptable degree of traumatic change, and material from patients coming to necropsy often shows changes due to the relatively long post–mortem intervals which also render them unsuitable for electron microscopy. Explanted hearts removed from recipients of cardiac allografts provide ideal material for the study of endothelium both over plaques and over lesion–free areas of the vessel since they can be perfused at physiological pressures and fixed within a few minutes of their removal. A study of coronary arteries from such explanted hearts shows that the surface changes seen in animal models are all reproduced in human material with the exception that platelet adhesion and activation (as shown by shape change) is regularly rather than occasionally seen (15) when defects in the endothelium over atherosclerotic plaques are present. These morphological observations do not provide support for the hypothesis that atherogenesis is initiated by micro–thrombi , but are certainly consistent with the view that platelets frequently do adhere to exposed areas of sub–endothelial intima in human coronary arteries and may thus make a contribution to plaque growth.

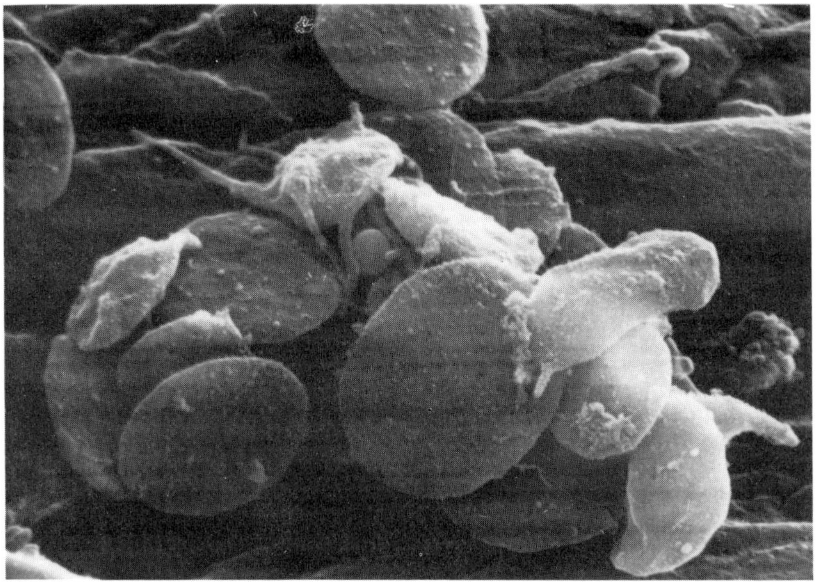

FIG.3. Scanning electron micrograph from at aorta following exposure to cigarette smoke. A small group of platelets can be seen adhering to the underlying endothelium. Some have preserved their normal disciform shape while others have clearly undergone shape change.

x 14000

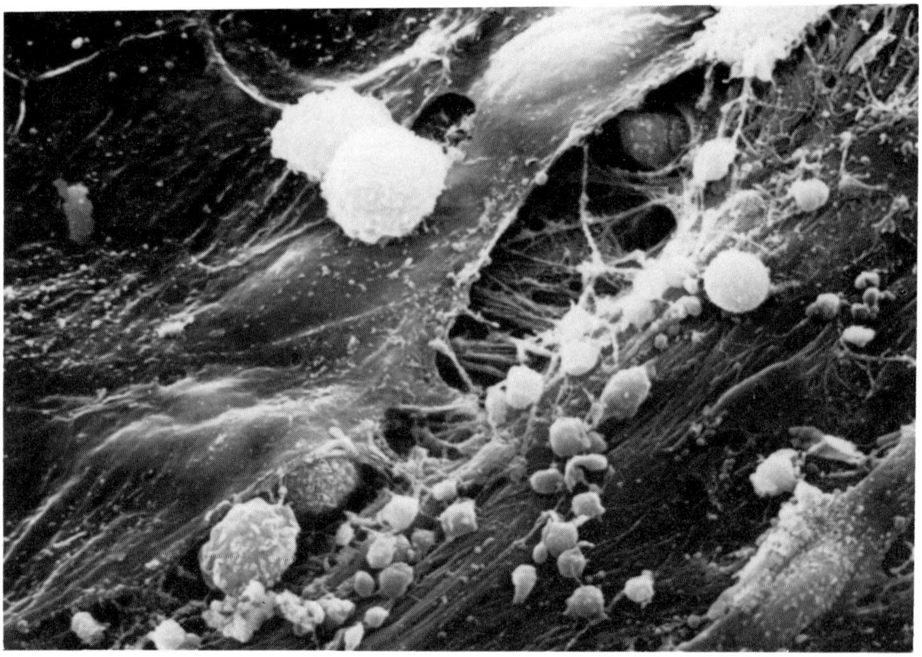

FIG. 4. Scanning electron micrograph of human coronary artery plaque . The right hand half of the image shows denudation of endothelium, this being intact over the left side. Two monocytes are adherent to the intact endothelium. The denuded area shows the presence of activated platelets and a few macrophages lying beneath the endothelium are also seen.

x 4400

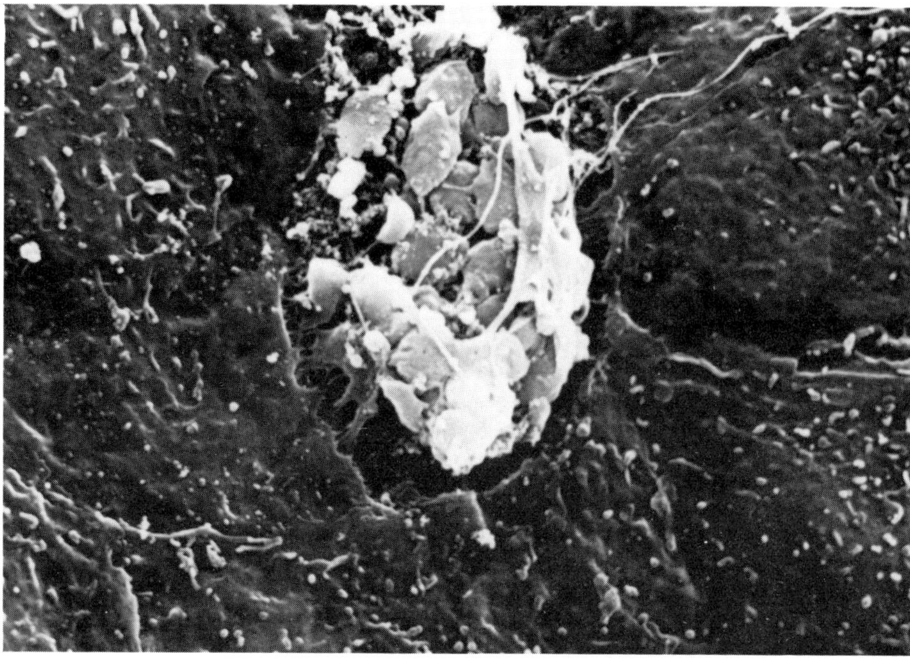

FIG. 5. Scanning electron micrograph of human coronary artery plaque. There is a small sharply demarcated defect in the endothelial surface and the resulting raw area is occupied by a mass of adherent and aggregated platelets which have all undergone shape change. The presence of a few fibrin strands is also noted.

x 9300

(ii) MICROSCOPICALLY IDENTIFIABLE THROMBI

Much of the interest in a role for thrombosis as a mediator of growth in atherosclerotic plaques stems, in the first instance, from the technologically simple but extremely perceptive morphological studies of the late J.B.Duguid (16,17) who put forward the view that many of the lesions regarded as being atherosclerotic are, at least in part, altered thrombi which have been transformed into plaque connective tissue by "organization". Duguid himself was at pains to point out that this represented , at least in part, a return to the view of atherogenesis espoused by Rokitansky in the middle of the last century. Of course, at the time of these observations of Duguid's ,the role of growth factors in relation , not only to atherogenesis but to wound healing and other processes involving connective tissue proliferation , was not known. Any valid assessment of the possible contribution of mural thrombosis to the growth of human atherosclerotic plaques must have as it's start, accurate identification of he presence of thrombus or its residua within the lesions.

Identification of Thrombotic Residua within Atherosclerotic Plaques

The recognition of the remains of thrombus on or within the arterial wall depends in the last analysis on demonstrating the presence of either fibrin or platelets either on the surface of plaques or within the substance of their connective tissue caps.

The use of conventional histological stains for identifying fibrin presents certain problems since, as fibrin ages, it loses it's ability to bind certain dyes and, in any event, dye binding is modified by the circumstances under which fibrinogen is cleaved and the fibrin cross–linked. There is no completely specific histological stain for platelets though the use of the Lendrum picro–Mallory stain in material which has been well fixed in formaldehyde saline enables one, in recent thrombi, to distinguish between fibrin which stains red and platelets which stain a lilac–blue colour. These objections do not apply in relation to immuno–histochemical methods. The use of polyclonal anti–fibrin sera has shown antibody binding to both fatty streaks and mature raised lesions (18,19,20). The material within plaques which binds anti–fibrin sera appears to be present in two distinct morphological forms. In the first of these, the antigen is diffusely distributed throughout the thickened intima . In the second,it appears in the form of discrete bands of material lying more or less parallel to the surface of the intima (21).It has been suggested that these two patterns are the expression of two different mechanisms of fibrin accumulation within the intima :–insudation of fibrinogen in the first instance and incorporation of mural thrombus in the second. This view gains some support from the fact that only lesions showing the "banded" pattern of fibrin deposition could be found to contain platelet antigens in the same areas.

Incorporated mural thrombi can be found in more than 40% of aortic atherosclerotic plaques (22). A study carried out at roughly the same time showed that there was a significant positive correlation between the proportion of aortic plaques showing thrombus incorporation and the presence of coronary artery occlusion (23). Whether this represents an increased pro–thrombotic tendency in the period before death or a decreased ability to clear thrombi by means of lysis remains a matter of speculation.

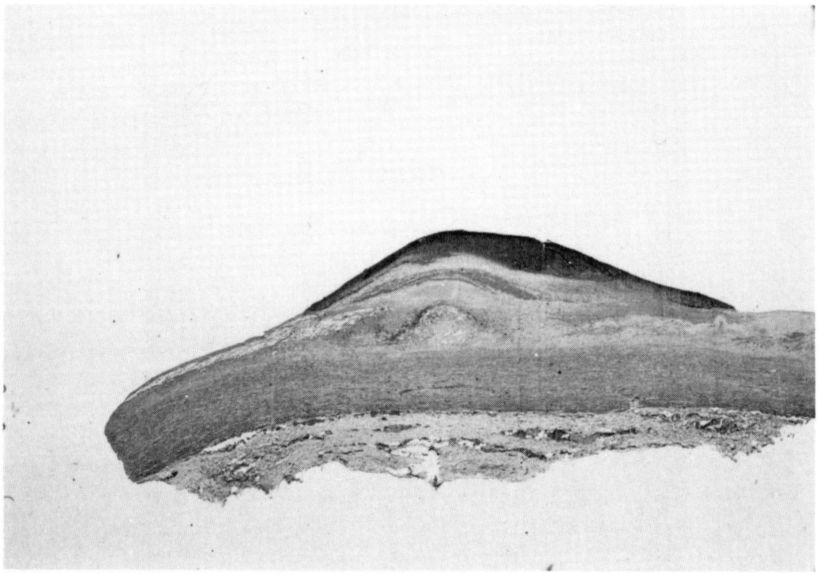

FIG. 6. Aortic atherosclerotic plaque. The surface of the plaque shows the presence of a darkly staining mural thrombus which is moulded to the outline of the atherosclerotic lesion. Deep to this , well within the substance of the plaque is a band of rather paler staining material which represents the residuum of a previous mural thrombus, now incorporated into the vessel wall.

Lendrum picro–Mallory x 15

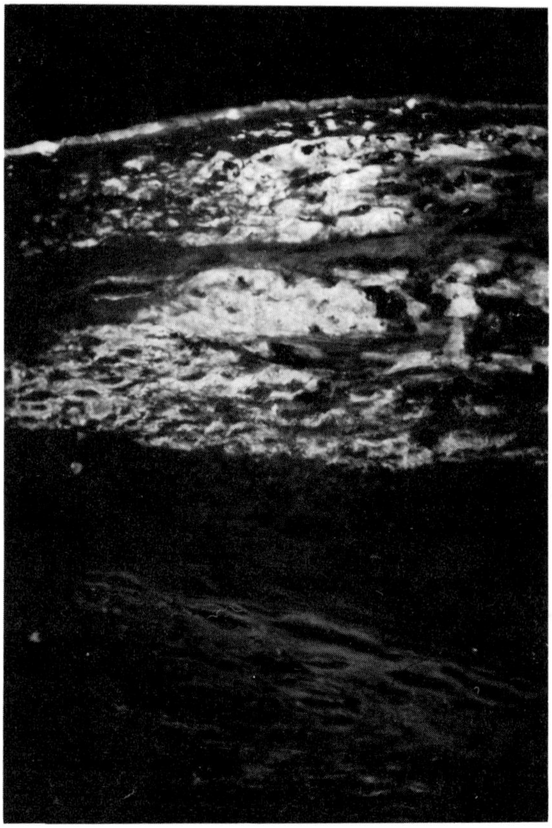

FIG. 7. Frozen section of a human aortic atherosclerotic plaque treated with a polyclonal, fluorescein–linked anti–human platelet antibody. The connective tissue cap of the plaque shows discrete bands of fluorescent material lying roughly parallel to the vessel surface in a manner to that seen in raised lesions treated with anti–fibrin sera.

U.V. light x 375

(iii) ANGIOGRAPHICALLY IDENTIFIABLE THROMBI IN THE CORONARY ARTERIES AND THEIR PATHOGENESIS

In the opening paragraph of the introduction, the importance of thrombosis in relation to the acute syndromes of ischaemic heart disease was emphasised. When populations are compared at necropsy there is a positive correlation (not very surprisingly) between the extent of atherosclerosis in the arterial tree and the risk of ischaemic heart disease.

Within populations and in the coronary artery tree, probably of greater importance are the

qualitative characteristics of individual lesions which may lead them to have a greater or lesser risk of acute thrombosis.Thus plaques which are at most risk of major acute thrombosis tend to have the following features: (1).

i. They are eccentric rather than concentric.

ii.They have a large, soft lipid–rich, easily deformable basal pool, and thus, a thinner , more easily disrupted connective tissue cap.

iii. The basal pool shows an absence of "struts" of collagen passing from the ablumenal aspect of the plaque "cap" across the basal pool to be inserted in the intact connective tissue layers deep to the pool.

iv. The collagen fibres which make up the bulk of the connective tissue plaque cap are separated from each other by large numbers of lipid–laden macrophages.

The first three of these histological features tend to be found particularly in association with deep intimal tears passing right through the thickness of the cap . In such lesions blood from the artery lumen flows rapidly into the atheromatous basal pool, the first part of the acute thrombus forming within the plaque substance itself. Cap disruption of this kind is found in association with about 75% of acute coronary artery thrombi.

It should be clear from the foregoing that the relative proportions of the connective tissue plaque cap and the underlying, lipid–rich, largely necrotic basal pool are major factors in relation to deep intimal injury. The nature of the lipid in the basal, atheromatous poll suggests , that at normal body temperature, it will be semi–liquid and thus easily deformable by haemodynamic factors and alterations in local vessel tone (1,24). This leads to a redistribution of mechanical stress during systole. Such stress appears, on computer modelling, to be maximal at the margins of the plaque cap where it abuts onto that part of the circumference of the artery wall where there is no underlying atheromatous pool of any significant size (25).Thus the mechanisms which lead to a large necrotic basal pool and a thin, easily ruptured plaque cap appear to be a key area for future study .

The last feature listed – **accumulation of lipid–filled, foamy macrophages between etiolated and separated collagen fibres within the upper layers of the plaque cap – is the histological correlate of superficial plaque injury** which is found in the remaining 25% of cases of acute coronary thrombosis.

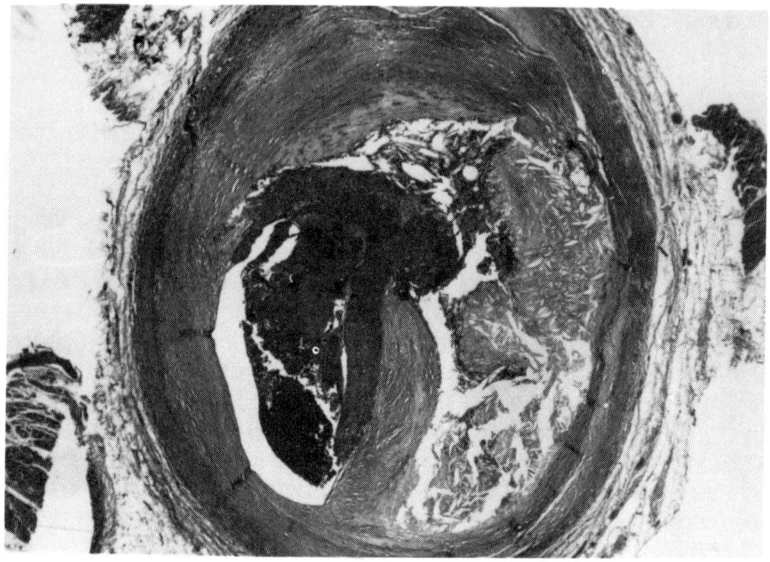

FIG. 8. Human coronary artery plaque. There is a deep intimal tear at the margin of the plaque cap where it abuts on intima in which there is no basal pool. which connects the vessel lumen with the soft atheromatous basal pool. A large, darkly staining mass of thrombus occupies the breach within the intima and extends into the vessel lumen.

Haematoxylin and Eosin x 35

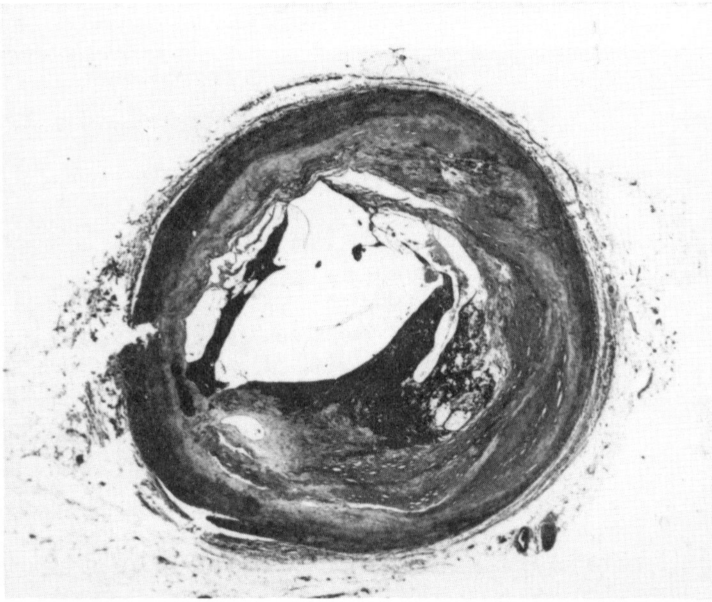

FIG. 9. Human coronary artery. The intimal surface in the lower portion of the vessel shows a darkly staining mural thrombus. There is no obvious trans–cap intimal tear and this thrombus has arisen on the basis of erosion of a large area of the plaque surface

Lendrum picro–mallory x 35

One might legitimately speculate as to whether this morphological appearance signifies breakdown of collagen by proteolysis or a reduction in collagen synthesis by smooth muscle cells which appear to be sparse under these circumstances. It is not without interest , in this connection, that Russell Ross (personal communication) has shown that macrophages expressing PDGF are not foam cells, while oxidized low density lipoprotein, which is recognized by the scavenger receptors on macrophages, inhibits the production of PDGF by macrophages which have taken up the altered LDL and have become "foam cells".

Significance of Thrombi in the Genesis of Ischaemic Heart Disease and the Progression of Atherosclerosis.

From all the foregoing it can be appreciated that ultra–microscopic thrombi and thrombi visible on optical microscopy might be expected to affect the natural history of atherosclerotic plaques purely as a result of their growth promoting functions. The third type of thrombus, as already stated above, is a major factor in the genesis of acute ischaemic syndromes but, in non–fatal cases, will also exert a growth promoting effect and leave the surviving patient with more severe lumenal narrowing in the affected segment than existed before the episode of plaque injury and acute thrombosis. .

Factors Likely to be Associated with an Increased Risk of Plaque–Related Thrombosis.

The classical triad of risk factors for thrombosis enunciated by Virchow :–

abnormalities in the vascular wall

abnormalities in the blood flow

abnormalities in the blood

still provides a useful theoretical template.

So far as the artery wall is concerned , atherosclerosis relates to the risk of thrombosis both in a quantitative and a qualitative sense. The first of these propositions is supported by the positive correlation that exists between the extent of atherosclerotic involvement of an arterial bed and the risk of one of the acute ischaemic syndromes listed at the beginning of this section and the second has been discussed in the immediately preceding section. .

"Pro–thrombotic " abnormalities in the blood can affect the platelets, the components of the clotting and fibrinolytic systems or all three. Platelets may be more aggregatable (as in familial hypercholesterolaemia) or more adhesive (as in diabetes mellitus) (26,27,28) and their behaviour may also be altered by diet (29,30,31). Raised plasma concentrations of fibrinogen and/or of factor VIIC are effective predictors of risk of acute coronary syndromes, the latter being strongly influenced by the lipid content of the diet .(32,33) Since we should be concerned , wherever possible, to relate pathological events to **modifiable** risk, it is not without interest that **cigarette smoking** appears to affect not only wall disease but also platelet function and the clotting system (34). It is associated with an increased amount of wall disease ; leads to an increase in plasma fibrinogen and factor VIIC and also appears to cause increased reactivity of platelets.

Thus attempts to modify the extremely high prevalence of atherosclerosis–related disease in many parts of Europe and North America must take cognizance both of factors which affect the extent and severity of atherosclerosis and those which may cause adverse changes in platelet function and clotting.

References

1. Davies, M.J. 1990. Morphology and natural history of atherosclerotic lesions in the human artery tree. In: Atheroma Vol.1, Atherosclerosis in ischaemic heart disease: The mechanisms, edited by Woolf, N. and Davies, M.J. Science Press, London,

pp 2:1 -2:52

2. Woolf, N. 1987.Thrombosis and atherosclerosis. In : Haemostasis and Thrombosis , edited by Bloom,A.L. and Thomas, D.P. Churchill Livingstone, Edinburgh,London,Melbourne and New York, pp651–678.

3. Ross, R., 1986. The pathogenesis of atherosclerosis – an update. New Engl. J. Med. 314, 488–500.

4. Woolf,N., Bradley, J.W.P., Crawford, T. and Carstairs, K.C. 1968. Experimental mural thrombosis in the pig aorta. The early natural history.Brit.J. Exper. Path., 49, 257.

5. Ross, R. 1989. Cellular Interactions in Atherosclerosis– The role of growth factors. In:Atherosclerosis VIII, edited by Crepaldi G. et al. Elsevier Science Publishers, pp21–24.

6. Ross, R., Raines, E.W. and Bowen–Pope, D.F. 1986. The biology of platelet–derived growth factor. Cell, 46, 155–169.

7. Waterfield, M.D., Scrace, G.T. Whittle, H. et al. 1983. Platelet derived growth factor is structurally related to the putative transforming protein $p28^{v-sis}$. Nature, 304, 35–39.

8. Doolittle, R.F.Hunkapiller, M.W., Hood, L.E. et al. 1983. Simian sarcoma virus oncogene v–sis is derived from the gene (or genes) encoding a platelet–derived growth factor. Science, 221, 275–277.

9. Smith, E.B. 1989. Human atherosclerotic lesions – an overview. In: Atherosclerosis VIII, edited by Crepaldi, G. et al. Elsevier Science Publishers, , pp13–19.

10. Walker, L., Reidy, M. and Bowyer, D. 11986. Morphology and cell kinetics of fatty streak lesion formation in the hypercholesterolaemic rabbit. Amer. J. Path., 125, 450–459.

11. Reidy, M. 1985. A reassessment of endothelial injury and arterial lesion formation. Lab. Invest., 53, 513–520.

12. Faggiotto, A., Ross, R. and Harker,L. 1984. Studies of hypercholesterolemia in the non–human primate I. Changes that lead to fatty streak formation. Arteriosclerosis, 4, 323–340.

13. Seddon, A.M., Woolf, N. , La Ville, A., et al. 1987. Hereditary hyperlipidemia and atherosclerosis in the rabbit due to overproduction of lipoproteins. II. Preliminary

report of arterial pathology. Arteriosclerosis, 7, 113–124.

14. Faggiotto, A. and Ross, R., 1984. Studies of hypercholesterolemia in the non-human primate. II> Fatty streak conversion to fibrous plaque. Arteriosclerosis, 4, 341–356.

15. Davies, M.J., Woolf,N., Rowles,P. and Pepper, J. 1988. Morphology of the endothelium over atherosclerotic plaques in human coronary arteries. Br Heart J., 60, 459–464.

16. Duguid, J.B. 1946. Thrombosis as a factor in the pathogenesis of coronary atherosclerosis. J Pathol. Bacteriol. 58, 207–212.

17. Duguid, J.B. 1948. Thrombosis as a factor in the pathogenesis of aortic atherosclerosis. J. Pathol. Bacteriol. 60, 57–61.

18. Woolf,N. and Crawford,T. 1960. Fatty streaks in aortic intima studied by an immuno–histochemical technique. J. Pathol. Bacteriol. 80, 205–208.

19. Woolf,N. 1961. The distribution of fibrin within the aortic intima: an immuno–histochemical study. Am J Pathol., 39, 521–532.

20. Walton,K and Williamson, N. 1968. Histological and immunofluorescent studies on the evolution of the human atheromatous plaque. J Atheroscl. Res. 8, 599–624.

21. Woolf,N. and Carstairs, K. 1967. Infiltration and thrombosis in atherogenesis – a study using immunofluorescent techniques. Am J Pathol , 51, 373–386.

22. Chandler, A.B. 1974. Mechanisms and frequency of thrombosis in the coronary circulation. Thromb. Res., 4, 3–23.

23. Woolf,N., Sacks,M.I. and Davies, M.J.,1969. Aortic plaque morphology in relation to coronary artery disease. Am. J. Pathol. 57, 187–197.

24. Lundberg, B. 1985. Chemical composition and physical state of lipid deposits in atherosclerosis. Atherosclerosis. 56, 93 – 110.

25. Richardson, P., Davies, M.J. and Born, G. 1989. Lancet, ii, 941–944.

26. Carvalho A.C.A., Colman, R.W. and Lees, R.S. 1974a. Platelet function in hyperlipoproteinaemia. New Engl. J. Med., 290, 434–438.

27. Carvalho, A.C.A., Colman, R.W. and Lees, R.S. 1974b. Clofibrate reversal of platelet hypersensitivity in hyperbetalipoproteinaemia. Circulation, 50, 570–574.

28. Lees, R.S. and Carvalho, A.C.A. 1978. Hypercholesterolaemia and platelets. In : The Thrombotic Process in Atherogenesis eds. Chandler, A.B., Eurenius, K., McMillan, G.C., Nelson, C.B., Schwartz, C.J. and Wessler, S. Plenum Press, New York, pp301–308.

29. Nordoy,A. 1976. Lipids as triggering factors in thrombosis. Thrombosis and Haemostasis, 35, 32–48.

30. Hornstra, G.and Lussenburg, R.N. 1975. Relationship between the type of dietary fatty acids and arterial thrombosis tendency in rats. Atherosclerosis, 22, 499–516.

31. Dyerberg,J. and Bang, H.O. 1979. Haemostatic function and platelet polyunsaturated fatty acids in Eskimos. Lancet, 2, 433–435.

32. Meade, T.W., Brozovic, M. and Chakrabarti, P. 1986. Haemostatic function and ischaemic heart disease: principal results of the Northwick Park Study. Lancet, 2, 533–537.

33. Meade, T.W. 1987. Thrombogenic Factors. In: Atherosclerosis: Biology and Clinical Science. edited by Olsson, A.G. Churchill Livingstone, pp 453–455.

34. Meade, T.W., Imeson, J. and Stirling, Y. 1987. Effects of changes in smoking and other characteristics on clotting factors and the risk of ischaemic heart disease. Lancet, 2, 986–988.

PHARMACOLOGICAL INHIBITION OF THE ADP-GP IIb/IIIa-FIBRINOGEN PATHWAY OF PLATELET AGGREGATION

J.-P. CAZENAVE, C. GACHET, F. LANZA

ABSTRACT. ADP plays a major role in hemostasis and in thrombosis. ADP binds to specific receptors on human platelets and has two distinct effects : i) induction of platelet shape change at low concentrations (0.1-0.5 μM), exposure of the GP IIb-IIIa fibrinogen receptor and platelet aggregation (1-5 μM); ii) inhibiton of PGE_1 or PGI_2 stimulated adenylate cyclase in intact platelets or platelet membranes. Fibrinogen binding to activated GP IIb-IIIa is the common pathway of platelet aggregation. Fibrinogen binds to the GP IIb-IIIa complex through RGDX sequences on Aα chain and through the γ 401-411 C-terminal peptide. The ADP-GP IIb-IIIa-fibrinogen pathway of platelet aggregation can be inhibited by pharmacological agents which are specific antagonists of the ADP receptor, which inhibit fibrinogen binding (monoclonal antibodies, synthetic peptides, desintegrins) to GP IIb-IIIa or which interfere with ADP-induced aggregation such as the thienopyridines. The thienopyridine, ticlopidine is a drug which has demonstrated in clinical trials efficacy in prevention of arterial thrombosis and its complications.

Platelet aggregation plays a major role in microvascular hemostasis and arterial thrombosis which occur in high flow and wall shear rate conditions when blood is in contact with a damaged vessel wall or with an artificial surface. Platelet aggregation is an active process requiring activation by an agonist such as adenosine-5'-diphosphate (ADP), metabolic energy, extracellular calcium ions, fibrinogen binding to the platelet membrane glycoprotein (GP) IIb-IIIa complex and platelet to platelet contact.

Thirty years ago in Norway, Hellem [1] observed that platelet adhesion to glass was mediated by a small heat-stable acid-soluble substance present in red cells, which was identified as ADP [2]. ADP was also found in platelets and was able to stimulate platelet aggregation [3]. The development of a simple turbidimetric method by Born [4] to follow quantitatively the aggregation of blood platelets *in vitro* made possible to study platelet function and its inhibition by pharmacological agents. Two years later, it was shown that fibrinogen was essential for the aggregation of platelets by ADP [5]. The binding of fibrinogen is mediated by the platelet membrane GP IIb-IIIa complex which acquires receptor function after induction by ADP [6,7]. The importance of the pathway of platelet aggregation mediated by ADP, fibrinogen and GP IIb-IIIa was clearly demonstrated by hereditary bleeding disorders of primary hemostasis such as Glanzmann's thrombasthenia where the platelet membrane GP IIb-IIIa complex is absent or abnormal and afibrinogenemia [8]. Platelet aggregation is also important in thrombosis occuring in high

A. G. Herman (ed.), Antithrombotics, 83–97.
© 1991 *Kluwer Academic Publishers. Printed in the Netherlands.*

flow systems and in the embolization of platelet-fibrin aggregates to the microcirculation of organs causing infarction [9].

In this review, we will consider some of the effects of ADP on platelet function and some aspects of the structure-function relationship between GP IIb-IIIa and fibrinogen in order to discuss the pharmacological agents which interfere specifically with the ADP-GP IIb/IIIa-fibrinogen pathway of aggregation. Some of these agents are already drugs which are used in patients to prevent the occurence and extension of arterial thrombosis or its complications.

1. Effects of ADP on Platelets

1.1 AGGREGATION

The addition of ADP to stirred human platelets suspended at 37°C in plasma or in a medium containing physiological concentrations of Ca^{2+} results in a series of responses [10,11] : i) fixation of ADP to a specific receptor; ii) rapid change of platelet shape from disc to sphere with emission of pseudopods; iii) induction and exposure of fibrinogen binding sites on the GP IIb-IIIa; iv) primary reversible platelet aggregation; v) inhibition of the ability of other agents to stimulate the synthesis of cAMP by adenylate cyclase.

In vitro, two types of platelet aggregation responses induced by ADP can be distinguished [12,13] : a primary or first phase aggregation that is reversible and occurs without the release reaction and a secondary phase of aggregation that is irreversible and associated with the release reaction. Primary, reversible human platelet aggregation is induced by low concentrations of ADP (0.5 to 1 μM) in the presence of physiological concentrations of Ca^{2+} and Mg^{2+} in plasma or suspending medium. Platelet aggregation and disaggregation is associated with fibrinogen binding to and dissociation from its receptor, the membrane GP IIb-IIIa complex [14]. When higher concentrations of ADP (2 to 10 μM) are added to citrated platelet rich plasma (cPRP), after a first wave of primary aggregation, a second wave of aggregation occurs which is related to the platelet release reaction (including secretion of ADP from platelet dense granules) triggered by the formation of prostaglandin endoperoxydes PGG_2 and PGH_2 and thromboxane A_2 (TXA_2) from membrane arachidonate. The second wave of aggregation is not reversible. The factors responsible for ADP-induced release reaction of human platelets have been extensively studied [15,94]. Addition of ADP to stirred platelets in a medium containing low concentrations of Ca^{2+} in the micromolar range induces the synthesis of TXA_2 by a mechanism not understood, the release of granule contents and extensive aggregation. Thus, ADP-induced release and secondary aggregation is an artefact of cPRP or artificial media to which Ca^{2+} has been omitted [16,17] and does not reflect the physiological *in vivo* response of platelets to ADP.

In vivo, the sources of ADP responsible for the aggregation of circulating platelets are coming either from external sources (damaged red blood cells or endothelium, plasma) or from internal sources, the platelet dense granules. When platelets are stimulated by agents such as collagen or thrombin they release ADP from dense granules which contribute to and reinforce aggregation. In addition, low concentrations of ADP potentiate the effects of all other aggregating agents [18], even weak agonists such as adrenaline and serotonin [19,20].

1.2. INHIBITION OF ACTIVATED ADENYLATE CYCLASE

Increasing the concentration of cAMP in platelets by activating the platelet membrane adenylate cyclase with PGI_2 or PGE_1 results in the inhibition of most platelet responses including aggregation to ADP and other agonists [21,22]. ADP, α_2-adrenergic agents and thrombin reduce the effects of prostaglandins on cAMP accumulation in intact platelets. The degree of inhibition of PGE1-stimulated cAMP by ADP in intact platelets is non competitive and about 90 %. The inhibition of the adenylate cyclase by ADP is not the cause of aggregation [10,23].

2. Activation of GP IIb-IIIa as a Fibrinogen Receptor

The platelet membrane GP IIb-IIIa complex is a cell-surface receptor, member of the family of integrins which mediate cell-cell and cell-substrate adhesions [24,25]. GP IIb-IIIa and the vitronectin receptor (VnR) are members of the group of cytoadhesins. They have a common β subunit (GP IIIa) and are classified as β_3 integrins [26]. The β_3 subunit can be associated with two different α subunits to form the VnR ($\alpha v\beta_3$) or the GP IIb-IIIa complex ($\alpha_{IIb}\beta_3$).

2.1. GP IIb-IIIa STRUCTURE [24,25]

A normal platelet contains about 50,000 copies of the GP IIb-IIIa complex, 2/3 are exposed randomly at the platelet surface and 1/3 is distributed with internal membranes of the surface connected canalicular system and the membranes of the cytoplasmic α-granules.

The GP IIb-IIIa complex is composed of one molecule of GP IIb (mol wt = 140,000) which consist of a large IIbα (mol wt = 125,000) and a small IIbβ (mol wt = 25,000) chain linked by disulfide bonding, and one molecule of GP IIIa (mol wt = 105,000), which is a single polypeptide chain. The complex requires micromolar Ca^{2+} concentrations to maintain its heterodimer structure and function in platelet aggregation [27,28].

Major progresses have been recently accomplished in understanding the structure and function relationships of GP IIb-IIIa by cloning and sequencing the cDNAs and the genes coding for GP IIb [29,30,31] and GP IIIa [32,33] and by sequencing the two proteins [15,34,35]. This new knowledge has made possible to study the functional domains of GP IIb, GP IIIa or the complex with the use of synthetic peptides and monoclonal antibodies (MoAb).

2.2. ACTIVATION OF GP IIb-IIIa

In the normal state, platelets circulate as isolated discs and do not bind on their surface fibrinogen although it is present in plasma at a concentration of 2-4 g/L. When platelets are activated by primary agonists for which they have specific receptors on their membrane they acquire adhesive properties and can bind fibrinogen [36]. Upon stimulation by ADP, specific binding sites for fibrinogen become available at the platelet surface and these new induced sites exhibit characteristics of a receptor system [7,37,38]. Fibrinogen binding is time and divalent cations dependent. It is saturable with respect to the concentration of ADP and fibrinogen. There is one class of binding site with an average number at steady state equilibrium of 38,000 ± 10,000 per platelet and affinity constant (Kd) of 5.10^{-7} M (0.2 g/L fibrinogen). Extracellular divalent cations, in particular Ca^{2+} are not required for receptor induction of adhesive properties but are necessary for fibrinogen-receptor interaction. When fibrinogen binding is measured under physiological conditions of ADP stimulation (during reversible ADP-induced aggregation) no more than 1,000 fibrinogen molecules bind reversibly per platelet [39].

A number of clinical and experimental evidences (Glanzmann's thrombasthenia, MoAb against GP IIb-IIIa complex, reconstitution of purified GP IIb-IIIa complex in phospholipid vesicles) have led to the conclusion that the platelet binding site for fibrinogen is the GP IIb-IIIa complex [24]. In addition to fibrinogen, the GP IIb-IIIa complex also can serve as a receptor for fibronectin, von Willebrand factor and vitronectin [40].

The mechanisms by which fibrinogen receptor function of GP IIb-IIIa is regulated by ADP or other agonists stimulation is not completely understood. It is possible that the increased concentration of cytoplasmic Ca^{2+} may transform directly the GP IIb-IIIa complex into a receptor active form. Indirectly, a guanine nucleotide binding protein (such as the G-proteins which regulate the activity of α_2-adrenoceptors) may be involved in coupling agonist interaction to the receptor function of GP IIb-IIIa required for aggregation [24]. The acquisition of GP IIb-IIIa upon platelet stimulation to become competent for binding fibrinogen may be due, either or both, to structural or conformational changes in the GP IIb-IIIa complex or in alterations of the microenvironment around GP IIb-IIIa [25].

Fibrinogen is the essential cofactor of platelet aggregation, implying that it must contain binding domains specifically recognized by GP IIb-IIIa. Two different types of amino acid sequences have been shown to mediate the binding of fibrinogen to GP IIb-IIIa. Two Arg-Gly-Asp (RGD) sequences are present in the Aα chain of fibrinogen. The first RGDS sequences at Aα 572-575 may not be necessary for fibrinogen binding to platelets [25,41], although a synthetic RGDS peptide inhibits the binding of fibrinogen as well as fibronectin and von Willebrand factor to GP IIb-IIIa [40]. A second RGDF sequence at Aα 95-98 is the potential fibrinogen recognition site implicated in binding to GP IIb-IIIa and platelet aggregation [41]. The C-terminus γ chain dodecapeptide of fibrinogen (γ 401-411, HHLGGAKQAGDV) is also implicated in fibrinogen binding to GP IIb-IIIa and platelet aggregation [41,42]. The site of recognition of the RGDX sequence, a general recognition sequence, has been localized on GP IIIa [43] and that of the γ chain, a specific helper sequence on GP IIb [44]. In order to aggregate to ADP, platelets need an intact GP IIb-IIIa complex able to bind fibrinogen.

3. Inhibition of ADP-Induced Platelet Aggregation

For many years, efforts have been focused on developing pharmacological agents which inhibit platelet aggregation induced by ADP, because the ADP-GP IIb-IIIa-fibrinogen pathway of aggregation is of major importance in hemostasis and thrombosis [45-48]. These pharmacological agents have contributed to understand the molecular mechanisms of action of ADP on platelets and the specific binding interactions of fibrinogen and other adhesive proteins to their induced receptor, the integrin GP IIb-IIIa complex. There are many pharmacological inhibitors of the ADP-GP IIb-IIIa-fibrinogen pathway of platelet aggregation which, for convenience, can be classified in two broad categories (Table 1). The most interesting category deals with agents which inhibit in a rather specific manner : i) the primary phase of ADP-induced aggregation by directly interfering with ADP, the ADP receptor or the ADP transduction system; ii) the binding of fibrinogen to the GP IIb-IIIa complex by competing with specific recognition sites or domains localized on the fibrinogen molecule or on the cytoadhesin. The second category of inhibitors is composed

TABLE 1. Classification of the pharmacological inhibitors of the ADP-GP IIb-IIIa-fibrinogen pathway of platelet aggregation

Mechanisms of action	Inhibitors
1. SPECIFIC EFFECTS	
Inhibit primary phase of ADP-induced aggregation	
i. Enzymes acting on ADP	ADPases, apyrase, CP/CPK
ii. ADP receptor antagonists	ATP, adenosine tetraphosphate, β,γ-methylene ATP, α,ω-diadenosine pentaphosphate, 2-methylthio ATP, 2-ethyltio ATP, AMP and 2-substituted analogs, 5'-p-fluorosulfonylbenzoyladenosine
iii. Thienopyridines	ticlopidine, PCR 4099, clopidogrel
iv. Others	penicillin G, cephalothin and related antibiotics, pyridoxal phosphate
Inhibit fibrinogen binding to GP IIb-IIIa	
i. MoAb against GP IIb-IIIa	AP-2, P_{37}, 7E3, 7E3-F(ab')$_2$
ii. GP IIb-IIIa-related peptides	GP IIb 296-306 (TDVNGDGRHDL) GP IIIa 211-222 (SVSRNRDAPEGG-NH_2)
iii. Fibrinogen-related peptides	RGD (Aα 95-97, 572-574), RGDV, RGDF, RGDW, RGD(Me) Y-NH_2, Ac-RGDS-NH_2, GRGDS, HHLGGAKQAGDV (γ 401-411), KQAGDV (γ 406-411)
iv. Desintegrins	trigramin, echistatin, bitistatin, applagin, albolabrin, elegantin, kistrin, batroxostatin, decorsin
2. GENERAL EFFECTS	
Increase cAMP levels :	
i. activate adenylate cyclase	adenosine, PGE_1, PGD_2, PGI_2 iloprost, taprostene, beraprost
ii. inhibit cAMP phosphodiesterase	dipyridamole, flavonoids, cilostamide, trequinsine
Chelation of Ca^{2+}	EDTA, EGTA
Inhibit calcium fluxes	verapamil, nicardipine, nifedipine, diltiazem
Inhibit calmodulin	chlorpromazine, trifluoperazine, W-7

of agents which interfere more generally with cytoplasmic transmission molecules acting as second messengers such as calcium or cAMP.

PGE_1 or PGI_2 and its stable analog iloprost stimulate platelet adenylate cyclase and increase cAMP levels [22]. This effect is potentiated and prolonged by phosphodiesterase inhibitors such as dipyridamole, flavonoids, cilostamide or trequinsine [46,47]. Inhibition of platelet activation is due to increased sequestration of Ca^{2+} and reduced binding of fibrinogen to unactivated GP IIb-IIIa leading to inhibition of aggregation [22]. Similarly drugs interfering with calmodulin (chlorpromazine, trifluoperazine, W-7) and with Ca^{2+} fluxes (verapamil, nicardipine, nifedipine, diltiazem) inhibit ADP-induced primary aggregation. Short term chelation of Ca^{2+} in the external medium inhibits fibrinogen binding to the GP IIb-IIIa complex and aggregation [13]. Prolonged incubation with EDTA at 37°C leads to dissociation of the complex which is unable to bind fibrinogen and platelets do not aggregate to ADP [28].

3.1. SPECIFIC INHIBITION OF ADP-INDUCED PRIMARY AGGREGATION

There are a number of compounds which specifically act on ADP itself, the ADP receptor or the primary phase of aggregation induced by ADP. These agents have been extremely useful tools to understand the mechanisms of action of ADP on platelets and the important role of ADP in platelet aggregation. Some of them, like the thienopyridines, are already antithrombotic drugs used in clinical medicine.

3.1.1. *Enzymes Acting On ADP*. Enzymes which hydrolyse ADP to AMP or adenosine such as ADPases in plasma or in snake venoms, potato apyrases and enzymatic systems such as creatine phosphate/creatine phosphokinase (CP/CPK) have been used in experiments to unravel the role of ADP from external sources or released from platelet dense granules in platelet aggregation [15,49], in platelet desensitization [50] and in preparing washed platelet suspensions [13,51].

3.1.2. *ADP Receptor Antagonists*. ADP binds to specific receptors on human platelets and has two distinct effects [10,11] : i) induction of platelet shape change, exposure of the fibrinogen receptor and aggregation, ii) inhibition of adenylate cyclase. These two effects of ADP on platelets appeared to be independent and unrelated events. The studies of ADP binding to intact platelets or isolated platelet membranes are complicated by several technical problems and have provided conflicting results as to whether there are two different receptors (one coupled to adenylate cyclase, the other responsible for aggregation) or one receptor with two binding sites for ADP or a common G-protein mediating both actions [10,11,52]. The platelet ADP receptors have a unique specificity : ADP is an agonist and ATP an antagonist. In the classical P_2 purinergic receptor, ADP and ATP are agonists [52].

A variety of analogs of ADP inhibit platelet aggregation by specifically interacting with ADP receptors. ATP is the best characterized competitive inhibitor of ADP-induced shape change and aggregation and cAMP accumulation [53]. A large number of competitive or non competitive antagonists of the ADP receptor which inhibit ADP-induced platelet aggregation have been studied [10,52] : adenosine tetraphosphate; β-γ-methylene ATP; α,ω-diadenosine pentaphosphate; 2-methylthioATP and 2-ethylthioATP; AMP, 2-methylthioAMP and 2-ethylthioAMP.

A reactive derivative of adenosine, 5'-p-fluorosulfonylbenzoyladenosine (FSBA) has been used as a stable ADP analog to label covalently the ADP-receptor [54]. FSBA is a non specific time-dependent inhibitor of ADP-induced shape change, fibrinogen binding and aggregation. FSBA does not prevent ADP to inhibit the adenylate cyclase and the accumulation of cAMP. FSBA labels covalently a single external platelet membrane protein of 100 kDa, aggregin. Aggregin may play a role in platelet activation by serving as the ADP receptor for shape change and aggregation and by modulating the latency of the fibrinogen receptor [55].

3.1.3. *Thienopyridines.* The thienopyridine ticlopidine [56,57] and its analogs PCR 4099 (racemic form of clopidogrel) and clopidogrel (SR 25990 C) are potent specific inhibitors of ADP-induced platelet aggregation. They also inhibit platelet aggregation induced by low concentrations of other agonists (thrombin for example), probably by blocking the amplification of platelet activation by ADP released from dense granules [58]. At higher concentrations of thrombin, platelet aggregation becomes less ADP-dependent and is no longer inhibited. Ticlopidine and its analogs exert their effects *ex vivo*, after oral administration, following at least three days of treatment to achieve optimal efficacy. The permanent inhibition of platelet functions, probably due to a metabolite, is dose related and the recovery of normal aggregation occurs at a rate consistent with platelet survival. The site and the mechanism of action of the thienopyridines are not yet clear. Ticlopidine [59] and PCR 4099 selectively inhibit ADP-induced platelet aggregation and fibrinogen binding without modifying quantitatively or qualitatively the membrane GP IIb-IIIa complex in rat and in man [60,61]. It does not seem that ticlopidine, which does not block ADP-induced shape change, exerts major effects on the ADP binding site on its receptor, although it inhibits ^{14}C-ADP binding but only to low affinity sites [62]. More recently, it was shown that ticlopidine selectively prevents the inhibitory effects of ADP but not of adrenaline on cAMP levels raised by stimulation of the adenylate cyclase of human platelets by PGE_1. These results suggested that ticlopidine or a metabolite impairs the coupling mechanism of the ADP aggregation pathway at an unknown level of the ADP signal transduction system involving or not an as yet unknown G-protein [63]. Similar observations were made with ticlopidine and clopidogrel in rats and rabbits [64].

3.1.4. *Other Drugs.* Penicillin G, cephalothin and related antibiotics inhibit *in vitro* and *in vivo* at high concentrations ADP-induced shape change, fibrinogen binding, primary aggregation and the release reaction. They also inhibit aggregation induced by other agonists. Their mechanism of action is not well understood, but they may coat permanently the platelet membrane and covalently modify receptors including the ADP and the fibrinogen receptors [65,66].

Pyridoxal phosphate [67,68] inhibits also aggregation induced by ADP and other agonists by a covalent modification of platelet membrane glycoproteins.

3.2. INHIBITION OF FIBRINOGEN BINDING TO GP IIb-IIIa

Platelet aggregation induced by ADP, as well as any known agonist, is essentially mediated by fibrinogen binding to its induced receptor, the GP IIb-IIIa complex. For this reason, GP IIb-IIIa-fibrinogen interactions are now important targets for the rational design of antiplatelet drugs inhibiting thrombosis.

3.2.1. *Monoclonal Antibodies Against GP IIb-IIIa.* Monoclonal antibodies (MoAbs) have been produced against human platelet membrane GP IIb-IIIa from whole platelets, purified proteins or derived peptides. This huge amount of work has resulted in an exponential growth of publications and books. MoAbs against GP IIb-IIIa can recognize the heterodimer complex, GP IIb or GP IIIa and can be mapped to peptidic epitopes on the GP [for review see 69,95]. These MoAbs are useful to determine the structure and function of platelet GP IIb-IIIa [25,69] and some of them inhibit fibrinogen binding and platelet aggregation.

AP-2 is a murine MoAb whose antigenic determinant resides and is specific for the GP IIb-IIIa Ca^{2+}-dependent heterodimer [70]. AP-2 binds in a specific and saturable manner to unstimulated and ADP-stimulated platelets. It is a non competitive potent antagonist of fibrinogen for binding to ADP-stimulated platelets. AP-2 exerts its effects by steric hindrance through binding to an epitope close to, but not identical with the fibrinogen binding site on GP IIb-IIIa. AP-2 is a potent inhibitor of platelet aggregation induced by ADP and other agonists. Incubation of human platelets with EDTA at 37°C is followed by dissociation of the GP IIb-IIIa complex, loss of AP-2 and fibrinogen binding to their receptor and lack of aggregation.

P_{37} [35] is a murine MoAb that inhibits fibrinogen binding and platelet aggregation induced by ADP. The epitope for P_{37} was found in the N-terminal region of GP III (peptide sequence 101-109) which is involved in fibrinogen binding through the Aα 94-99 peptide containing an RGD domain.

Another murine MoAb, 7E3 [71] binds to the intact GP IIb-IIIa complex and inhibits completely fibrinogen binding and platelet aggregation. 7E3 binds three times faster to activated than unactivated platelets. The $F(ab')_2$ fragment of 7E3 binds more rapidly than the intact 7E3 antibody to unactivated platelets.

3.2.2. *GP IIb-IIIa-Related Peptides.* Binding of fibrinogen to GP IIb-IIIa is necessary for platelet aggregation to occur and is mediated through discrete sequences in the integrin which are ligand recognition sites. A synthetic peptide of 12 amino acids (GP IIIa 211-222, SVSRNRDAPEGG-NH_2) derived from the sequences of the N-terminal region of GP IIIa blocks the binding of fibrinogen, fibronectin, vitronectin and von Willebrand factor to GP IIb-IIIa. A polyclonal antibody to GP IIIa 211-222 blocks fibrinogen binding to GP IIb-IIIa and ADP-induced human platelet aggregation [72]. Similarly, a peptide of 11 amino acids corresponding to residues 296-306 of GP IIb (TDVNGDGRHDL, designated B12) inhibits human platelet aggregation induced by ADP and binding of fibrinogen to platelets and to purified GP IIb-IIIa. B12 interacts directly with the C-terminus of the γ chain of fibrinogen [73].

These synthetic peptides corresponding to discrete sequences in GP IIb or GP IIIa have antiaggregating properties. It is difficult at the present time to use them as pharmacological agents because they have a low affinity for GP IIb-IIIa, they are unstable *in vivo* and not active orally, large amounts have to be administered intravenously and they are potentially immunogenic [74].

3.2.3. *Fibrinogen-Related Peptides.* Arg-Gly-Asp (RGD) amino acid sequence, present in position 95-97 and 572-574 of the Aα chains of fibrinogen, is a basic recognition specificity to GP IIb-IIIa. Synthetic RGDX tetrapeptides inhibit competitively fibrinogen binding to GP IIb-IIIa (IC_{50} : 10 nM to 50 μM) and ADP-induced platelet aggregation. A number of RGD peptides (Table 1) have shown antithrombotic activity after intravenous administration of large amounts because they are unstable and have a short half-life [25,41,74]. Similarly, synthetic dodecapeptide (γ 401-411, HHLGGAKQAGDV) and hexapeptide (γ 406-411, KQAGDV) inhibit binding of fibrinogen and platelet aggregation [42,74].

3.2.4. *Desintegrins.* RGD containing peptides of 49 to 83 amino acids have been isolated from snake venoms and are powerful inhibitors of fibrinogen binding to platelet GP IIB-IIIA (IC_{50} : 30 to 300 nM) and of platelet aggregation. The platelet GP IIb-IIIa protein antagonists that have been isolated from viper venoms (trigramin, echistatin, bitistatin, applagin, albolabrin, elegantin, kistrin, batroxostatin) and leeches (decorsin) form a family of platelet aggregation inhibitors named desintegrins [75-80].

4. Clinical Implications

Platelet aggregation by ADP has a major role in the development and extension of arterial thrombosis and thrombosis of artificial surfaces and their complications. Under these pathological conditions, thrombin generated and bound to the vascular and artificial surfaces is important and contributes further to release ADP from platelet dense granules.

Clinical trials have been recently conducted with ticlopidine [81,82] and give further evidence that the ADP-GP IIb-IIIa-fibrinogen pathway is important. Ticlopidine prevents fatal and non fatal major ischemic events in heart, brain and peripheral arteries of patients at risk of thrombotic accidents as demonstrated by two large North-American studies conducted in patients with cerebrovascular disease : the Canadian-American Ticlopidine Study, CATS [83] and the Ticlopidine Aspirin Stroke Study, TASS [84]; the Swedish Multicentre Study (STIMS) in patients with intermittent claudication [85] and the italian Studio della Ticlopidina nell' angina Instable (STAI) in patients with unstable angina [86]. Ticlopidine has also proved to be useful in diabetic retinopathy, hemodialysis and coronary artery by-pass graft [81].

Recent experimental and clinical studies with the new protein inhibitors of fibrinogen binding to platelet GP IIb-IIIa demonstrate that specific inhibition of platelet aggregation might be useful in acute thrombosis. Intravenous injection of the MoAb 7E3 or the 7E3 $F(ab')_2$ abolishes experimental thrombus formation and increases lysis of coronary artery thrombus by recombinant tissue plasminogen activator [87,88]. In man, it inhibits platelet aggregation [89,90] and reduces angina pectoris [91]. The desintegrins, RGD-containing peptides from pit vipers were also administered intravenously to animals to inhibit platelet deposition to surfaces of extracorporeal circuits [92] and to enhance and sustain coronary arterial thrombolysis with recombinant tissue-type plasminogen activator [93]. Although MoAbs, RGD peptides and desintegrins appear as promising antithrombotic agents, they need further evaluation in patients. Limitations to their use may come from their cost, *in vivo* reduced stability and half-life and potential immunogenicity. Nethertheless they are powerful tools to unravel the mechanisms of platelet aggregation through the ADP-GP IIb-IIIa-fibrinogen pathway and they will help to design and synthesize new antithrombotic molecules.

5. References

1. Hellem, A.J. (1960) 'The adhesiveness of human blood platelets in vitro', Scand. J. Clin. Lab. Invest. 12 (Suppl.51).
2. Gaarder, A., Jonsen, J., Hellem, A. and Owren, P.A. (1961) 'Adenosine diphosphate in red cells as a factor in the adhesiveness of human blood platelets', Nature 191, 513-532.
3. Ollgaard, E. (1961) 'Macroscopic studies of platelet aggregation : nature of an aggregating factor in red blood cells and platelets', Thromb. Diath. Haemorrh. 6, 86-97.
4. Born, G.V.R. (1962) 'Aggregation of blood platelets by adenosine diphosphate and its reversal', Nature 194, 927-929.

5. Cross, M.J. (1964) 'Effect of fibrinogen on the aggregation of platelets by adenosine diphosphate', Thromb. Diath. Haemorrh. 12, 524-527.
6. Mustard, J.F., Packham, M.A., Kinlough-Rathbone, R.L. (1978) 'Fibrinogen and ADP-induced platelet aggregation', Blood 54, 453-466.
7. Marguerie, G.A., Plow, E.F. and Edgington, T.S. (1979) 'Human platelets possess an inducible and saturable receptor specific for fibrinogen', J. Biol. Chem. 254, 5357-5363.
8. George, J.N., Nurden, A.T. and Phillips, D.R. (1984) 'Molecular defects in interactions of platelets with vessel wall', N. Engl. J. Med. 311, 1084-1098.
9. Mustard, J.F., Murphy, E.A., Rowsell, H.C. and Downie, H.G. (1962) 'Factors influencing thrombus formation in vivo', Amer. J. Med. 33, 621-647.
10. Macfarlane, D.E. (1987) 'Agonists and receptors : adenosine diphosphate' in H. Holmsen (ed.), Platelet Responses and Metabolism, Vol.2, Receptors and Metabolism, CRC Press, Boca Raton, pp. 19-36.
11. Siess, W. (1989) 'Molecular mechanisms of platelet activation', Physiol. Rev. 69, 58-178.
12. Kinlough-Rathbone, R.L., Mustard, J.F., Packham, M.A., Perry, D.W., Reimers, H.J. and Cazenave, J.-P. (1977) 'Properties of washed human platelets', Thromb. Haemostas. 37, 291-308.
13. Cazenave, J.-P., Hemmendinger, S., Beretz, A., Sutter-Bay, A. and Launay, J. (1983) 'L'agrégation plaquettaire : outil d'investigation clinique et d'étude pharmacologique. Méthodologie', Ann. Biol. Clin. 41, 167-179.
14. Kinlough-Rathbone, R.L., Mustard, J.F., Perry, D.W., Dejana, E., Cazenave, J.-P., Packham, M.A. and Harfenist, E.J. (1983) 'Factors influencing the deaggregation of human and rabbit platelets', Thromb. Haemostas. 49, 162-167.
15. Mustard, J.F., Perry, D.W., Kinlough-Rathbone, R.L. and Packham, M.A. (1975) 'Factors responsible for ADP-induced release reaction of human platelets', Amer. J. Physiol. 228, 1757-1765.
16. Lages, B. and Weiss, H.J. (1981) 'Dependence of human platelet functional responses on divalent cations : aggregation and secretion in heparin- and hirudin-anticoagulated, platelet-rich plasma and the effects of chelating agents' Thromb. Haemostas. 45, 173-179.
17. Packham, M.A., Kinlough-Rathbone, R.L. and Mustard, J.F. (1987) 'Thromboxane A_2 causes feedback amplification involving extensive thromboxane A_2 formation on close contact of human platelets in media with a low concentration of ionized calcium', Blood 70, 647-651.
18. Kinlough-Rathbone, R.L. and Mustard, J.F. (1986) 'Synergism of agonists' in H. Holmsen (ed.), Platelet Responses and Metabolism, Vol. 1, Responses, CRC Press, Boca Raton, pp. 193-207.
19. Lanza, F., Beretz, A., Stierlé, A., Hanau, D., Kubina, M. and Cazenave, J.-P. (1988) 'Epinephrine potentiates human platelet activation but is not an aggregating agent', Amer. J. Physiol. 255, H1276-H1288.
20. De Clerck, F., David, J.L. and Janssen, P.A.J. (1982) 'Inhibition of 5-hydroxytryptamine-induced and amplified human platelet aggregation by ketanserin (R 41468), a selective 5-HT_2 receptor antagonist', Agents Actions 12, 388-397.
21. Haslam, R.J., Davidson, M.M.L., Davies, T., Lynham, J.A. and McClenaghan, M.D. (1978) 'Regulation of blood platelet function by cyclic nucleotides', Adv. Cyclic Nucleotide Res. 9, 533-552.
22. Kerins, D.M., Murray, R. and FitzGerald, G.A. (1991) 'Prostacyclin and prostaglandin E_1 : molecular mechanisms and therapeutic utility', Progr. Hemostas. Thromb. 10, 307-337.

23. Haslam, R.J. (1973) 'Interactions of the pharmacological receptors of blood platelets with adenylate cyclase', Ser. Haematol. 6, 333-350.
24. Phillips, D.R., Charo, I.F., Parise, L.V. and Fitzgerald, L.A. (1988) 'The platelet membrane glycoprotein IIb-IIIa complex', Blood 71, 831-843.
25. Plow, E.F. and Ginsberg, M.H. (1989) 'Cellular adhesion : GP IIb-IIIa as a prototypic adhesion receptor', Progr. Hemostas. Thromb. 9, 117-156.
26. Albelda, S.M.and Buck, C.A. (1990) 'Integrins and other cell adhesion molecules', FASEB J. 4, 2868-2880.
27. Fitzgerald, L.A. and Phillips, D.R. (1985) 'Calcium regulation of the platelet membrane glycoprotein IIb-IIIa complex', J. Biol. Chem. 260, 11366-11374.
28. Pidard, D., Rosa, J.-P., Kunicki, T.J. and Nurden, A.T. (1986) 'Temperature-dependent effects of EDTA on the membrane glycoprotein IIb-IIIa complex and platelet aggregability', Blood 67, 604-611.
29. Poncz, M., Eisman, R., Heidenreich, R., Silver, S.M., Vilaire, G., Surrey, S., Schwartz, E.and Bennett, J.S. (1987) 'Structure of the platelet membrane glycoprotein IIb : homology of the alpha subunits of the vitronectin and fibronectin membrane receptors', J. Biol. Chem. 262, 8476-8482.
30. Loftus, J.C., Plow, E.F., Frelinger, A.L.III, D'Souza, S.E., Dixon, D., Lacy, J., Sorge, J. and Ginsberg, M.H. (1987) 'Molecular cloning and chemical synthesis of a region of platelet GIIb involved in adhesive function', Proc. Natl. Acad. Sci. USA 84, 7114-7118.
31. Uzan, G., Frachet, P., Lajmanovich, A., Prandini, M.H., Denarier, E., Duperray, A., Loftus, J., Ginsberg, M., Plow, E. and Marguerie, G. (1988) 'Molecular cloning of human platelet GPIIb from mRNA megakaryocytes and erythroleukemic cells : evidence for a unique gene product with extensive homology to other Arg-Gly-Asp adhesion receptors', Eur. J. Biochem. 171, 87-93.
32. Fitzgerald, L.A., Steiner, B., Rall, S.C.Jr, Lo, S.S. and Phillips, D.R. (1987) 'Protein sequence of endothelial glycoprotein IIIa derived from a cDNA clone. Identity with platelet glycoprotein III and similarity to integrin', J. Biol. Chem. 262, 3936-3939.
33. Lanza, F., Kieffer, N., Phillips, D.R. and Fitzgerald L.A. (1990) 'Characterization of the human platelet glycoprotein IIIa gene. Comparison with the fibronectin receptor β-subunit gene', J. Biol. Chem. 265, 18098-18103.
34. Calvete, J.J., Henschen, A. and Gonzalez-Rodriguez, J. (1991) 'Assignment of disulphide bonds in human platelet GPIIIa. A disulphide pattern for the β-subunits of the integrin family', Biochem. J. 274, 63-71.
35. Calvete, J.J., Arias, J., Alvarez, M.V., Lopez, M.M., Henschen, A. and Gonzalez-Rodriguez, J. (1991) 'Further studies on the topography of the N-terminal region of human platelet glycoprotein IIIa. Localization of monoclonal antibody epitopes and the putative fibrinogen-binding sites', Biochem. J. 274, 457-463.
36. Colman, R.W. and Walsh, P.N. (1987) 'Mechanisms of platelet aggregation', in R.W. Colman, J. Hirsh, V.J. Marder and E.W. Salzman (eds.), Hemostasis and Thrombosis, 2nd edition, J.B. Lippincott Company, Philadelphia, pp. 594-605.
37. Marguerie, G.A., Edgington, T.S. and Plow, E.P. (1980) 'Interaction of fibrinogen with its platelet receptor as part of a multi-step reaction in ADP-induced platelet aggregation', J. Biol. Chem. 255, 154-161.
38. Peerschke, E.I.B. (1985) 'The platelet fibrinogen receptor', Semin. Hematol. 22, 241-249.
39. Harfenist, E.J., Packham, M.A. and Mustard, J.F. (1980) 'Reversibility of the association of fibrinogen with rabbit platelets exposed to ADP', Blood 56, 189-198.

40. Plow, E.F., Ginsberg, M.H. and Marguerie, G.A. (1986) 'Expression and function of adhesive proteins on the platelet surface' in D.R. Phillips, M.A. Shuman (eds.), Biochemistry of Platelets, Academic Press, Orlando, pp. 226-256/
41. Andrieux, A., Hudry-Clergeon, G., Ryckewaert, J.-J., Chapel, A., Ginsberg, M.H., Plow, E.F. and Marguerie, G. (1989) 'Amino acid sequences in fibrinogen mediating its interaction with its platelet receptor, GP IIb-IIIa', J. Biol. Chem. 264, 9258-9265.
42. Kloczewiak, M., Timmons, S., Lukas, T.J. and Hawiger, J. (1984) 'Platelet receptor recognition site on human fibrinogen. Synthesis and structure-function relationship of peptides corresponding to the carboxy-terminal segment of the γ chain', Biochemistry 23, 1767-1774.
43. D'Souza, S.E., Ginsberg, M.H., Lam, S.C.T. and Plow, E.F. (1988) 'Chemical crosslinking of arginyl-glycyl-aspartic acid peptides to an adhesion receptor on platelets', J. Biol. Chem. 263, 3943-3951.
44. D'Souza, S.E., Ginsberg, M.H., Burke, T.A.and Plow, E.F. (1990) 'The ligand binding site of the platelet integrin receptor GP IIb-IIIa is proximal to the 2nd calcium binding domain of its alpha-subunit', J. Biol. Chem. 265, 3440-3446.
45. Mustard, J.F. and Packham, M.A. (1970) 'Factors influencing platelet function : adhesion, release and aggregation', Pharmacol. Rev. 22, 97-187.
46. Cazenave, J.-P., Wiesel, M.-L., and Hemmendinger, S. (1984) 'Current treatment for thrombotic diseases', Agents Actions 15 (suppl.), 24-49.
47. Maffrand, J.-P. (1990) 'Nouvelles thérapeutiques antiagrégantes', Sang Thrombose Vaisseaux 2, 175-177.
48. Cazenave, J.-P. and Beretz, A. (1991) 'Médicaments inhibiteurs des fonctions plaquettaires' in M. Schorderet (ed.), Pharmacologie : des Concepts Fondamentaux aux Applications Thérapeutiques, 2nd edition, Editions Slatkine, Genève, pp. 287-299.
49. Haslam, R.J. (1967) 'Mechanisms of blood platelet aggregation' in S.A. Johnson and W.H. Seegers (eds.), Physiology of Hemostasis and Thrombosis, C.C. Thomas, Springfield, pp. 88-112.
50. Holme, S. and Holmsen, H. (1975) 'ADP-induced refractory state of platelets in vitro. I. Methodological studies on aggregation in platelet rich plasma', Scand. J. Haematol. 15, 96-103.
51. Ardlie, N.G., Perry, D.W., Packham, M.A. and Mustard, J.F. (1971) 'Influence of apyrase on stability of suspensions of washed rabbit platelets', Proc. Soc. Exp. Biol. Med. 136, 1021-1023.
52. Haslam, R.J. and Cusack, N.J. (1981) 'Blood platelet receptors for ADP and for adenosine' in G. Burnstock (ed.), Purinergic Receptors, Chapman and Hall, London, Chapter 7.
53. Macfarlane, D.E. and Mills, D.C.B. (1975)'The effect of ATP on platelets : evidence against the central role of released ADP on primary aggregation', Blood 46, 309-320.
54. Mills, D.C.B., Figures, W.R., Scearce, L.M., Stewart, G.J., Colman, R.F. and Colman, R.W. (1985) 'Two mechanisms for inhibition of ADP-induced platelet shape change by 5'-p-fluorosulfonylbenzoyladenosine. Conversion to adenosine, and covalent modification at an ADP binding site distinct from that which inhibits adenylate cyclase', J. Biol. Chem. 260, 8078-8083.
55. Colman, R.W. (1990) 'Aggregin : a platelet ADP receptor that mediates activation', FASEB J. 4, 1425-1435.

56. Panak, E., Maffrand, J.-P., Picard-Fraire, C., Vallée, E., Blanchard, J. and Roncucci, R. (1983) 'Ticlopidine : a promise for the prevention and treatment of thrombosis and its complications', Haemostasis 13 (suppl.1), 1-54.
57. Maffrand, J.-P., Defreyn, G., Bernat, A., Delebassée, D. and Tissinier, A.M. (1988) 'Reviewed pharmacology of ticlopidine', Angiologie 77; 6-13.
58. Féliste, R., Delebassée, D., Simon, M.F., Chap, H., Defreyn, G., Vallée, E., Douste-Blazy, L. and Maffrand, J.-P. (1987) 'Broad spectrum anti-platelet activity of ticlopidine and PCR 4099 involves the suppression of the effects of released ADP', Thromb. Res. 48, 403-415.
59. Dunn, F.W., Soria, J., Soria, C., Thomaidis, A., Lee, H. and Caen, J.P. (1984) 'In vivo effect of ticlopidine on fibrinogen-platelet cofactor activity and binding of fibrinogen to platelets', Agents Actions 15 (suppl.), 97-103.
60. Gachet, C., Stierlé, A., Cazenave, J.-P., Ohlmann, P., Lanza, F., Bouloux, C., Maffrand, J.-P. (1990) 'The thienopyridine PCR 4099 selectively inhibits ADP-induced platelet aggregation and fibrinogen binding without modifying the membrane glycoprotein IIb-IIIa complex in rat and in man', Biochem. Pharmacol. 40, 229-238.
61. Hardisty, R.M., Powling, M.J. and Nokes, T.J. (1990) 'The action of ticlopidine on human platelets. Studies on aggregation, secretion, calcium mobilization and membrane glycoproteins', Thromb. Haemostas. 62, 150-155.
62. Lips, J.P.M., Sixma, J.J. and Schiphorst, M.E. (1980) 'The effect of ticlopidine administration to humans on the binding of adenosine diphosphate to blood platelets', Thromb. Res. 17, 19-27.
63. Gachet, C., Cazenave, J.-P., Ohlmann, P., Bouloux, C., Defreyn, G., Driot, F. and Maffrand, J.-P. (1990) 'The thienopyridine ticlopidine selectively prevents the inhibitory effects of ADP but not of adrenaline on cAMP levels raised by stimulation of the adenylate cyclase of human platelets by PGE_1', Biochem. Pharmacol. 40, 2683-2687.
64. Defreyn, G., Gachet, C., Savi, P., Driot, F., Cazenave, J.-P. and Maffrand, J.-P. (1991) 'Ticlopidine and clopidogrel (SR 25990 C) selectively neutralize ADP inhibition of PGE_1-activated platelet adenylate cyclase in rats and rabbits', Thromb. Haemostas. 65, 186-190.
65. Cazenave, J.-P., Packham, M.A., Guccione, M.A. and Mustard, J.F (1973) 'Effects of penicillin G on platelet aggregation, release and adherence to collagen', Proc. Soc. Exp. Biol. Med. 142, 159-166.
66. Cazenave, J.-P., Guccione, M.A., Packham, M.A. and Mustard, J.F. (1977) 'Effects of cephalothin and penicillin G on platelet function in vitro', Brit. J. Haematol. 35, 135-152.
67. Subbarao, K.I., Kuchibhotla, J. and Kakkar, V.Y. (1979) 'Pyridoxal 5'-phosphate. A new physiological inhibitor of blood coagulation and platelet function', Biochem. Pharmacol. 28, 531-534.
68. Cazenave, J.-P., Hemmendinger, S., Wiesel, M.-L., Sutter-Bay, A. and Beretz, A. (1983) 'Pyridoxal phosphate (PALP) inhibits three majors steps involved in thrombus formation : adhesion to collagen, aggregation by ADP and the effects of thrombin on human platelets. Eur. Heart J. 4 (suppl.B), 8.
69. McGregor, J.L. (1986) 'Monoclonal antibodies and human blood platelets', INSERM Symposium N° 27, Elsevier Science Publishers, Amsterdam.
70. Pidard, D., Montgomery, R.R., Bennett, J.S., Kunicki, T.J. (1983) 'Interaction of AP-2, a monoclonal antibody specific for the human platelet glycoprotein IIb-IIIa complex, with intact platelets', J. Biol. Chem. 258, 12582-12586.

71. Coller, B.S. (1985) 'A new murine monoclonal antibody reports an activation-dependent change in the conformation and/or microenvironment of the platelet glycoprotein IIb/IIIa complex', J. Clin. Invest. 76, 101-108.
72. Charo, I.F., Nannizzi, L., Phillips, D.R., Hsu, M.A. and Scarborough, R.M. (1991) 'Inhibition of fibrinogen binding to GP II-IIIa by a GP IIIa peptide', J. Biol. Chem. 266, 1415-1421.
73. D'Souza, S.E., Ginsberg, M.H., Matsueda, G.R. and Plow, E.F. (1991) 'A discrete sequence in a platelet integrin is involved in ligand recognition', Nature 350, 66-68.
74. Marguerie, G. (1990) 'La GP IIb-IIIa plaquettaire : nouvelle cible pour de nouveaux agents antithrombotiques', Sang Thrombose Vaisseaux 2, 309-314.
75. Dennis, M.S., Henzel, W.J., Pitti, R.M., Lipari, M.T., Napier, M.A., Deisher, T.A., Bunting, S., Lazarus, R.A. (1990) 'Platelet glycoprotein-IIb-IIIa protein antagonists from snake venoms. Evidence for a family of platelet-aggregation inhibitors. Proc. Natl. Acad. Sci. USA 87, 2471-2475.
76. Huang, T.-F., Holt, J.C., Kirby, E.P., Niewiarowski, S. (1989) 'Trigramin : primary structure and its inhibition of von Willebrand factor binding to glycoprotein IIb/IIIa complex on human platelets', Biochemistry 28, 661-666.
77. Savage, B., Marzec, U.M., Chao, B.H., Harker, L.A., Maraganore, J.M. and Ruggeri, Z.M. (1990) 'Binding of the snake venom-derived proteins applagin and echistatin to the arginine-glycine-aspartic acid recognition site(s) on platelet glycoprotein-IIB-IIIa complex inhibits receptor function', J. Biol. Chem. 265, 11766-11772.
78. Garsky, V.M., Lumma, P.K., Freidinger, R.M., Pitzenberger, S.M., Randall, W.C., Veber, D.F., Gould, R.J. and Friedman, P.A. (1989) 'Chemical synthesis of echistatin, a potent inhibitor of platelet aggregation from *Echis carinatus* : synthesis and biological activity of selected analogs', Proc. Natl. Acad. Sci. USA 86, 4022-4026.
79. Seymour, J.L., Henzel, W.J., Nevins, B. Stultz, J.T. and Lazarus, R.A. (1990) 'Decorsin, a potent glycoprotein-IIb-IIIa antagonist and platelet aggregation inhibitor from the leech *Macrobdella decora*', J. Biol. Chem. 265, 10143-10147.
80. Rucinski, B., Niewiarowski, S., Holt, J.C., Soszka, T. and Knudsen, K.A. (1990) 'Batroxostatin, an Arg-Gly-Asp-containing peptide from *Bothrops atrox*, is a potent inhibitor of platelet aggregation and cell interaction with fibronectin', Biochim. Biophys. Acta 1054, 257-262.
81. McTavish, D., Faulds, D. and Goa, K.L. (1990) 'Ticlopidine. An updated review of its pharmacology and therapeutic use in platelet-dependent disorders', Drugs 40, 238-259.
82. Editorial (1991) 'Ticlopidine', Lancet 337, 459-460.
83. Gent, M., Blakeley, J.A., Baston, J.D. and the CATS Group (1989) 'The Canadian-American Ticlopidine Study (CATS) in thromboembolic stroke', Lancet i, 1215-1220.
84. Hass, W.K., Easton, J.D., Adams, H.P. et al for the Ticlopidine Aspirin Study Group (1989) 'A randomised trial comparing ticlopidine hydrochloride with aspirin for the prevention of stroke in high risk patients', N. Engl. J. Med. 321, 501-507.
85. Janzon, L., Bergquist, D., Boberg, J. et al (1990) 'Prevention of myocardial infarction and stroke in patients with intermittent claudication : effects of ticlopidine. Results from STIMS, the Swedish Ticlopidine Multicentre Study', J. Intern. Med. 227, 301-308.
86. Balsano, F., Rizzon, P., Violi, F. et al and the STAI Group (1990) 'Antiplatelet treatment with ticlopidine in unstable angina : a controlled multicenter clinical trial', Circulation 82, 17-26.

87. Coller, B.S., Folts, J.D., Smith, S.R., Scudder, L.E. and Jordan, R. (1989) 'Abolition of in vivo platelet thrombus formation in primates with monoclonal antibodies to the platelet GP IIb-IIIa receptor. Correlation with bleeding time, platelet aggregation and blockade of GP IIb-IIIa receptors', Circulation 80, 1766-1774.
88. Easuda, T., Gold, H.K., Leinbach, R.C., Saito, T., Guerrero, J.L., Jang, I.K., Holt, R., Fallon, J.T. and Collen, D. (1990) 'Lysis of plasminogen activator-resistant platelet-rich coronary artery thrombus with combined bolus injection of recombinant tissue-type plasminogen activator and antiplatelet GP IIb/IIIa antibody', J. Amer. Coll. Cardiol. 16, 1728-1735.
89. Coller, B.S., Scudder, L.E., Berger, H.J. and Iuliucci, J.D. (1988) 'Inhibition of human platelet function in vivo with a monoclonal antibody : with observations on the newly dead as experimental subjects', Ann. Intern. Med. 109, 635-638.
90. Coller, B.S. and Scudder, L.E. (1985) 'Inhibition of dog platelet function by in vivo infusion of $F(ab')_2$ fragments of a monoclonal antibody to the platelet glycoprotein IIb/IIIa receptor', Blood 66, 1456-1459.
91. Gold, H.K., Gimple, L.W., Yasuda, T., Leinbach, R.C. Werner, W., Holt, R., Jordan, R., Berger, H., Collen, D. and Coller, B.S. (1990) 'Pharmacodynamic study of F(ab')2 fragments of murine monoclonal antibody-7E3 directed against human platelet glycoprotein IIb/IIIa in patients with unstable angina pectoris', J. Clin. Invest. 86, 651-659.
92. Musial, J., Niewiarowski, S., Rucinski, B., Stewart, G.J., Cook, J.J., Williams, J.A. and Edmunds, L.H. (1990) 'Inhibition of platelet adhesion to surfaces of extracorporeal circuits by disintegrins - RGD - containing peptides from viper venoms', Circulation 82, 261-273.
93. Yasuda, T., Gold, H.K., Leinbach, R.C., Yaoita, H., Fallon, J.T., Guerrero, L., Napier, M.A., Bunting, S. and Collen, D. (1991) 'Kistrin, a polypeptide platelet GP IIb/IIIa receptor antagonist, enhances and sustains coronary arterial thrombolysis with recombinant tissue-type plasminogen activator in a canine preparation', Circulation 83, 1038-1047.
94. Packham, M.A., Bryant, N.L., Guccione, M.A., Kinlough-Rathbone, R.L. and Mustard, J.F. (1989) 'Effect of concentration of Ca^{2+} in the suspending medium on the responses of human and rabbit platelets to aggregating agents', Thromb. Haemostas. 62, 968-976.
95. Knapp, W., Dörken, B., Gilks, W.R., Rieber, E.P., Schmidt, R.E., Stein, H. and von dem Borne, A.E.G.Kr (1989) 'Leucocyte Typing IV. White Cell Differentiation Antigens', Part 6, Oxford University Press, Oxford, pp. 951-1046.

CALCIUM FLUXES IN PLATELETS AND ENDOTHELIAL CELLS; MECHANISMS AND FUNCTIONAL SIGNIFICANCE

TREVOR J. HALLAM

ABSTRACT Elevation of cytosolic $[Ca^{2+}]$, $[Ca^{2+}]_i$, is a key excitatory event in both platelet and endothelial cell activation, and hence, may play functionally opposing roles in the pathophysiological mechanisms underlying thrombosis, i.e. elevated platelet $[Ca^{2+}]_i$ is pro-aggregatory while elevated endothelial cell $[Ca^{2+}]_i$ is anti-aggregatory leading to increased production of prostacyclin and NO. Recent evidence has shown that $[Ca^{2+}]_i$ is raised in both cell types by release of Ca^{2+} from internal stores and by influx via a receptor-mediated Ca^{2+} entry mechanism distinct from classical voltage-gated Ca^{2+} channels for which there are many pharmacologial ligands. Furthermore, these Ca^{2+} influx mechanisms in platelets and endothelial cells are distinguishable, probably reflecting the nature of each cellular response. These developments will be reviewed here in conjunction with other studies which challenge the role of elevated $[Ca^{2+}]_i$ as the central, or even necessary, signal for cell activation. Potential consequences of inhibition of Ca^{2+} flux are considered.

1. INTRODUCTION

The aim of this chapter is to consider whether inhibition of calcium fluxes in platelets or endothelial cells can be of benefit by controlling the pathophysiological conditions underlying thrombosis. In order to properly consider this it is important to note that platelets and endothelial cells are non-excitable cells and cannot be stimulated by spontaneous or imposed changes in the membrane potential [1-4]. Consequently one would not expect to find membrane potential sensitive calcium channels present in the membrane of either cell. However, several clinical reports have suggested that membrane potential sensitive "L"-type calcium channel blockers such as the dihydropyridine series of compounds can have inhibitory effects on platelet function [5,6]. It is important, therefore, to

A. G. Herman (ed.), Antithrombotics, 99–119.
© 1991 Kluwer Academic Publishers. Printed in the Netherlands.

understand whether these effects are likely to be selective and specific to the inhibition of Ca^{2+} flux.

Prior to 1981 the available technologies for measuring the prevailing concentration of divalent cations inside cells and for measuring the requirement of elevated cytosolic free calcium concentration, $[Ca^{2+}]_i$, for a particular physiological response were limited to the use of two techniques. Measurement of $[Ca^{2+}]_i$ was made by specific ion selective micro-electrodes [7], the limitation being the size of the cell that was to be impaled. With platelets this technology was albeit impossible. The major way of determining the level of $[Ca^{2+}]_i$ required to stimulate a particular response fell at that time to the use of permeabilised cell preparations, either by using crude detergents which complex with cholesterol present in the plasma membrane, such as saponin or digitonin, or by using high voltage electric discharge to produce pores or holes in the plasma membrane giving access to the cytoplasmic space [8]. This technique has been used in conjuction with varying Ca^{2+} buffers which set intracellular $[Ca^{2+}]$, allowing the determination of the $[Ca^{2+}]$ threshold for particular physiological responses, most notably in platelets by Knight and Scrutton [8,9] to work out $[Ca^{2+}]_i$ requirements for α, dense and lysosomal granule content exocytosis.

In the early 1980s two new technologies became available for studying the mechanisms underlying Ca^{2+} movement and of its actions. The first was the introduction in 1982 of fluorescent Ca^{2+} indicators, e.g. quin2 [10]. The second was the development of high resolution patch clamp electrophysiological techniques allowing the direct measurment of ion flux through a patch of plasma membrane [11]. Fluorescent Ca^{2+} indicators, broadly based on the divalent cation chelator EGTA were designed to produce a simple way of measuring $[Ca^{2+}]_i$ in intact cells without the need for difficult manipulation, i.e. impalement on micro-electrodes.

The dyes were developed to preserve the selectivity of EGTA for Ca^{2+} over Mg^{2+} with a Kd for Ca^{2+} around 100nM, but to give a fluorescent change which would report changes in $[Ca^{2+}]$. The dyes are very hydrophilic similar to EGTA since they contain four carboxylic acid groups. To circumvent the problem of cell accessibility and avoid the need to inject cells with such hydrophilic molecules into the cytosol of cells, Roger Tsien esterified the acid moieties with acetoxymethyl groups [10], a technique first used in the pharmaceutical industry to improve the absorption of penicillins across the gastro-intestinal tract. By making the dyes more hydrophobic in this way enough dye now gains access to the cytosol where esterases facilitate the loss of the acetoxymethyl groups leaving the free acid of the fluorescent dye free in the cytosol. In this way the dyes are trapped and accumulate within the cell. Measurements of $[Ca^{2+}]_i$ in many cells with many different stimuli using this technique have been made over the last 10 years with refinements over that period to allow firstly average

$[Ca^{2+}]_i$ measurement in populations of cells in suspension [12], then in monolayer [13]; and then of single cells using epifluorescence microscopy [14]. Further developments in the last five years have allowed for Ca^{2+} imaging showing temporal changes of $[Ca^{2+}]_i$ within individual or adjacent endothelial cells [4] or platelets [15] over several frames and more recently spatial resolution should become achievable when combined with confocal microscopy. The success of the latter technique awaits development of further ratio dyes with longer excitation wavelength amenable to excitation by lasers.

The original dye, quin2, has several major drawbacks but, nevertheless used appropriately, proved to be a valuable tool in determining what Ca^{2+} could and could not do. First, the fluorescence yield from quin2 is low and so a large amount of dye is reqired to give sufficient signal/noise over background autofluorescence of cells. Consequently, concentrations of quin2 of around millimolar were not uncommon, inevitably leading to increased buffering of the cell cytoplasm thus subsequent stimulation of cells with this amount of buffering often result in only a very small rise in $[Ca^{2+}]_i$ on stimulation [3]. This can of course be useful if it is wished to determine whether elevated $[Ca^{2+}]_i$ alone is a sufficient and necessary trigger for a particular physiological response (see below). The Kd for quin2 for Ca^{2+} in conditions similar to that found in the cytosol is typically 115nM. While this allows for accurate measurment of cytosolic $[Ca^{2+}]$ in resting or unstimulated cells, around 100nM, in stimulated cells the Kd is too low to accurately measure peak $[Ca^{2+}]_i$ transients over 1μM. A third drawback with quin2 is that the excitation or emission spectra show only an increase in intensity with increased $[Ca^{2+}]$; there is no shift in spectra. This can be problematic when used to measure $[Ca^{2+}]_i$ in contracting cells or fibres or single cells because movement artefacts or an increase in the intensity of light due to increased concentration of dye in the light path can be confused with an increase in $[Ca^{2+}]_i$. Subsequent developments have been made to get around some of these difficulties, noteably with the introduction of the ratio dyes fura-2 and indo-1 [14]. The optimal excitation wavelenghths for fura-2 for monitoring an increase in $[Ca^{2+}]$ are 340nm for an increase in fluorescence and 380nm for decrease in fluorescence intensity. The isosbestic point, i.e. the excitation wavelength where there is no change in fluorescence with change in $[Ca^{2+}]$ concentration, is 360nm. Measurement of fura-2 fluorescence in intact cells monitored at the isosbestic point has been particularly useful to report the influx of quenching divalent cations such as Mn^{2+} [16]. These studies will be described in more detail below.

While patch clamp electrophysiological analyses have predominantly been made using excitable cells, non-excitable cells such as platelets and endothelial cells have also been studied. Some of the key studies using this technology is discussed below with particular emphasis to receptor-mediated Ca^{2+} movements.

The following sections will discuss how these technologies have been applied to answer a) how Ca^{2+} is moved on stimulation in platelets and endothelial cells, and how do these cells differ in their Ca^{2+} handling; b) what Ca^{2+} can and cannot do functionally; and c) what the available pharmacological ligands can do to receptor-stimulated Ca^{2+} fluxes and to physiological responses in vitro and what they are likely to be useful for, if anything, in disease states.

2. HOW IS Ca^{2+} MOVED?

In platelets and in endothelial cells, in common with many other sorts of cells, receptor-stimulated $[Ca^{2+}]_i$ transients are larger in the presence of, than in the absence of, extracellular Ca^{2+} [3, 17]. There is a simple conclusion to be made, i.e. that receptor stimulation results in the release of Ca^{2+} from an intracellular store while the larger or longer maintained rise observed in the presence of extracellular Ca^{2+} is due to a stimulated influx of Ca^{2+} across the plasma membrane.

2.1. Release of Ca^{2+} from Intracellular Stores

The most widely accepted mechanism for the stimulated release of Ca^{2+} from intracellular stores centres on the activation of the phosphatidylinositol 4,5-biphosphate-specific phospholipase C. The resulting formation of inositol 1,4,5-trisphosphate, IP_3, then acts on specific receptors located in the membrane of the intracellular organelle charged with storing Ca^{2+} [18, 19]. The major organelle responsible for storing agonist-releasable Ca^{2+} appears to be an endoplasmic reticular membrane system analogous to the sarcoplasmic reticulum in muscle and in platelets likely to be the dense tubular system. IP_3 concentrations of 1-2μM have been shown to be required for half-maximal release [20, 21]. Here, in platelets we meet our first paradox. ADP acting on cell surface receptors causes both the release of Ca^{2+} from intracellular stores and, since a larger transient is stimulated in the presence of extracellular Ca, it is likely that ADP also stimulates Ca^{2+} influx [3]. However, in several studies [22, 23], little or no IP_3 has been measurable on stimulation with ADP despite the measurable release of Ca^{2+} from intracellular stores. The possibility that there may be a mechanism for stimulating the release of Ca^{2+} from intracellular organelles other than by the production and actions of IP_3 on stimulation by ADP [3] appeared to be further substantiated by the inability of ADP to stimulate secretion under these conditions (i.e. in the presence of aspirin), an event that requires the activation of protein kinase C by endogenously produced diacylglycerol from the other half of the PIP_2 molecule [24]. If IP_3 is responsible for ADP-stimulated Ca^{2+} discharge then one would have to assume that very low levels of IP_3 are required since no protein kinase C activation is apparent, suggesting that the diacylglycerol levels never accumulate sufficiently to activate the enzyme. Since the two molecules are generated simultaneously this appears to be unlikely, although not impossible.

Another physiologically relevant stimulus further complicates the picture. Collagen is able to stimulate the production of diacylglycerol and consequent activation of protein kinase C and slow secretory response without any detectable $[Ca^{2+}]_i$ transient [25, 26]. This suggests that diacylglycerol is produced but no IP_3. It is conceivable that the endogenously-produced diacylglycerol derives from a mechanism other than the actions of a PIP_2-specific phosphoinositidase C, i.e. by the actions of a phospholipase C that hydrolyses PI, PIP or indeed another membrane phospholipid such as phosphatidyl choline or phosphatidyl ethanolamine. Alternatively, diacylglycerol may be derived from stimulated phospholipase D followed by the actions of a phosphatase on the resulting phosphatidic acid. However, most platelet stimuli, namely PAF, thrombin, TxA_2, 5-HT and vasopressin all produce Ca^{2+} discharge and generate IP_3 and diacylglycerol, suggesting that the major cause of the release of Ca^{2+} from intracellular stores is the generation and actions of IP_3.

In endothelial cells there are no known exceptions, i.e. thrombin, PAF, histame H_1, and bradykinin receptors all appear to be linked to conventional PIP_2-hydrolysing G-protein linked phosphodiesterases with concomitant $Ca^{2+}]_i$ transients. It is not clear whether the nature of the Ca^{2+} store in platelets and endothelial cells is similar or different. There has been evidence to suggest that the Ca^{2+} store in some cells can be distinct from endoplasmic reticular membrane systems; this distinct organelle has been termed the calciosome [27]. The available evidence at present suggest that there is one common intracellular store shared by the various stimuli that can elicit Ca^{2+} discharge. This evidence comes from experiments using intracellular dyes. Stimulation with agonist in the presence of EGTA causes complete discharge of the internal store, and despite some re-filling eventually $[Ca^{2+}]_i$ falls to the pre-stimulated near-basal level as the cell becomes Ca^{2+}-depleted. Subsequently, if a second stimulus, a different agonist, is given in the presence or absence of the initial stimulus, there is little, if any, further effect on $[Ca^{2+}]_i$ [13, 17].

However, a subsequent challenge with a membrane permeant Ca^{2+} ionophore such as iononycin or A23187 will often result in a further smaller rise in $[Ca^{2+}]_i$, suggesting that there are membrane-bounded intracellular stores which are not releasable by the messenger(s) produced as a result of stimulation by agonists. Similar studies on platelets have not been possible due to the nature of the platelet and its response to Ca^{2+} mobilising stimuli. It is relatively simple experimentally to repeatedly challenge an endothelial cell since it is naturally, and for the purpose of these studies, immobilised on matrix. However, platelets exist by nature in suspension and in Ca^{2+}-measuring experiments using fluorescent indicators are also in suspension. Repeated stimulation of platelets is not achievable without stimulating aggregation which interferes with fluorescence intensity and therefore $[Ca^{2+}]_i$ measurement.

2.2. Ca^{2+} Influx

In endothelial cells loaded with fura-2, the initial $[Ca^{2+}]_i$ transient stimulated by thrombin, histamine, bradykinin and ATP is very similar in the presence or in the absence of extracellular Ca^{2+}, presumably representing discharge from intracellular stores [13, 17, 28, 29]. However, beyond 2-3 minutes, stimulation in the presence of extracellular Ca^{2+} causes $[Ca^{2+}]_i$ to be maintained elevated above the pre-stimulated levels at a steady-state of several hundred nanomolar; the absolute level dependent on the particular agonist. The simplest explanation is that the continued presence of agonist results in a nett influx of Ca^{2+} ions into the cytosol, either by an agonist-evoked decreased ability of the Ca^{2+} ATPases in the plasma membrane to extrude Ca^{2+} (but only in the presence of extracellular Ca^{2+}, or, by an increase in the influx of Ca^{2+} across the plasma membrane. While there is no evidence that suggests agonists can compromise the ability of plasma membrane Ca^{2+}-ATPases the converse appears to be true. Sage and Rink [30] have examined the extrusion mechanism of cells by treating with Ca^{2+}-ionophore to continually discharge internal stores in the presence of extracellular EGTA. In platelets, the restoration of $[Ca^{2+}]_i$ towards basal levels is slow, however addition of thrombin or protein kinase C stimulants cause a more rapid recovery. This suggests that agonists can stimulate Ca^{2+} pumping via activiation of protein kinase C.

There are precedents for receptor-stimulated Ca^{2+} entry, e.g. the NMDA receptor-operated channel in neurones [31]. The removal of extracellular Ca^{2+} by chelation using EGTA, or by removal of the agonist or by blockade of the receptor using a selective antagonist all result in a rapid decline of $[Ca^{2+}]_i$ back to resting pre-stimulated levels [29]. Re-constitution of the "influx" component can be achieved by first stimulating complete discharge of internal stores and then adding back extracellular Ca^{2+} in the continued presence of agonist [28]. Therefore, the maintained level appears to be dependent on both the presence of extracellular Ca^{2+} and stimulus.

These simple manipulations and interpretations of ion flux are made using fluorescent Ca^{2+} indicators which report $[Ca^{2+}]_i$ and do not directly measure ion flux across membranes. Patch electrode measurements have been made on cultured endothelial cells showing non-specific cation channels activated by stretch [32] and thrombin or bradykinin [33, 34] and more recently histamine [35]. It appears that all these channels display poor selectivity for cations and thus Ca^{2+} may permeate sufficiently to account for the influx component of $[Ca^{2+}]_i$ transients reported by dyes, although these studies are inconclusive. Mahaut-Smith et al [36] showed that intact human platelets could be successfully patched and went on to characterise an ADP-induced inward cation current. However, Zschauer et al [37] have isolated channels from thrombin-stimulated platelets that are very selective for divalent over monovalent cations. These important studies demonstrate that endothelial and platelet agonists are able to stimulate cation influx by activation of plasma membrane channels, but their mechanism of control and functional significance is still unclear.

Fluorescent Ca^{2+} indicators can also be used to measure flux and have provided valuable information as to the different controlling mechanisms that exist for divalent cation entry in platelets and endothelial cells. We first showed that the fluorescent Ca^{2+} indicator quin2 could be used in conjuction with the quenching divalent cation Mn^{2+} to demonstrate receptor-mediated divalent cation influx into intact human platelets [16]. Mn^{2+} binds quin2 approximately 40-fold more avidly than Ca^{2+} and consequently micromolar $[Mn^{2+}]_i$ will displace cytosolic Ca^{2+} from intracellular quin2. By stimulating quin2-loaded human platelets in the absence of extracellular Ca^{2+} or chelators, but in the presence of 1mM Mn^{2+}, ADP, PAF and thrombin were all able to cause a stimulated quench of the quin2 fluoresence. This result suggested that either Mn^{2+} influx could be stimulated by these agonists or that the intracellular dye was released on stimulation to be quenched by extracellular Mn^{2+}. Use of the divalent cation chelator DTPA, which is not cell permeant, did not reverse the quench of the quin2 fluorescence by Mn^{2+}; lysis of the cells with 0.1% Triton X-100 under these conditions did reverse the quin2 fluorescence. This evidence demonstrates that the quenched quin2 was still within the cells and that agonists had successfully stimulated the influx of Mn^{2+} across the plasma membrane. The stimulated quench of the intracellular dye appears to be irreversible suggesting that Mn^{2+} cannot be extruded by plasma membrane Ca^{2+}-ATPases [16]. These data are consistent with receptor mediated divalent cation entry rather than agonist-evoked inhibition of Ca^{2+}-ATPases being responsible for nett influx. Similar experiments have been more recently performed on endothelial cells showing that both thrombin and histamine can stimulate Mn^{2+} influx into the cytosol [28].

The use of Mn^{2+} as a surrogate for extracellular Ca^{2+} and a reporter for divalent cation flux has demonstrated some differences between endothelial cells and platelets suggesting that different transduction mechanisms may be in play. First, stopped-flow detailed kinetic studies of $[Ca^{2+}]_i$ transients stimulated by ADP and thrombin have shown that $[Ca^{2+}]_i$ transients in the presence of extracellular Ca^{2+} commence with less delay than the elevated $[Ca^{2+}]_i$ response observed with the same agonist in the absence of extracellular Ca^{2+} [38]. With ADP the onset of the $[Ca^{2+}]_i$ transient in the presence of extracellular Ca^{2+} is very rapid - approximately 20ms. The simplest explanation is that stimulated influx is evoked prior to discharge from internal stores. This conclusion is further substantiated by stopped-flow studies using Mn^{2+} which show that stimulated quenching of intracellular dye due to influx occurs within 20ms while the release of Ca^{2+} from internal stores requires 200-300ms [39], probably reflecting the time taken for the generation of sufficient soluble messengers, e.g. IP_3, to activate the export mechanism in the intracellular organelle membrane. It is not known how ADP stimulates influx; both Ca^{2+} and Mn^{2+} influx are inhibited by similar concentrations of Ni^{2+} or Zn^{2+}, competing divalent cations that do not gain access to the cytosol, providing some supportive evidence that the mechanism of entry for Ca^{2+} and Mn^{2+} is similar [16].

Whatever the mechanism, it is likely to be closely coupled to the ADP-receptor and unlikely to require the generation of soluble second messengers such as IP_3, although Penner et al [40] have reported that this molecule can activate Ca^{2+} influx in rat mast cells by simultaneous patch clamp and fura-2 measurments. This Ca^{2+} entry was enhanced by hyperpolarising the membrane, as expected for Ca^{2+} influx through channels not gated by membrane potential.

Powling and Hardisty [41] using monoclonal antibodies to the fibrinogen receptor, glycoprotein IIb/IIIa on the platelet surface showed that stimulated increases in $[Ca^{2+}]_i$ were compromised in the presence of their antibody. This suggests that a "Ca^{2+}-channel" may be closely associated with glycoprotein IIb/IIIa. More recent studies have shown that RGDS containing peptides, analogous to residues 572-576 of the fibrinogen A α-chain and which are much smaller molecules than monoclonal antibodies also affect Ca^{2+} flux suggesting that glycoprotein IIb/IIIa itself may be closely associated with Ca^{2+} movement [42].

In endothelial cells the time-course of onset of stimulated influx and its relationship to the discharge of Ca^{2+} from internal stores appears to be somewhat different. The onset of thrombin-stimulated divalent cation influx as reported by stimulated Mn^{2+}-quenching is delayed by several hundred milliseconds and occurs only after discharge of Ca^{2+} from the internal store [28]. This suggests that in endothelial cells Ca^{2+} influx occurs as a consequence of the prior discharge of Ca^{2+} from the internal store and may not be under the direct control of receptor stimulation [29]. A similar re-filling model for Ca^{2+} entry has been proposed in pancreatic acinar cells [43] and in rat parotid acinar cells [44]. This proposed mechanism has been tested in endothelial cells by measuring the ability of intracellular stores to re-fill or Mn^{2+} influx rates under conditions where the store has been depleted but the stimulus subsequently removed [29]. Complete discharge of the intracellular store with histamine in the absence of extracellular Ca^{2+} can be attained so that there is little further dischargeable Ca^{2+} when challenged with a subsequent addition of thrombin, even if the histamine stimulation is curtailed by the addition of excess H_1-antagonist mepyramine. If extracellular Ca^{2+} is added back for a short period after the brief period of stimulation with histamine, following addition of mepyramine, then firstly a brief $[Ca^{2+}]_i$ transient occurs, an event which is not observed when extracellular Ca^{2+} is added back to endothelial cells which have not been previously stimulated and have intact internal stores, and secondly the internal store has now re-filled as evidenced by the ability of subsequent thrombin addition to cause Ca^{2+} discharge from the internal store [29]. Under similar conditions if Mn^{2+} is added, a stimulated rate of Mn^{2+} entry is apparent, reported by quenching of the intracellular fura-2 fluorescence at 360nm excitation, even though the histamine stimulus has been completely blocked [29]. These data provide strong evidence to suggest that stimulated divalent cation influx can occur as a consequence of the state of the intracellular store and independent of whether the cell surface receptors are continually stimulated. Elegant experiments on single human umbilical vein endothelial cells using triple wavelength photometric recordings of fura-2 fluorescence (using such a protocol) have shown that the rate of Mn^{2+} entry is inversely proportional to the state of fullness of the intracellular store [36]. Just how the state of the intracellular store signals to a surface membrane influx mechanism is unclear [45]. Conceptually this is very difficult since we know that Mn^{2+} fluxes into the cytoplasm appearing to discount an intracellular "gap-junction" between internal Ca^{2+} containing organelle and plasma membrane which is negatively gated by intracellular store $[Ca^{2+}]$. However it is conceivable that Mn^{2+} first enters via an intracellular store and is then released into the cytosol.

While the examples chosen here exemplify the two major routes for divalent cation entry as a consequence of receptor stimulation, namely a rapid ADP receptor-operated ion channel in the platelet and a "re-filling influx" in the endothelial cell, the evidence does not rule out that more than one mechanism may be active in either cell. Sage and co-workers [47] have recently published evidence to suggest that ADP causes two phases of divalent cation entry, the later phase being attributable to a "re-filling influx." Takeda and co-workers [35], using patch electrodes have provided evidence for histamine-stimulated non-selective cation channels in endothelial cells, the activity of which are directly dependent on receptor stimulation. This suggests that these channels are unlikely to account for the "re-filling flux" although even in isolated patches of plasma membrane it is dangerous to assume that the membrane is completely free of closely-associated intracellular membrane systems which may normally constitute part of the internal store and gating mechanism.

3. WHAT DOES $[Ca^{2+}]$ DO?

3.1. In Platelets:

Ca^{2+} has been implicated for many years as the central and major second messenger common to all excitatory agonists. However, much of the evidence which supported this view has been circumstantial until the development of fluorescent Ca^{2+} indicators. Early studies showed that the removal of extracellular Ca^{2+} could compromise the ability of agonists to produce physiological responses such as aggregation and secretory exocytosis. The interpretation that the only consequence of stimulating cells in the absence of extracellular Ca^{2+} was to remove the major source of a key intracellular messenger is complicated by the fact that there are extracellular requirements for divalent cations, for example for the binding of fibrinogen to the platelet surface glycoprotein IIb/IIIa [48]. Studies using Ca^{2+} ionophores such as A23187 which effectively mimicked the actions of most excitatory agonists provided further circumstantial evidence that a rise in $[Ca^{2+}]_i$ is a key physiological messenger [49]. However, use of ionophores in the presence of physiological concentrations of extracellular divalent cations can easily produce very large non-physiological elevations in $[Ca^{2+}]_i$ which may non-selectively stimulate the cell. Use of permeabilised cell preparations with Ca^{2+}-buffers provided the first data defining the minimal levels of cytosolic $[Ca^{2+}]$ required to elicit secretory exocytosis, i.e. 1-3μM [8]. Use of fluorescent Ca^{2+} indicators with agents that act selectively to increase $[Ca^{2+}]_i$, i.e. ionophores such as ionomycin, defined further $[Ca^{2+}]_i$ thresholds for key physiological responses of platelets. Shape change required elevations of $[Ca^{2+}]_i$ to 300nM while both platelet aggregation and secretory exocytosis require elevations of $[Ca^{2+}]_i$ to around 1μM [26, 50], the latter response being in close agreement with data produced in permeabilised cells.

One of the most important applications of the Ca^{2+} indicator quin2 was to buffer the cytosol to such an extent that $[Ca^{2+}]_i$ remained below the $[Ca^{2+}]_i$ threshold when cells are stimulated in the absence of extracellular Ca^{2+}. In this way it was possible to determine whether elevated $[Ca^{2+}]_i$ is the major excitatory messenger responsible for a particular response. Early studies using quin2 to increase the cytosolic buffering several fold such that, in the absence of extracellular Ca^{2+}, the agonist-evoked discharge of Ca^{2+} from intracellular stores could only evoke a very small change in $[Ca^{2+}]_i$ to around double the basal level, well below the Ca^{2+} threshold for any response, showed that secretory exocytosis could occur at levels of $[Ca^{2+}]_i$ near the normal prestimulated resting level of 100nM [50]. These secretory processes are now well characterised and attributable to the activation of protein kinase C [25]. Activation of the enzyme is brought about by receptor-stimulated generation of endogenous diacylglycerols, at least part of which derive from inositol phospholipids. Exogenously applied protein kinase C stimulants such as phorbol esters and oleoylacetylglycerol were shown to effectively stimulate protein kinase C in intact cells and cause exocytosis of granular contents with no increase in $[Ca^{2+}]_i$ [25, 26].

Similar studies on shape change responses showed that ADP, PAF and thrombin could all cause shape change with peak stimulated $[Ca^{2+}]_i$ lower than the $[Ca^{2+}]_i$ threshold using ionomycin [3, 51]. Platelets loaded with several millimolar quin2, in the absence of extracellular Ca^{2+}, were stimulated with a maximal dose of ionomycin, typically around 100nM, to completely discharge all membrane-bounded internal stores. $[Ca^{2+}]_i$ increased under these conditions from around 80nM to a maximum of 200nM. Simultaneous measurements of optical density revealed no shape change as expected since ionomycin driven shape change required a peak $[Ca^{2+}]_i$ threshold of at least 300nM. Addition of agonists such as ADP, PAF or thrombin to these ionophore-treated cells caused no further change in $[Ca^{2+}]_i$ since there was no source of extracellular or intracellular Ca^{2+} but a rapid shape change response was evoked by all of these agonists. This data strongly suggested that there are second messengers, other than $[Ca^{2+}]_i$, that can elicit shape change. Shape change is a complicated response reflecting an initial polymerisation of actin to form microfilamentous pseudopodia formation followed by the disassembly of the peripheral bands of microtubules. These events are followed by phosphorylation of myosin 20kDa light chains by Ca^{2+}/calmodulin-dependent myosin light chain kinase, MLCK, which causes a contractile response moving the secretory granules to the centre of the cell, and culminating with the activation of gelsolin which disassembles the actin microfilaments. Hallam and co-workers [51] showed that at least one of these responses, the activation of MLCK, classically thought to be stimulated by elevation of $[Ca^{2+}]_i$, could be stimulated by platelet agonists in the absence of any increase in $[Ca^{2+}]_i$. Since myosin light chains and MLCK are widely distributed throughout the cell it is likely that some form of soluble messenger is responsible but the nature of this stimulus remains uncharacterised. Further experiments showed that low doses of the thromboxane A_2 mimetic, U46619, could elicit shape change with no detectable change in $[Ca^{2+}]_i$ under normal physiological extracellular Ca^{2+} concentrations [52].

Stimulatory pathways for platelet aggregation are equally intriguing. Elevations of $[Ca^{2+}]_i$ to around 600nM with ionomycin is insufficient to cause platelet aggregation yet the subsequent addition of ADP causes a rapid aggregatory response without any further elevation in $[Ca^{2+}]_i$ suggesting that the activating conformational change of glycoprotein IIb/IIIa which then binds fibrinogen leading to aggregation is stimulated by ADP-receptor activation by a route other than just an elevation in $[Ca^{2+}]_i$ [3]. Other workers [53] have shown that thrombin could induce aggregation of platelets suspended in a high K^+-containing medium even though the depolarising effect reduces the maximal $[Ca^{2+}]_i$ transient, as predicted in non-voltage gated channels against suggesting excitatory mechanisms other than elevated $[Ca^{2+}]_i$.

Although these data suggest that there are multiple, as yet unknown, additional mechanisms for stimulating cells it is clear that physiologically attainable elevations in $[Ca^{2+}]_i$ can cause these responses and so the role of $[Ca^{2+}]_i$ rises are likely to play a role in synergy with other mechanisms. However, the precise consequence of inhibition of Ca^{2+} fluxes remains unpredictable.

3.2. In Endothelial Cells:

A number of key responses of endothelial cells are thought to require elevations in $[Ca^{2+}]_i$. Two such responses that are most pertinent are stimulation of PGI_2 production and of NO release. $[Ca^{2+}]_i$-activation curves for PGI_2 production constructed using Ca^{2+}-ionophores in conjunction with fluorescent indicators have shown $[Ca^{2+}]_i$ thresholds of 800-1000nM are required [17], presumably to activate the rate-limiting enzyme, phospholipase A_2. Similar $[Ca^{2+}]_i$-activation curves for thrombin and ATP stimulation showed identical $[Ca^{2+}]_i$ thresholds suggesting that elevated $[Ca^{2+}]_i$ is both a sufficient and probably the major physiological trigger for PGI_2 production [17, 56]. Ca^{2+}-depletion experiments where cells are stimulated in the absence of extracellular Ca^{2+} and where internal stores have been previously discharged with ionophores show that thrombin is subsequently unable to cause further increases in $[Ca^{2+}]_i$ or to stimulate PGI_2 production showing that elevated $[Ca^{2+}]_i$ is a necessary stimulus [17].

These results are in contrast to similar studies in platelets where activation of arachidonic acid mobilising enzymes with consequent production of thromboxane A_2 can occur in the absence of an increase in $[Ca^{2+}]_i$. In aspirin-treated platelets both collagen, and adrenaline acting through an α2-adrenoceptor, can stimulate the production of TxA_2 without prior increase in $[Ca^{2+}]_i$ above basal [55]. $[Ca^{2+}]_i$ rises will occur with these stimuli but only secondary to released excitatory agonists acting back on cell surface receptors. Interestingly, in endothelial cells, although elevations in $[Ca^{2+}]_i$ appear to be the only route for PGI_2 production, activators of protein kinase C cause a significant shift to the left of the $[Ca^{2+}]_i$-activation curve although they have no affect on resting cells [56]. Paradoxically, PKC activation inhibits rises in $[Ca^{2+}]_i$ stimulated by thrombin. It is unclear why thrombin does not appear to sufficiently activate PKC through endogenously produced diacylglycerol to shift the PGI_2 production $[Ca^{2+}]_i$-activation curve to the left of that for ionomycin. It may be that exogenously applied PKC stimulants such as phorbol esters and diacylglycerols activate PKC to significantly greater levels than activatable physiologically.

The release of endothelium-derived relaxing factor, EDRF, recently characterised as NO [57, 58], appears to require the presence of extracellular Ca^{2+}. Endothelium-dependent relaxations following stimulation by Ca^{2+}-ionophore A23187 and a variety of agonists have all ben abrogated by the removal of external Ca^{2+} from the media [59-61] and it has been assumed that Ca^{2+} influx is necessary. The fact that several agonists cause the synthesis and release of both PGI_2 and NO concomitantly suggests that the stimulatory mechanisms are very similar. However, PGI_2 release is not so critically dependent on the presence of extracellular Ca^{2+}, possibly because a simultaneous activation of protein kinase C enhances PGI_2 production but blocks NO release [62].

3.3. $[Ca^{2+}]_i$ spiking

When considering the likely effects of increased $[Ca^{2+}]_i$ on stimulation with agonists one has to take into account the characteristics of low level stimulation revealed by single cell epi-fluorescence photometry. It is clear that maintained rises in $[Ca^{2+}]_i$ evoked by maximal concentrations of agonists is simplistic. In endothelial cells stimulated with sub-optimal doses of histamine, 0.1-3.0μM, oscillations of $[Ca^{2+}]_i$ are observed where the frequency is dose-dependent [4]. More recent observations have revealed that under certain conditions, perhaps related to the existence of gap junctions between individual cells in monolayer, some agonists can induce oscillating increases in $[Ca^{2+}]_i$ in monolayers that are synchronised [63]. The spikes in $[Ca^{2+}]_i$ appear to be caused by incomplete Ca^{2+} discharge from internal stores, but both frequencey and amplitude require the continued presence of extracellular Ca^{2+}. The functional significance of this spiking behaviour is presently unclear. Given that the $[Ca^{2+}]_i$-activation curve for many responses is so steep it may be that rises in $[Ca^{2+}]_i$ act as a switch and that frequency-modulation is the key to evoking physiological responses rather than amplitude of $[Ca^{2+}]_i$ transients. If the on-rate of a particular Ca^{2+}-activated mechanism, e.g. phosphorylation, is relatively fast compared with off-rate, e.g. de-phosphorylation, then frequency-modulation may be both sufficient and the most energy-efficient controlled stimulus. A maintained high level $[Ca^{2+}]_i$ is energy consuming given constantly activated plasma membrane Ca^{2+}-ATPases. Until efficient methods exist for measuring cell responses of individual cells simultaneously with $[Ca^{2+}]_i$ spikes, the precise inter-relationship will remain unclear.

It is not clear whether spiking $[Ca^{2+}]_i$ responses are stimulated in platelets. Early imaging experiments designed to determine whether thrombin and ADP act on discrete platelet sub-populations failed to reveal any longer term $[Ca^{2+}]_i$ spiking activity [15]. It may be the lack of spiking activity observed reflects the suicidal "all-or-nothing" nature of platelet responses; it is not a cell well disposed for chronic low-level responsiveness.

4. INHIBITORS OF RECEPTOR-MEDIATED Ca^{2+} ENTRY

Considerable progress has been made in elucidating mechanisms of entry of Ca^{2+} via voltage-gated Ca^{2+} channels in excitable cells [64, 65]. This progress has been greatly helped by the availability of high affinity ligands, noteably the organic "calcium antagonists" and toxins. It has proved harder to elucidate the mechanisms and functional significance of receptor-mediated calcium entry, RMCE, since electro-physiological studies have proved difficult and a serious impediment is the lack of suitable ligands [45]. There have been reports that successful blockade of stimulated Ca^{2+} entry into human platelets can be accomplished with selective voltage-gated calcium channel antagonists such as verapamil and the dihydropyridine, nicardipine [e.g. 66], however, the concentrations of ligands used in these studies is considerably higher than the concentrations required to give complete blockade of voltage-gated channels. This suggests that these ligands are acting in a non-selective manner, a view further substantiated by the similar inhibitory activity on platelets of the dihydropyridine "calcium agonist" Bay K8644 at high concentrations.

Indirect results for and against voltage-gated Ca^{2+} currents stimulating EDRF release from endothelial cells have been presented. Singer and Peach [59] reported that verapamil and nifedipine antagonised EDRF-responses in rabbit aorta yet Spedding et al [67] inferred the converse when Ca^{2+} entry blockers had no effect on EDRF release in rat aorta and BAY K8644 was an ineffective simulus.

Recently a novel compound has been reported, SK+F 96365, which is structurally distinct from classical calcium antagonists and which shows selectivity in blocking RMCE compared with internal Ca^{2+} release in platelets and endothelial cells [68]. The IC_{50} for inhibition of RMCE by SK+F 96365 in platelets stimulated with ADP or thrombin was around 10μM, concentrations that did not affect internal Ca^{2+} release. Similar effects with SK+F 96365 were observed in endothelial cells. The compound also inhibited agonist-stimulated Mn^{2+} entry in both platelets and endothelial cells with similar IC_{50}'s. The effects of SK+F 96365 were independent of cell type and agonist as would be expected from a compound that modulates post-receptor events. Voltage-gated Ca^{2+} entry in two preparations, i.e. GH_3 pituitary cells and rabbit ear artery smooth muscle cells, were also inhibited by SK+F 96365. However, ATP-stimulated divalent cation channels in rabbit ear artery smooth muscle were unaffected. Therefore, SK+F 96365 shows no selectivity between RMCE and voltage-gated Ca^{2+} entry unlike the classic calcium antagonists.

The effects of SK+F 96365 on functional responses of platelets and endothelial cells thought to be driven by RMCE were studied by Meritt and co-workers [68]. Under conditions where platelet aggregation is dependent on stimulated Ca^{2+} influx, the response was blocked by

SK+F 96365 with similar IC_{50}'s to those for inhibition of $[Ca^{2+}]_i$ transients and Mn^{2+} flux. Hence, SK+F 96365 is a useful tool to distinguish RMCE from internal Ca^{2+} release and to probe the role of Ca^{2+} influx in mediating functional responses. However, it is not a potent tool and it is not selective since it also blocks voltage-gated Ca^{2+} entry.

In attempting to interpret the likely effects of blocking Ca^{2+} influx in terms of disease states one has to take great care. For example, SK+F 96365 is able to inhibit platelet aggregation under conditions where the cytosol is heavily buffered, i.e. loaded with quin2, because the internal Ca^{2+} release is unable to overcome the excessive cytosolic Ca^{2+}-buffering and the response is driven by Ca^{2+} influx. However, in unloaded cells, SK+F 96365 has little effect on the aggregatory response; the internal Ca^{2+} release in an unbuffered system more analogous to the physiological state causes a rise in $[Ca^{2+}]_i$ sufficiently to stimulate the response. With an acute response such as aggregation it is sufficient for $[Ca^{2+}]_i$ to be elevated over 1μM for only a few seconds. In more chronic state of stimulation and responses, e.g. in endothelial cells, it is likely that inhibition of Ca^{2+} influx will affect responsiveness since intracellular Ca^{2+} stores will gradually become depleted. In endothelial cells, SK+F 96365 decreases the plateau phase of a histamine-evoked maximal $[Ca^{2+}]_i$ response and has predictable effects on $[Ca^{2+}]_i$ spiking stimulated with sub-optimal concentrations of histamine or thrombin analogous to removal of external Ca^{2+}. SK+F 96365 immediately and reversibly abrogates $[Ca^{2+}]$-spiking consistent with the role of Ca^{2+} entry for maintenance of frequency and amplitude of spiking. It will be intriguing to determine the effects of SK+F 96365 on PGI_2 production and on EDRF release.

5. CONCLUSION

Although the key roles of elevated $[Ca^{2+}]_i$ in platelet and endothelial responses have been exemplified here, it is clear that the hypothesis that inhibition of Ca^{2+} fluxes could, if selectivity can be assured, be beneficial in thrombosis is a complex issue. Selective inhibition of Ca^{2+} fluxes in the platelet leaving endothelial cell $[Ca^{2+}]_i$ transients unaffected would perhaps be the first step to a useable tool. However, aggregation may be unaffected by blockade of Ca^{2+} influx alone without modifying the release of Ca^{2+} from internal stores. Nevertheless, abnormal Ca^{2+} handling resulting in higher resting $[Ca^{2+}]_i$ levels in arterial and venous thrombotic patients has been reported to be reversed by verapamil [6] despite the lack of evidence for voltage-gated channels. It remains to be seen why such beneficial effects appear to occur: proposed interpretations have suggested that platelets from thrombotics are less robust giving rise to excessive leakage of Ca^{2+} into the cell and the high levels of verapamil used may imply non-selective mechanisms of action.

Perhaps more fundamental to the issue is to ask what role $[Ca^{2+}]_i$ plays physiologically. It is clear elevated $[Ca^{2+}]_i$ can evoke many, if not all, of the functional responses produced by agonists but evidence with dyes suggest it may not be the major or even necessary excitatory pathway under some circumstances. The only way to determine whether inhibition of Ca^{2+} flux can be of benefit in thrombotic disorders is inevitably to test selective and specific agents, of which, to my knowledge there are none.

ACKNOWLEDGEMENT

I thank Ann Salisbury Davies for secretarial assistance.

REFERENCES

[1]. MacIntyre, D.E. and Rink, T.J. (1982) 'The role of platelet membrane potential in the initiation of platelet aggregation', Thromb. Haemostas. (Stuttgart) 47, 22.

[2]. Doyle, V.M. and Ruegg, U.T. (1985), 'Lack of evidence for voltage dependent calcium channels on platelets', Biochem. Biophys. Res. Commun. 127, 161.

[3]. Hallam, T.J. and Rink, T.J. (1985), 'Responses to adenosine diphosphate in human platelets loaded with the fluorescent calcium indicator quin2', J. Physiol. 368, 131-146.

[4]. Jacob, R., Merritt, J.E., Hallam, T.J. and Rink, T.J. (1988), 'Repetitive spikes in cytoplasmic calcium evoked by histamine in human endothelial cells', Nature 335, 40-45.

[5.] Jy, W., Ahn, Y.S., Shanbaky, N., Fernandez, L.F., Harrington, W.J. and Brown, H.E. (1984), 'Calcium channel blockade for thrombosis and other disorders', Clin. Res. 32, 494a.

[6]. Jy, W., Ahn, Y.S., Shanbaky, N., Fernandez, L.F., Harrington, W.J. and Haynes, D.H. (1987), 'Abnormal calcium handling by platelets in thrombotic disorders', Circulation Res. 60, 346-335

[7]. Thomas, R.C. (1981), 'Ion-selective micro-electrodes. In: Techniques in Cellular Physiology' (Baker P.F. ed.), Vol. P1/11, p125, pp1-12, Elsevier.

[8]. Knight, D.E. and Scrutton, M.C. (1980), 'Direct evidence for a role for Ca^{2+} in amine storage granule secretion by human platelets', Thrombosis Res. 20, 437-446.

[9]. Knight, D.E. and Scrutton, M.C. (1980), 'Gaining access to the cytosol: the technique and applications of electropermeabilization', Biochem. J. 234, 497-506.

[10]. Tsien, R.Y., Pozzan, T. and Rink, T.J. (1982), 'Calcium homeostasis in intact lymphocytes: cytoplasmic free calcium monitored with a new, intracellularly trapped fluorescent indicator', J. Cell. Biol. 94, 335-340.

[11]. Hamill, O.P., Marty, A., Neher, E., Sakmann, B. and Sigwall, F.J. (1981), "Improved patch-clamp techniques for high-resolution current recordings from cells and cell-free membrane patches', Pflugers Arch. 391, 85-100.

[12]. Rink T.J. and Pozzan, T. (1985), 'Using quin2 in cell suspensions', Cell Calcium 6, 133.

[13]. Hallam, T.J. and Pearson, J.D. (1986), 'Exogenous ATP raises cytoplasmic free calcium in fura-2 loaded piglet aortic endothelial cells', FEBS Letts. 207, 95-99.

[14]. Tsien, R.Y., Rink, T.J. and Poenie, M. (1985), 'Measurement of cytosolic free Ca^{2+} in individual small cells using fluorescence microscopy with dual excitation wavelengths', Cell Calcium 6, 145.

[15]. Hallam, T.J., Poenie, M. and Tsien, R.Y. (1986), 'Homogeneity of ADP- and thrombin-stimulated rises in $[Ca^{2+}]_i$ in fura-2 loaded human platelet populations revealed by fluorescence ratio image processing', J. Physiol. 377, 123P.

[16]. Hallam, T.J. and Rink, T.J. (1985), 'Agonists stimulate divalent cation channels in the plasma membrane of human platelets', FEBS Letts, 186, 175-179.

[17]. Hallam, T.J., Pearson, J.D and Needham, L.A. (1988), 'Thrombin-stimulated elevation of human endothelial cell cytoplasmic free calcium concentration causes prostacyclin production', Biochem. J. 251, 243-250.

[18]. Streb, H., Irvine, R.F., Berridge, M.J. and Schulz, I. (1983), 'Release of Ca^{2+} from a non-mitochondrial intracellular store in pancreatic acinar cells by inositol, 1,4,5-triphosphate', Nature 306, 67-69.

[19]. Magocsi, M., Enyedi, A., Sarkadi, B. and Gardos, G. (1988), 'Effects of phosphoinositides on calcium movements in human platelet membrane vesicles', Biochim. Biophys. Acta 944, 202-212.

[20]. O'Rourke, F.A., Halenda, S.P., Zavoico, G.B. and Feinstein, M.B. (1985), 'IP_3 release Ca^{2+} from a Ca^{2+}-transporting membrane vesicle fraction derived from human platelets', J. Biol. Chem. 260, 956-950.

[21]. Rittenhouse, S.E. and Sasson, J.P. (1985), 'Mass changes in IP_3 in human platelets stimulated by thrombin', J. Biol. Chem. 260, 8657-8662.

[22]. Fisher, G.J, Bakshian, S. and Baldassare, J.J. (1985), 'Activation of human platelets by ADP causes a rapid rise in cytosolic free calcium without hydrolysis of phosphatidylinositol 4,5-bisphosphate', Biochem. Biophys. Res. Commun. 129, 958.

[23]. Vickers, J.C., Kinlough-Rathbone, R.L. and Mustard, J.F. (1986), 'The decrease in phosphatidylinositol 4,5-bisphosphate in ADP-stimulated washed rabbit platelets is not primarily due to phsopholipase C activation', Biochem. J. 237, 327-332.

[24]. Hallam, T.J., Simpson, A.W.M., O'Connor, N. and Rink, T.J. (1985), 'Control and inter-relation of aggregation and secretion; the roles of Ca^{2+}, diacylglycerol and thromboxane with particular reference to ADP stimulation, In: "Mechanisms of stimulus-response coupling in platelets", (J. Westwick, M.F. Scully, D.E. MacIntyre and V.V. Kakkar, eds.), Plenum, N.Y., pp145-162.

[25]. Rink, T.J., Sanchez, A. and Hallam, T.J. (1983), 'Diacylglycerol and phorbol ester stimulate secretion without raising cytoplasmic free calcium in human platelets', Nature 305, 317-319.

[26]. Rink T.J. and Hallam, T.J. (1984), 'What turns platelets on?', Trends Biochem. Sci. 9, 215-219.

[27]. Volpe, P. , Krause, K., Hashimoto, S., Zorzato, F., Pozzan, T., Meldolesi, J. and Lew, D.P. (1987), 'Calciosome, a cytoplasmic organelle: The IP_3-sensitive Ca^{2+} store of non-muscle cells?', Proc. Natl. Acad. Sci (U.S.A.) 85, 1081-1095.

[28]. Hallam, T.J., Jacob, R. and Merritt, J.E. (1988), 'Evidence that agonists stimulate divalent cation influx into human endothelial cells', Biochem. J. 255, 179-184.

[29]. Hallam, T.J., Jacob, R. and Merritt, J.E. (1989), 'Influx of divalent cations can be independent of receptor stimulation in human endothelial cells', Biochem. J. 259, 125-129.

[30]. Rink, T.J. and Sage, S.O. (1987), 'Stimulated Ca^{2+} efflux from fura-2 loaded human platelets', J. Physiol. 393, 513-524.

[31]. Mayer, M.L. and Westbrook, G.L. (1987), 'Permeation and block of N-methyl D-Aspartic acid receptor channels by divalent cations in mouse cultured central neurones', J. Physiol. 394, 501-527.

[32]. Lansman, J.B., Hallam, T.J. and Rink, T.J. (1987), 'Single stretch-activated ion channels in vascular endothelial cells as mechanotransducers', Nature 325, 811-813.

[33]. Adams, D.J., Lategan, T.W., Lodge, N.J. and van Breemen, C. (1987), 'Inward rectifying K^+-channels and thrombin-activated cation channels in cultured endothelial cells from bovine pulmonary artery', J. Physiol. 394, 45P.

[34]. Johns, A., Lategan, T.W., Lodge, N.J., Ryan, U.S., van Breemen, C. and Adams, D.J. (1987), 'Calcium entry through receptor-operated channels in bovine pulmonary artery endothelial cells', Tissue Cell 19, 733-746.

[35]. Bregestovski, P., Bakhramov, S., Danilov, A., Moldobaeva, A. and Takeda, K. (1988), 'Histamine-induced inward currents in cultured endothelial cells from human umbilical vein', Br. J. Pharmacol 95, 429-436.

[36]. Mahaut-Smith, M.P., Rink, T.J. and Sage, S.O. (1989), 'Single channels in human platelets activated by ADP', J. Physiol. 415, 24P.

[37]. Zschauer, A., van Breemen, C., Buhler, F.R. and Nelson, M.T. (1988), 'Calcium channels in thrombin-activated human platelet membranes', Nature 334, 703-705.

[38]. Sage, S.O. and Rink, T.J. (1986), 'Kinetic differences between thrombin-induced and ADP-induced calcium influx and release from internal stores in fura-2 loaded human platelets', Biochem, Biophys, Res. Commun. 136, 1124-1129.

[39]. Sage, S.O., Merritt, J.E., Hallam, T.J. and Rink, T.J. (1989), 'Receptor-mediated calcium entry in fura-2 loaded human platelets stimulated with ADP and thrombin. Dual wavelength studies with Mn^{2+}', Biochem. J. 258, 923-926.

[40]. Penner, R., Mathews, G and Neher, E (1988), 'Regulation of calcium influx by second messengers in rat mast cells', Nature 334, 449-504.

[41]. Powling, M.J. and Hardisty, R.M. (1985), 'GPIIb/IIIa complex and Ca^{2+} influx into stimulated platelets', Blood 66, 731-734.

[42]. Sinigaglia, F., Bisio, A., Torti, M., Balduini, C.L., Bertolino, G. and Balduini, C. (1988), 'Effect of GPIIb/IIIa complex ligands on calcium movement and cytoskeleton organisation in activated platelets', Biochem. Biophys. Res. Commun. 154, 258-264.

[43]. Pandol, S.J., Schoffield, M.S., Fimmel, C.J. and Muallem, S. (1987), 'The agonist-sensitive calcium pool in the pancreatic acinar cell. Activation of plasma membrane Ca^{2+} influx mechanism', J. Biol. Chem. 262, 16963-16968.

[44]. Putney, J.W. (1986), 'A model for receptor-regulated calcium entry', Cell Calcium 7, 1-12.

[45]. Hallam, T.J. and Rink, T.J. (1989), 'Receptor-mediated Ca^{2+} entry: diversity of function and mechanism', Trends Pharmacol. Sci. 10, 8-10.

[46]. Jacob, R. (1990), 'Agonist-stimulated divalent cation entry into single cultured human umbilical vein endothelial cells', J. Physiol. 421, 55-77.

[47]. Sage, S.O., Reast, R. and Rink, T.J. (1990), 'ADP evokes biphasic Ca^{2+} influx in fura-2 loaded human platelets: evidence for Ca^{2+} entry regulated by the intracellular Ca^{2+} store', Biochem. J. 265, 675-680.

[48]. Fujimura, K. and Phillips, D.R. (1983), 'Calcium cation regulation of glycoprotein IIb/IIIa complex formation in platelet plasma membranes', J. Biol. Chem. 258, 10247-10252.

[49]. Packham, M.A., Guccione, M.A., Greenberg, J.P., Kinlough-Rathbone, R.L. and Mustard, J.F. (1977), 'Release of [^{14}C]-5HT during initial platelet changes induced by thrombin, collagen or A23187', Blood 50, 915.

[50]. Rink, T.J., Smith, S.W. and Tsien, R.Y. (1982), 'Cytoplasmic free Ca^{2+} in human platelets: Ca^{2+} thresholds and Ca^{2+}-independent activation for shape-change and secretion', FEBS Letts. 148, 21.

[51]. Hallam, T.J., Daniel, J.L. Kendrick-Jones, J. and Rink, T.J. (1985), 'Relationship between cytoplasmic free calcium and myosin light chain phosophorylation in intact platelets', Biochem. J. 232, 373-377.

[52]. Simpson, A.W.M., Hallam, T.J. and Rink, T.J. (1986), 'Low concentrations of the stable prostaglandin endoperoxide U44069 stimulate shape change in quin2-loaded platelets without a measurable increase in $[Ca^{2+}]_i$', FEBS Letts. 201, 301-305.

[53]. Sage, S.O. and Rink, T.J. (1986), 'Effects of ionic substitution on $[Ca^{2+}]_i$ rises evoked by thrombin and PAF in human platelets', Eur. J. Pharmacol. 128, 99-107.

[54]. Carter, T.D., Hallam, T.J., Cusack, N.J. and Pearson, J.D. (1988), 'Regulation of P2Y-purinoceptor-mediated prostacyclin release from human endothelial cells by cytosolic calcium concentration', Br. J. Pharmacol. 95, 1181-1190.

[55]. Pollock, W.K., Irvine, R.F. and Rink, T.J. (1986), 'Free Ca^{2+}-requirements of agonist-induced thromboxane A_2 synthesis in human platelets', Eur. J. Pharmac. 132, 309-313.

[56]. Carter, T.D., Hallam, T.J. and Pearson, J.D. (1989), 'Protein kinase C activation alters the sensitivity of agonist-stimulated endothelial-cell prostacyclin production to intracellular Ca^{2+}', Biochem, J. 262, 431-437.

[57]. Palmer, R.M.J., Ferrige, A.G. and Moncada, S. (1987), 'Nitric oxide release accounts for the biological actitivity of EDRF', Nature 327, 524-526.

[58]. Palmer, R.M.J., Ashton, D.S. and Moncada, S. (1988), 'Vascular endothelial cells synthesise nitric oxide from L-arginine', Nature 333, 664-666.

[59]. Singer, H.A. and Peach, M.J. (1982), 'Calcium- and endothelial-mediated vascular smooth muscle relaxation in rabbit aorta', Hypertension 4 (Suppl. II), 19-25.

[60]. Gordon, J.L. and Martin, W. (1983), 'Endothelium-dependent relaxation of the pig aorta: relationship to stimulation of ^{86}Rb efflux from isolated endothelial cells', Br. J. Pharmacol. 79, 531-541.

[61]. Griffith, T.M., Edwards, D.H., Lewis, M.J., Newby, A.C., Lewis, M.J. and Henderson, A.H. (1986), 'Production of EDRF is dependent on oxidative phosphorylation and extracellular calcium', Cardiovasc, Res. 20, 7-12.

[62]. Lewis, M.J. and Henderson, A.H. (1987), 'A phorbol ester inhibits the release of EDRF', Eur. J. Pharmacol. 137, 167-171.

[63]. Sage. S.O., Adams, D.J. and van Breemen, C. (1989), 'Synchronised oscillations in cytoplasmic free calcium concentration in confluent bradykinin-stimulated bovine pulmonary artery endothelial cell monolayers', J. Biol. Chem. 264, 6-9.

[64]. Campbell, K.P, Leung, A.T. and Sharp, A.H. (1988), 'The biochemistry and molecular biology of the dihydropyridine-sensitive Ca^{2+} channel', Trends Neurosci. 11, 425-430.

[65]. Tsien, R.W., Lipscombe, D., Madison, D.V., Bley, K.R. and Fox, A.P. (1988), 'Multiple types of neuronal calcium channels and their selective modulation', Trends Neurosci. 11, 431-438.

[66]. Avdonin, P.V., Merishikov, M.Y., Svitina-Ulitina, I.V. and Tkachuk, V.A. (1988), 'Blocking of the receptor-stimulated calcium entry into human platelets by verapamil and nicardipine', Thrombos Res. 52, 587-597.

[67]. Spedding, M., Schini, V., Schoeffter, P. and Miller, R.C. (1986), 'Calcium channel activation does not increase release of EDRF in rat aorta although tonic release of EDRF may modulate calcium channel activity in smooth muscle', J. Cardiovasc. Pharmacol. 8, 1130-1137.

[68]. Merritt, J.E., Armstrong, W.P., Benham, C.D., Hallam, T.J., Jacob, R., Jaxa-Chamiec, A.A., Leigh, B.K., McCarthy, S.A., Moores, K.E. and Rink, T.J. (1990) 'SK+F 96365, a novel inhibitor of receptor-mediated calcium entry', Biochem. J. 271, 515-522.

INHIBITION OF PLATELET FUNCTION BY CYCLIC NUCLEOTIDES AND CYCLIC NUCLEOTIDE-DEPENDENT PROTEIN KINASES

U. WALTER, C. NOLTE, J. GEIGER,
P. SCHANZENBÄCHER and K. KOCHSIEK

ABSTRACT. Platelets and their interaction with the vessel wall are very important for the regulation of vascular tone and hemostasis. The vessel wall-platelet interaction and the activation state of platelets appear to be altered in vascular diseases such as atherosclerosis, hypertension and thrombosis. In these diseases, it is often desirable to inhibit the activation of platelets and the associated adhesion, aggregation and release of platelet-derived vasoactive factors. Therefore, it is of considerable interest to understand the nature and mechanism of action of platelet inhibitors. Two very important physiological platelet inhibitors are produced by endothelial cells, prostacyclin (PG-I_2) and the endothelium-derived relaxing factor (EDRF). PG-I_2 and nitric oxide-generating agents such as EDRF and other nitrovasodilators stimulate in human platelets the stoichiometric and reversible phosphorylation of several proteins mediated by either cAMP/cAMP-dependent protein kinase or cGMP/cGMP-dependent protein kinase, respectively. The platelet pathways affected by both cGMP/cGMP-dependent protein kinase and cAMP/cAMP-dependent protein kinase result in the inhibition of platelet activation, most likely due to the inhibition of agonist-induced calcium mobilization. Some current concepts concerning the mechanisms of action of cyclic nucleotide-elevating platelet inhibitors will be discussed.

1. Introduction

Platelets and platelet-derived vasoactive agents are important physiological regulators of vascular tone and hemostasis. Many lines of evidence suggest that platelet activation significantly contributes to the pathogenesis of atherosclerosis, myocardial infarction, unstable angina pectoris and thrombosis [1-4]. The role of platelets in the pathogenesis of cardiovascular disorders including coronary disease is also supported by the increasing evidence that platelet inhibitors such as aspirin are beneficial in the treatment of unstable angina pectoris, for the secondary prevention of vascular events in patients with coronary heart and cerebrovascular disease, and probably even for the primary prevention of cardiovascular disease in individuals at high risk [5].

A. G. Herman (ed.), Antithrombotics, 121–138.
© 1991 *Kluwer Academic Publishers. Printed in the Netherlands.*

Class	Substance	Vascular Smooth Muscle Cells: Contraction	Vascular Smooth Muscle Cells: Proliferation	Vascular Smooth Muscle Cells: Endothel-dep. Vasodilation	Platelet Activation: Adhesion, Secretion, Aggregation	Intracellular Messengers
Primary Vasoconstrictors	Endothelin	+++	?	–	–	Ca^{++}, IP_3, DG
	Thromboxane A_2	+++	+	–	+++	Ca^{++}, IP_3, DG
	Vasopressin (V_1)	++	+	–	++	Ca^{++}, IP_3, DG
	Norepinephrine (α_1)	+++	+	–	–	Ca^{++}, IP_3, DG
	Angiotensin II	+++	++	–	–	Ca^{++}, IP_3, DG
Growth-factors	PDGF	+	+++	–	–	Tyrosin-(P), Ca^{++}, IP_3
Endothel-dep. Vasodilators	Serotonin	+	++	+++	+	Ca^{++}, IP_3, DG
	Histamine	+	+	+++	–	Ca^{++}, IP_3, DG
	Bradykinin		+	+++	–	Ca^{++}, IP_3, DG
	ADP			++	+++	Ca^{++}
	Acetylcholine	+		+++	–	Ca^{++}, IP_3, DG
	Thrombin			+++	+++	Ca^{++}, IP_3, Tyrosin-(P)
Direct Vasodilators	Catecholamines (β_1)	↓		–	↓	cAMP / cAMP-PK
	$PG\text{-}I_2$ / $PG\text{-}E_1$	↓	↓	–	↓	cAMP / cAMP-PK
	EDRF / NO-Vasodil.	↓	↓	–	↓	cGMP / cGMP-PK / PDE
	ANF	↓	↓	–	–	cGMP / cGMP-PK / PDE

Fig. 1. Regulation of platelets and vascular smooth muscle cells by vasoactive substances

Four different classes of vasoactive substances, their effects on vascular smooth muscle cells and platelets, and their intracellular signal transduction systems are listed. The effects are stimulatory (+), negligible or absent (–), or inhibitory (↓). Ca^{++}, intracellular free calcium; IP_3, inositol trisphosphate; DG, 1,2-diacyglycerol; Tyrosine-(P), tyrosine-phosphorylation; cAMP-PK, cAMP-regulated protein kinase, cGMP-PK, cGMP-regulated protein kinase; PDE, phosphodiesterase; PDGF, platelet-derived growth factor; EDRF, endothelium-derived relaxing factor; ANF, atrial natriuretic factor.

Activation of platelets results in increased adhesion of platelets to components of the vessel wall, aggregation, release of vasoactive agents from platelet dense granules (i.e. ADP, serotonin) and from platelet alpha granules (i.e. platelet-derived growth factor PDGF, platelet factor 4, fibrinogen etc.), as well as in the increased production and release of thromboxane A_2. Activation of platelets may not only lead to acute vascular complications such as thrombosis but also, perhaps due to the release of growth factors, to longterm effects such as neointimal hyperplasia and smooth muscle proliferation, one of the hallmarks of atherosclerosis [1,3]. Therefore, understanding the pathways responsible for platelet activation and platelet inhibition is of considerable interest and potential importance for the development of future strategies with respect to the prevention and treatment of diseases in which a pathophysiological participation of activated platelets appears likely. This chapter will review the intracellular pathways responsible for the regulation of platelet activation, particularly the pathways mediating the effects of platelet inhibitors.

2. Regulation of platelet activation

Multiple vasoactive agents stimulate or inhibit the activation of human platelets (Fig.1). Some potent vasoconstrictors (i.e. thromboxane A_2 and vasopressin) and some potent endothelium-dependent vasodilators (i.e. thrombin, ADP and serotonin) are also potent platelet activators. Some substances released from activated platelets are either potent activators of both platelets and vascular smooth muscle cells (i.e. thromboxane A_2) or function as endothelium-dependent vasodilators and platelet activators (i.e. ADP, serotonin). However, endothelium-dependent vasodilators may also directly activate vascular smooth muscle cells and cause vasoconstriction which appears to be pathophysiologically important in vascular areas with a deficient, injured or absent endothelial cell layer. In such areas of diseased arteries, one observes paradoxical vasoconstriction in response to endothelium-dependent vasodilators and increased vasoconstriction in response to aggregating platelets [4]. Vasoconstrictors and important vascular cell growth factors have overlapping activities with respect to the regulation of smooth muscle contraction, smooth muscle proliferation and platelet activation (6 - 8). Interestingly, most direct vasoconstrictors, endothelium-dependent vasodilators and platelet activators appear to use as their intracellular signal transduction system inositoltrisphosphate (IP_3), Ca^{++}, 1,2-diacylglycerol (DG), and the subsequent activation of Ca^{++}-dependent protein kinases and protein kinase C as indicated in Figures 1 and 2 [6,9,10]. Many platelet activators increase the activity of phospholipase C resulting in elevated IP_3 and DG levels, an increased cytosolic Ca^{++} level (due to IP_3-induced Ca^{++}-discharge from intracellular vesicles), and the activation of protein kinase C and Ca^{++}/calmodulin-dependent protein kinases such as myosin light chain kinase (MLCK). More recently, it was shown that platelet activators also increase tyrosine phosphorylation in platelets [11,12] and that tyrosine phosphorylation of phospholipase C-γ1 (PLC-γ1) increases the activity of this PLC isozyme [13]. However, whether tyrosine phosphorylation of PLC is an important mechanism for the activation of platelets remains to be elucidated.

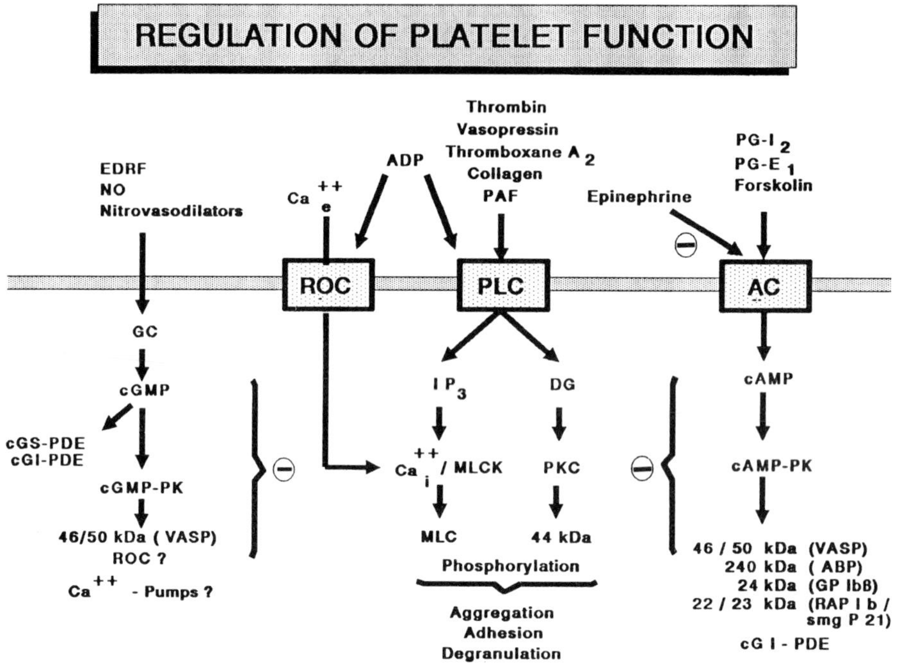

Fig. 2. Regulatory pathways in platelet function

Vasoactive substances and their intracellular pathways resulting in platelet activation (aggregation, adhesion, degranulation, etc.) are shown. Substances which elevate cGMP or cAMP levels activate cGMP- or cAMP-dependent protein kinases (cGMP-PK, cAMP-PK) and prevent the activation of platelets by inhibiting the activation pathways. Other abbreviations: PAF, platelet activating factor; ROC, receptor-operated calcium channel; PLC, phospholipase C; AC, adenylyl cyclase; GC, guanylyl cyclase; IP_3, inositol-trisphosphate; DG, 1,2-diacylglycerol; cGS-PDE, cGMP-stimulated phosphodiesterase; cGI-PDE, cGMP-inhibited phosphodiesterase; MLCK, myosin light chain kinase; PKC, protein kinase C. Substrates for the different protein kinases are VASP (vasodilator-stimulated phosphoprotein), MLC (myosin light chains) or other proteins indicated by their apparent molecular mass (in kilodalton, kDa).

Some platelet activators stimulate the influx of extracellular Ca^{++} via receptor-operated calcium channels (as observed with ADP) or lower the intracellular cAMP level (as observed with epinephrine via $alpha_2$-receptors). Activation of platelets and the increased intracellular Ca^{++} also stimulates phospholipase A_2 resulting in increased production and release of thromboxane A_2. Release of thromboxane A_2, ADP and serotonin by activated platelets further stimulates platelet activation and is responsible for the secondary phase of aggregation. Direct vasodilators and platelet inhibitors such as prostaglandin I_2 (PG-I_2), prostaglandin E_1 (PG-E_1) and EDRF (probably identical with nitric oxide NO) appear to use an intracellular signal transduction system consisting of the cyclic nucleotides cAMP, cGMP and their corresponding protein kinases as indicated in Figures 1 and 2 [14,15]. The intracellular pathways involved in platelet activation and their modulation by inhibitory pathways are no doubt more complex than the network shown in Fig. 2. However, this simplified scheme will be used to consider some potential mechanisms of action of platelet inhibitors.

3. Inhibition of platelet activation

Platelets are not only activated by multiple factors, they are also inhibited by a variety of different agents and pathways as indicated in Table 1 [4,5].

Table 1. Some mechanisms of platelet inhibition

1) Inhibition of synthesis and release of Thromboxane A_2
(Aspirin; Indomethacin; Imidazole?; Sulfinpyrazone ?)

2) Antagonism of platelet activators
(Ticlopidin for ADP; Thromboxane antagonists)

3) Inhibition of thrombin generation or function
(Heparin; Hirudin)

4) Inhibition of calcium influx
(calcium antagonists)

5) Elevation of platelet cAMP levels

6) Elevation of platelet cGMP levels

Here, the regulation of platelet cAMP and cGMP levels and the posssible mechanisms of action of these cyclic nucleotides will be considered. It is now well established that agents which elevate either platelet cAMP levels (i.e. PG-I_2, PG-E_1 etc.) or cGMP levels (EDRF, nitroprusside etc.) are powerful inhibitors of platelet activation [16-18]. Two of the physiologically most important cyclic nucleotide-elevating platelet inhibitors, PG-I_2 and EDRF, are produced by vascular endothelial cells which are central to a very important, if not the most important, antithrombotic mechanism. In addition to PG-I_2, related prostaglandins and other agents regulate the level of platelet cAMP as summarized in Table 2 [19,20].

Table 2. Regulation of platelet cAMP levels

1) Increase via stimulatory G-proteins (Gs)
(PG-I_2, PG-E_1, PG-E_2, Adenosine (A_2), Catecholamines (ß))

2) Increase via inhibition of cAMP phosphodiesterases (PDE)
(inhibition of cGI- PDE by cGMP, Milrinone, Amrinone, Cilostamide, Anagrelide; inhibition of low Km PDE by Dipyridamole)

3) Decrease via inhibitory G-proteins (Gi)
(Catecholamines α_2, ADP, Thrombin, PAF, Vasopressin)

4) Decrease via stimulation of phosphodiesterases (PDE)
(activation of cGI-PDE by cAMP-mediated phosphorylation; activation of cGS-PDE by cGMP)

The principle platelet enzyme responsible for the synthesis of cGMP is the heme-containing guanylyl cyclase, which, in contrast to the adenylyl cyclase, is a cytosolic protein. This enzyme is the target and "intracellular receptor" for EDRF and other nitrovasodilators. EDRF and NO derived from other nitrovasodilators (i.e. Nitroprusside, Nitrates, Molsidomin) are thought to bind to the prosthetic group heme, which is involved in an activation of the soluble guanylyl cyclase. The particulate guanylyl cyclase, the receptor for the atrial natriuretic factor (ANF) is present in endothelial cells, vascular smooth muscle cells and other tissues, but not in human platelets. Platelet cGMP levels can therefore be regulated by the activation of the soluble guanylyl cyclase or by the regulation of cGMP-hydrolyzing phosphodiesterases [15,21] as shown in Table 3.

Table 3. Elevation of platelet cGMP levels

1) Activation of the soluble guanylyl cyclase
(EDRF and other NO-generating nitrovasodilators)

2) Inhibition of the cGMP-specific phosphodiesterase
(Dipyridamole, Zaprinast (M&B 22948))

Agents which are powerful activators of the soluble guanylyl cyclase (EDRF and other NO-generating agents) are potent inhibitors of platelet activation. However agents which elevate cytosolic calcium and activate platelets are also known to moderately elevate platelet cGMP levels [22] but this is now thought to be due to the stimulation of the Ca^{++}-dependent EDRF-synthase

in activated platelets and to represent a possible feed-back inhibition of platelet activation [23].
Platelet cyclic nucleotide levels are not only regulated by synthesizing enzymes (adenylyl and guanylyl cyclases) but also by specific cyclic nucleotide phosphodiesterases (PDEs). Degradation of the cyclic nucleotides cAMP and cGMP is known to be catalyzed by a large, still growing number of enzymes representing at least 5 different isozyme families [20,24,25].
In Table 4, some properties of these families of isozymes are summarized.

Table 4. Cyclic nucleotide phosphodiesterase isozymes (n.s., not significant; cA, cAMP; cG, cGMP)

	Isozyme Family	Substrate	Selective Inhibitors	Present in Human Platelets
I	Ca^{++}/calmodulin-dependent	cA + cG	Phenothiazines	n.s.
II	cGMP-stimulated	cA + cG	none known	+
III	cGMP-inhibited	cA >> cG	Milrinone, Amrinone, Anagrelide etc. cGMP	+++
IV	cAMP-specific	cA >>> cG	RO 201724 Rolipram	n.s.
V	cGMP-specific	cG >>> cA	Dipyridamole, Zaprinast (M&B 22948)	+++

Inhibitors of the phosphodiesterase isozyme families III and V raise platelet cAMP and cGMP levels, respectively, inhibit platelet aggregation and therefore demonstrate potential as antiplatelet drugs. Inhibitors of the type V family may be of particular interest since they are poor vasodilators [25]. A recent study demonstrated that anagrelide, an inhibitor of the phosphodiesterease family type III and powerful inhibitor of platelet aggregation, looks promising for the treatment of thrombocytosis [26]. However, the precise mechanism of action for this effect is still uncertain.
From all of the results briefly reviewed here, it can be clearly concluded that elevation of platelet cAMP or cGMP levels, either by stimulation of adenylyl or guanylyl cyclases or by inhibition of phosphodiesterases, inhibits platelet activation and aggregation.

4. Mechanisms of action of cAMP and cGMP in platelets.

Whereas the intracellular effects of cAMP are primarily mediated by cAMP-dependent protein kinases, there is now substantial evidence that the intracellular effects of cGMP are mediated by more than one pathway [15,24,27-29] as shown in Fig. 3.

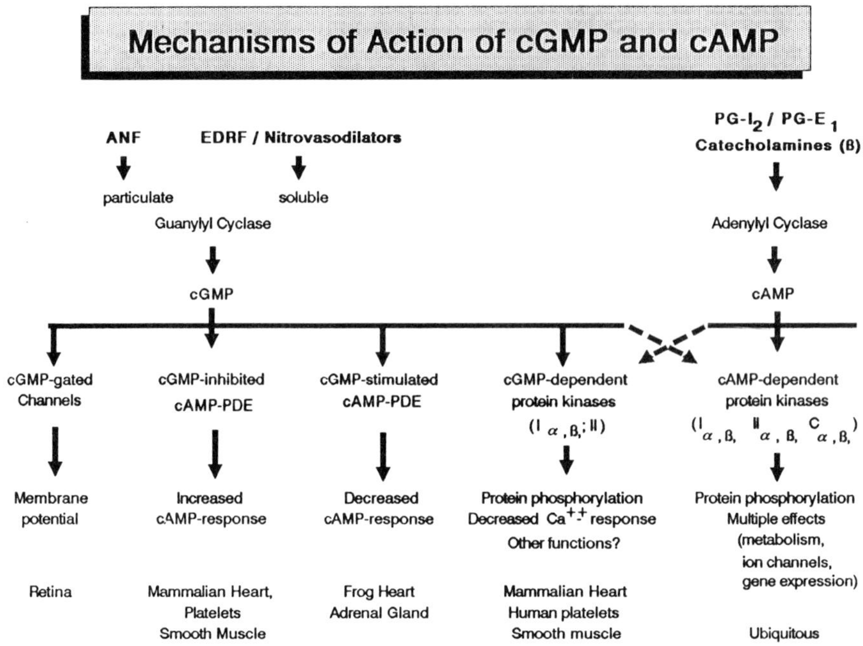

Fig. 3. Some current concepts concerning the intracellular mechanisms of action of cGMP and cAMP. The cyclic nucleotides are elevated in response to extracellular stimuli such as ANF, nitrovasodilators (e.g. EDRF), prostaglandins and catecholamines.

Each of the cyclic nucleotide-regulated proteins shown in Fig. 3 (cGMP-gated channels, cGMP-regulated phosphodiesterases, and cGMP- and cAMP-dependent protein kinases) represents a family of closely related but distinct regulatory proteins, and the physiological significance of this diversity is the subject of intense current investigation. While at present there is no evidence that platelets contain cGMP- or cAMP-gated ion channels, human platelets are known to contain significant levels of cGMP-inhibited and cGMP-stimulated phosphodiesterases [20,24,25,30], cGMP-dependent protein kinase type I [31,32] and cAMP-dependent protein kinases type I, II_{β} and II_{α} [32,33; S.M. Lohmann, M. Halbrügge and U. Walter, unpublished experiments]. Of considerable interest is the increasing evidence that a cAMP-mediated response can be modulated by cGMP-regulated phosphodiesterases. The effects of cGMP on cAMP-regulated events may be inhibitory (antagonistic) or stimulatory (synergistic) depending on whether cGS-PDE or cGI-PDE is the major cGMP-regulated PDE (Fig.3). The cGS-PDE has been shown to mediate the inhibition of cGMP on two cAMP-stimulated effects, the L-type calcium current in frog cardiac myocytes [34] and aldosterone secretion in bovine adrenal glomerulosa cells [35]. A cGI-PDE appears to participate in mediating the synergistic actions of nitrovasodilators with respect to the effects of cAMP-elevating drugs in rabbit platelets [36,37] and rat aortic smooth muscle [38]. Many cells of the cardiovascular system including cardiac myocytes, vascular smooth muscle cells and platelets contain the two types of cGMP-regulated phosphodiesterases as well as cGMP-dependent protein kinases and cAMP-dependent protein kinases. This diversity in cyclic-nucleotide-regulated enzymes often makes it difficult to determine the exact contribution of each protein to the regulation of a complex cellular function. In cardiac myocytes, cGMP and cGMP-dependent protein kinase antagonize the positive inotropic effects of cAMP and cAMP-dependent protein kinase [39], whereas vascular smooth muscle cells and platelets are inhibited by the apparently synergistic effects of cGMP/cGMP-dependent protein kinase and cAMP/cAMP-dependent protein kinase [14,15,40].

Human platelets, when compared to other mammalian cell types, contain some of the highest concentration of both cGMP- and cAMP-dependent protein kinase [32; Eigenthaler et al., manuscript submitted]. Considerable evidence supports the view that these two protein kinases mediate the effects of cGMP- and cAMP-elevating platelet inhibitors. In intact human platelets, cAMP-elevating prostaglandins or cGMP-elevating nitrovasodilators cause the inhibitory effects on platelet activation (including agonist-induced PLC activation, calcium mobilization, Ca^{++}-dependent protein phosphorylation, adhesion and aggregation), as well as stimulatory effects on the phosphorylation of certain proteins, which can be mimicked by specific, cell-membrane permeable activators of the cAMP-PK or cGMP-PK, respectively [10,15,41-45]. As shown in Fig. 4, ADP-induced calcium mobilization in intact human platelets is strongly inhibited by the cGMP-elevating agent sodium nitroprusside (SNP), and by the specific, cell-membrane-permeable cGMP analog 8-CPT-cGMP. The data shown in Fig. 4 and other experimental data (no effect of 8-CPT-cGMP on the activity of the cGMP-regulated phosphodiesterases, activation of cGMP-dependent protein kinase by 8-CPT-cGMP in intact human platelets etc.) strongly suggest that the cGMP-dependent protein kinase mediates the nitrovasodilator inhibition of ADP-induced calcium elevation and platelet activation. ADP is known to elevate platelet Ca^{++}-levels by increased calcium influx (via a receptor-operated calcium channel) and by increased calcium mobilization from intracellular vesicles [46,47], and both events appear to be inhibited by the cGMP-dependent protein kinase (J.Geiger et al., manuscript in preparation). There is also considerable evidence that cAMP and the cAMP-dependent protein kinase inhibit agonist-induced calcium mobilization in human platelets [10,15,47,48]. Inhibition of agonist-induced calcium mobilization in human platelets appears to be an important effect of cyclic nucleotides and cyclic nucleotide-regulated protein kinases, but additional functions and effects have been considered [10,15,47-54], as indicated in Table 5.

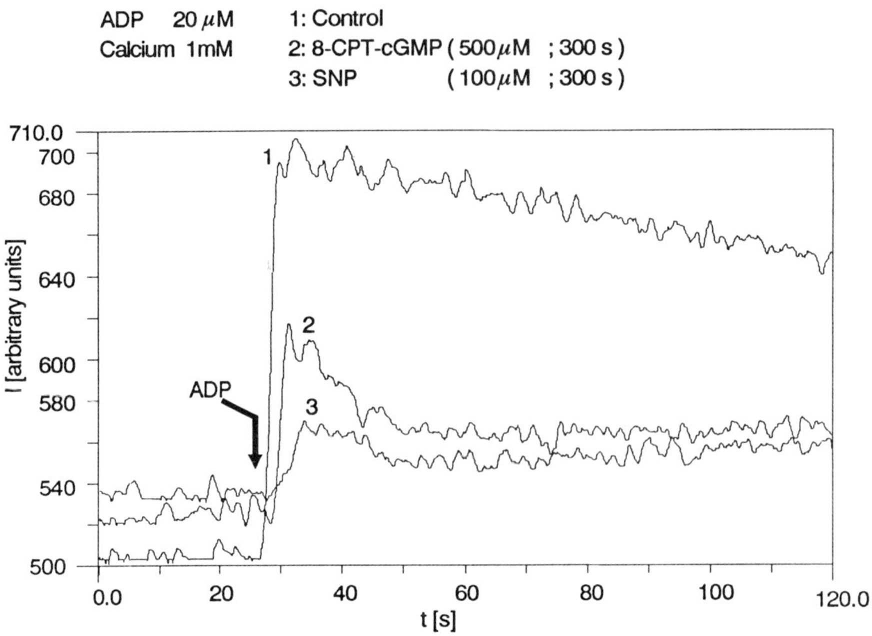

Fig. 4. Inhibition of the ADP-induced calcium mobilization by sodium nitroprusside (SNP) and 8-CPT-cGMP in intact human platelets. Intact Fura-2-loaded human platelets, preincubated for 5 min in the absence or presence of SNP or 8-CPT-cGMP as indicated, were stimulated with 20 µM ADP in the presence of 1 mM extracellular calcium. The time course of the ADP-induced elevation of intracellular calcium (indicated by the increased fluorescence intensity I) is shown.

At present, it is not possible to decide which of the potential mechanisms shown in Table 5 is actually the major one responsible for cyclic nucleotide-induced inhibition of platelet activation. Several of these platelet functions may be the target for the inhibitory effects of cAMP and cGMP, however, some of these pathways may be differentially regulated by cAMP/cAMP-dependent protein kinase and cGMP/cGMP-dependent protein kinase. It appears likely that the inhibition of agonist-mediated phospholipase C activation as well as receptor-operated calcium channels is a major site of cyclic nucleotide action in human platelets. However, the molecular details of these effects are presently unclear. Although one subtype of phospholipase C (PLC-γ) was recently shown to be phosphorylated by the cAMP-dependent protein kinase in intact fibroblasts, no change in its enzymatic activity was noted [55], suggesting that the cyclic nucleotide regulation of PLC activity may be more complex (requiring regulation of the interaction between G-Proteins and receptors, or G-Proteins and PLC ?).

Table 5. Possible mechanisms for the inhibition of platelet activation by cyclic nucleotides and cyclic-nucleotide-regulated protein kinases

1) Inhibition of the phosphatidylinositol cycle
   a) at the level of phospholipase C activation
   b) at the level of PIP_2-resynthesis

2) Inhibition of the inositoltrisphosphate-induced calcium release from intracellular vesicles

3) Inhibition of receptor-operated calcium channel activation and calcium influx from the extracellular space

4) Activation of calcium removal from the cytoplasm
   a) at the level of intracellular calcium pumps
   b) at the level of plasmalemmal calcium pumps

5) Inhibition of calcium-dependent protein kinases (inactivation of myosin light chain kinase by cAMP- dependent phosphorylation)

6) Activation of a protein phosphatase capable of reversing calcium-mediated protein phosphorylation

7) Inhibition of the rapid agonist-induced reorganization of the platelet cytoskeleton during activation

8) Inhibition of exposure of fibrinogen binding sites.

Another approach for elucidating the molecular mechanism of action of cyclic nucleotides is to search for specific substrates of cAMP-dependent protein kinase or cGMP-dependent protein kinase. Studies with both intact human platelets as well as platelet extracts provided evidence that several proteins are phosphorylated by the cAMP-dependent protein kinase in intact cells (see also Fig. 2) including a 240 kDa actin binding protein (ABP), a 46/50 kDa membrane-associated protein termed vasodilator-stimulated phosphoprotein (VASP), myosin light chain kinase (MLCK), a small GTP-binding protein (smg p21 or Rap 1b), the cell membrane-bound glycoprotein Ibß, the cGMP-inhibited phosphodiesterase (cGI-PDE), a 24 kDa plasma membrane-bound protein associated with a Ca^{++}-ATPase, and a few other proteins of unknown identity [15,45,56,57]. In contrast, the 46/50 kDa protein termed VASP is the only protein known to be specifically phosphorylated by the cGMP-dependent protein kinase in extracts and intact human platelets [41-45]. Considerable research is underway to define the functional significance of these phosphorylation events. Our group has characterized and purified the 46/50 kDa protein VASP since it is the only protein known to be phosphorylated by both cAMP- and cGMP-dependent protein kinase in platelet membranes and intact platelets in response to cAMP- as well as cGMP-elevating platelet inhibitors [41,43,44]. Although the cellular function of VASP is not yet known, phosphorylation of this protein correlates very well with the inhibition of platelet activation [15,41-45], a finding which has been recently confirmed by another group [56]. Phosphorylation of one site alters the apparent molecular mass of VASP in gel electrophoresis, a property which has been used for the convenient quantitative analysis of VASP phosphorylation in intact platelets [44]. Furthermore, the phosphorylation-induced shift was used to demonstrate that platelet VASP is phosphorylated in endothelial cell-platelet coincubations as shown in Fig. 5.

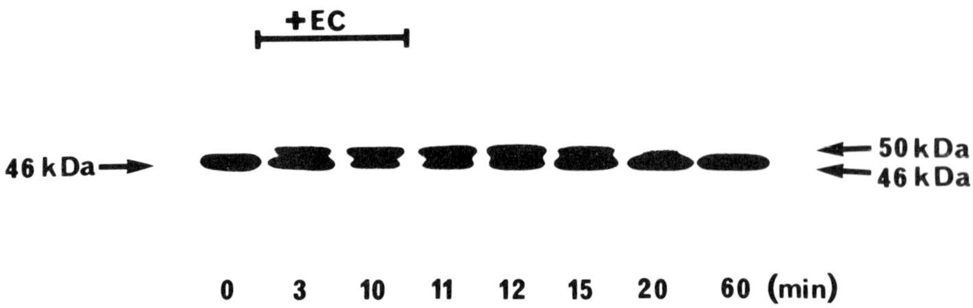

Fig.5. Endothelial cell-dependent phosphorylation of the vasodilator-stimulated phosphoprotein (VASP) in intact platelets. Isolated, washed human platelets were added to a monolayer of human umbilical cord endothelial cells (EC) as indicated. Platelet aliquots were removed and analyzed for the state of VASP phosphorylation. The shift of VASP from a 46 to a 50 kilodalton (kDa) protein indicates the phosphorylation of VASP. Endothelial cells caused the almost complete shift of VASP to the 50 kDa phosphoform, an effect which was completely reversible when platelets and endothelial cells were separated.

Other experiments indicated that the endothelial-dependent phosphorylation of platelet VASP was caused by the endothelial factors EDRF and PG-I_2 whose effects on VASP phosphorylation were mediated by the pathways using cGMP/cGMP-dependent protein kinase or cAMP/cAMP-dependent protein kinases, respectively, as summarized in Fig. 6.

Ongoing experiments appear to indicate that this endothelial cell - platelet interaction and endothelial cell-dependent phosphorylation of platelet proteins mediated by cyclic nucleotide signal transduction pathways can be demonstrated *in vivo* in man.

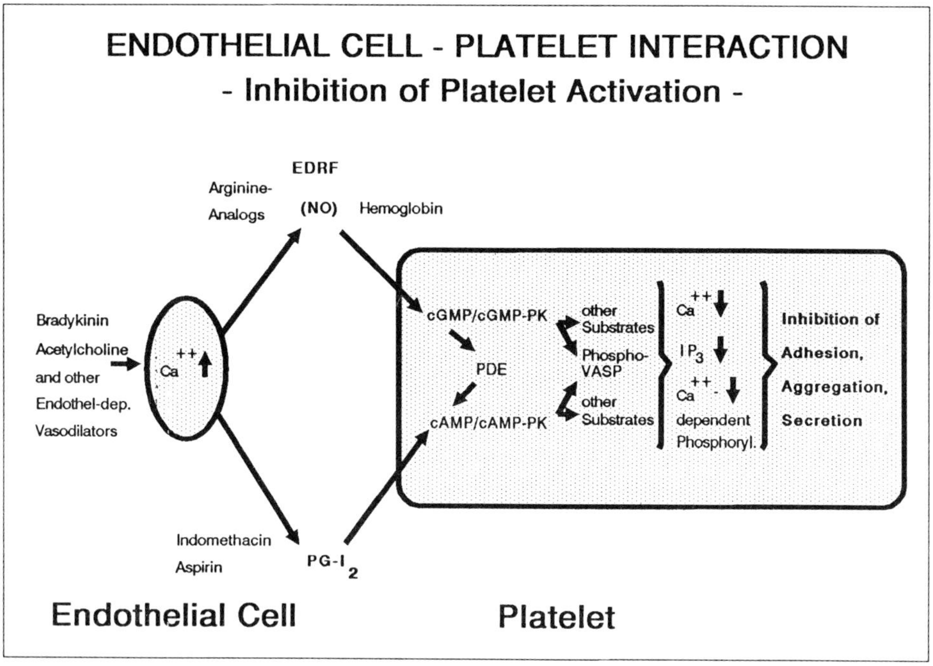

Fig.6. Model summarizing the regulation of platelet protein phosphorylation by endothelial cells. Human endothelial cells, stimulated by endothelium-dependent vasodilators, produce EDRF and PG-I_2, which cause the stimulation of protein phosphorylation mediated by cGMP/cGMP-dependent protein kinase or cAMP/ cAMP-dependent protein kinase, respectively, and inhibit platelet activation. Phosphorylation of certain proteins, including the 46/50 kDa vasodilator-stimulated phosphoprotein (VASP), appears to be an important component in this reaction cascade which can be modulated by drugs such as aspirin and indomethacin.

5. Concluding remarks

Considerable evidence indicates that activation of human platelets is inhibited by two intracellular pathways regulated by either cAMP or cGMP. This is in agreement with data demonstrating that the inhibition of platelet activation by cAMP-elevating agents (e.g. PG-I_2, PG-E_1, etc.) and cGMP-elevating agents (e.g. EDRF and other nitrovasodilators) is synergistic [58-61]. This synergism may derive from several different mechanisms. For example, nitrovasodilators which elevate cGMP can cause cGMP-dependent inhibition

of the type III phosphodiesterase (cGI-PDE), and thereby raise cAMP levels [20,36-38]. Also, cAMP- and cGMP-elevating agents may cause synergistic phosphorylation of substrate proteins by activation of cAMP- and cGMP-dependent protein kinases, respectively [15,44]. Furthermore, the cAMP- and cGMP-dependent protein kinases may each have distinct substrates which have independent effects on the various platelet activation pathways [15]. The current knowledge concerning cyclic nucleotide regulation of platelets suggests that the simultaneous use of cAMP-elevating inhibitors and cGMP-elevating nitrovasodilators as antithrombotic drugs would be useful.
The action of nitrovasodilators could be increased by the use of inhibitors for the type V (cGMP-specific) phosphodiesterase, whereas the effects of cAMP-elevating agents could be potentiated by inhibitors of type III (cGMP-inhibited) phosphodiesterase. However, it is also necessary to unravel the molecular details of cyclic nucleotide action in platelets, in particular the function and physiological role of the specific substrates for the cAMP- and cGMP-dependent protein kinase and their interaction with other proteins. In this respect it is of interest to note that the elucidation of a critical protein-protein interaction important for the activity of 5-lipoxygenase, an enzyme involved in the synthesis of leukotrienes, led to the development of a new and potent inhibitor of this enyzme which may have potential in the treatment of allergy and inflammation [62]. It is hoped that an understanding of the molecular events involved in platelet activation and inhibition will also contribute to the development of new and safe antithrombotic drugs.

Acknowledgements. The research of our laboratory is supported by the Deutsche Forschungsgemeinschaft (Ko 210/ 11-1). The authors thank S. Ebert for the skillful preparation of the manuscript.

6. Selected references

1) Ross, R. (1986) The pathogenesis of atherosclerosis - an update. N. Engl. J. Med. 314, 488 - 500
2) Hirsh, J. (1987) Hyperreactive platelets and complications of coronary artery disease. N. Engl. J. Med. 316, 1543 - 1544
3) Schwartz, S.M., Heimark, R.L., and Majesky, M.W. (1990) Developmental mechanisms underlying pathology of arteries. Physiol. Rev. 70, 1177 - 1209
4) Dinerman, J.L., and Mehta, J.L. (1990) Endothelial, platelet and leucocyte interactions in ischemic heart disease: Insights into potential mechanisms and their clinical relevance. J. Am. Coll. Cardiol. 16, 207 - 222
5) Stein, B., Fuster, V., Israel, D.H., Cohen, M., Badimon, L., Badimon, J.J., and Chesebro, J.H. (1989) Platelet inhibitor agents in cardiovascular disease: an update. J. Am. Coll. Cardiol. 14, 813 - 836
6) Hathaway, D.R., and March, K.L. (1989) Molecular cardiology: new avenues for the diagnosis and treatment of cardiovascular disease. J. Am. Coll. Cardiol. 13, 265 - 282

7) Ip, J.H., Fuster, V., Badimon, L., Badimon, J., Traubman, M.B., and Chesebro, J.H. (1990) Syndromes of accelerated atherosclerosis: role of vascular injury and smooth muscle proliferation. J. Am. Coll. Cardiol. 15, 1667 - 1687

8) Berk, B.C., and Alexander, R.W. (1989) Vasoactive effects of growth factors. Biochem. Pharmacol. 38, 219 - 225

9) Hathaway, D.R., March, K.L., Lash, J.A., Adam, L.P., and Wilensky, R.L. (1991) Vascular smooth muscle: a review of the molecular basis of contractility. Circulation 83, 382 - 390

10) Siess, W. (1989) Molecular mechanisms of platelet activation. Physiol. Rev. 69, 58 - 178

11) Ferrell, jr J.E., and Martin, S.G. (1988) Platelet tyrosine phosphorylation is regulated by thrombin. Mol. Cell. Biol. 8, 3603- 3610

12) Golden, A., and Brugge, J.S. (1989) Thrombin treatment induces rapid changes in tyrosine phosphorylation in platelets. Proc. Natl. Acad. Sci. USA 86, 901 - 905

13) Nishibe, S., Wahl, M.I., Hernandez-Sotomayor, S.M.T., Tonks, N.K., Rhee, S.G., and Carpenter, G. (1990) Increase of the catalytic activity of phospholipase C-γ1 by tyrosine phosphorylation. Science 250, 1253 - 1256

14) Walter, U., Waldmann, R., and Nieberding, M. (1988) Intracellular mechanism of action of vasodilators. Eur. Heart J. 9 (Suppl. H), 1 - 6

15) Walter, U. (1989) Physiological role of cGMP and cGMP-dependent protein kinase in the cardiovascular system. Rev. Physiol. Biochem. Pharmacol. 113, 42 - 88

16) Moncada, S., Radomski, M.W., and Palmer, R.M.J. (1988) Endothelium-derived relaxing factor. Identification as nitric oxide and role in the control of vascular tone and platelet function. Biochem. Pharmacol. 37, 2495 - 2501

17) Vane, J.R., Äanggard, E.E., and Botting, R.M. (1990) Regulatory functions of the vascular endothelium. N. Engl. J. Med. 323, 27 - 36

18) Ignarro, L.J. (1991) Signal transduction mechanisms involving nitric oxide. Biochem. Pharmacol. 41, 485 - 490

19) Aktories, K., and Jakobs, K.H. (1985) 'Regulation of platelet cAMP formation', in G.L. Longenecker (ed.), The platelets: physiology and pharmacology, Academic Press, New York, pp 271 - 288

20) Beavo, J.A., and Reifsnyder, D.H. (1990) Primary sequence of cyclic nucleotide phosphodiesterase isozymes and the design of selective inhibitors. Trends Pharmacol. Sci. 11, 150 - 155

21) Tremblay, J., Gerzer, R., and Hamet, P. (1988) Cyclic GMP and cell function. Adv. Second Messenger and Phosphoprotein Res. 22, 319 - 383

22) Goldberg, N.D., and Haddox, M.K. (1977) Cyclic GMP metabolism and involvement in biological regulation. Annu. Rev. Biochem. 46, 823 - 896

23) Radomski, M.W., Palmer, R.M.J., and Moncada, S. (1990) An L-arginine/nitric oxide pathway present in human platelets regulates aggregation. Proc. Natl. Acad. Sci. USA 87, 5193 - 5197

24) Beavo, J.A.(1988) Multiple isoenzymes of cyclic nucleotide phosphodiesterase. Adv. Second Messenger and Phosphoprotein Res. 22, 1 - 38

25) Nicholson, C.D., Challiss, R.A.J., and Shahid, M. (1991) Differential modulation of tissue function and therapeutic potential of selective inhibitors of cyclic nucleotide phosphodiesterase isoenzymes. Trends Pharmacol. Sci. 12, 19 - 27

26) Silverstein, M.N., Petitt, R.M., Solberg, L.A., Fleming, J.S., Knight, R.C., Schachter, L.P. (1988) Anagrelide: a new drug for treating thrombocytosis. N. Engl. J. Med. 318, 1292 - 1294

27) Beebe, S.J., and Corbin, J.D. (1986) 'Cyclic nucleotide-dependent protein kinases' in P.D. Boyer, E.G. Krebs (eds.) The Enzymes, third edition, Vol. 17, Academic Press, New York, pp 43 - 111

28) Meinecke, M., Büchler, W., Fischer, L., Lohmann, S.M., and Walter, U. (1990) 'cAMP-dependent protein kinase: subunit diversity and functional role in gene expression' in G. Jeserich, H.H. Althaus, and T.V. Waehneldt (eds.) Cellular and molecular biology of myelination. NATO ASI Series H, Vol. 43, Springer-Verlag, Heidelberg, pp 201 - 215

29) Taylor, S.S., Buechler, J.A., and Yonemoto, W. (1990) cAMP-dependent protein kinase: framework for a diverse family of regulator enzymes. Annu. Rev. Biochem. 59, 971 - 1005

30) Grant, P.G., Mannarino, A.F., and Colman, R.W. (1990) Purification and characterization of a cyclic GMP-stimulated nucleotide phosphodiesterase from the cytosol of human platelets. Thromb. Res. 59, 105 119

31) Waldmann, R., Bauer, S., Göbel, C., Hofmann, F., Jakobs, K.H., and Walter, U. (1986) Demonstration of cGMP-dependent protein kinase and cGMP-dependent protein phosphorylation in cell-free extracts of platelets. Eur. J. Biochem. 158, 203 - 210

32) Eigenthaler, M., Friedrich, C., Schanzenbächer, P., and Walter, U. (1990) Concentration and regulation of cyclic nucleotides, vasodilator-regulated protein kinases and one of their substrates in human platelets. Eur. J. Clin. Invest. 20 (2), A16

33) Salama, S.E., and Haslam, R.J. (1984) Characterization of the protein kinase activities of human platelet supernatant and particulate fractions. Biochem. J. 218, 285 - 294

34) Hartzell, H.C., and Fischmeister, R. (1986) Opposite effects of cyclic GMP and and cyclic AMP on Ca^{++} current in single heart cells. Nature 323, 273 - 275

35) MacFarland, R.T., Zelus, B.D., and Beavo, J.A. (1991) High concentrations of a cGMP-stimulated phosphodiesterase mediate ANP-induced decreases in cAMP and steroidogenesis in adrenal glomerulosa cells. J. Biol. Chem. 266, 136 - 142

36) Maurice, D.H., and Haslam, R.J. (1990) Molecular basis of the synergistic inhibition of platelet function by nitrovasodilators and activators of adenylate cyclase: inhibition of cyclic AMP breakdown by cyclic GMP. Mol. Pharmacol. 37, 671 - 681

37) Bowen, R., and Haslam, R.J. (1991) Effects of nitrovasodilators on platelet cyclic nucleotide levels in rabbit blood; role for cyclic AMP in synergistic inhibition of platelet function by sin-1 and prostaglandin E_1. J. Cardiovascul. Pharmacol. 17, 424 - 433

38) Maurice, D.H., Crankshaw, D., and Haslam, R.J. (1991) Synergistic actions of nitrovasodilators and isoprenaline on rat aortic smooth muscle. Eur. J. Pharmacol. 192, 235-242
39) Mery, P.-F., Lohmann, S.M., Walter, U., and Fischmeister, R. (1991) Ca^{++}-current is regulated by cyclic GMP-dependent protein kinase in cardiac myocytes. Proc. Natl. Acad. Sci. USA 88, 1197 - 1201.
40) Lincoln, T.M. (1989) Cyclic GMP and the mechanism of vasodilation. Pharmacol. Ther. 41, 479 - 502
41) Waldmann, R., Nieberding, M., and Walter, U. (1987) Vasodilator-stimulated protein phosphorylation is mediated by cAMP- and cGMP-dependent protein kinases. Eur. J. Biochem. 167, 441 - 448
42) Waldmann, R., and Walter, U. (1989) Cyclic nucleotide-elevating vasodilators inhibit platelet aggregation at an early step of the activation cascade. Eur. J. Pharmacol. 159, 317-320
43) Halbrügge, M., and Walter, U. (1989) Purification of a vasodilator-regulated phosphoprotein from human platelets. Eur. J. Biochem. 185, 41 - 50
44) Halbrügge, M., Friedrich, C., Eigenthaler, M., Schanzenbächer, P., and Walter, U. (1990) Stoichiometric and reversible phosphorylation of a 46 kDa protein in human platelets in response to cGMP- and cAMP-elevating vasodilators. J. Biol. Chem. 265, 3088 - 3093
45) Halbrügge, M., Friedrich, C., Eigenthaler, M., Meszaros, G., Kochsiek, K., and Walter, U. (1990) 'Nitrovasodilator-regulated protein phosphorylation in human platelets' in S. Moncada, E.A. Higgs (eds.) Nitric oxide from L-arginine: a bioregulatory system. Elsevier Science Publisher, Amsterdam, pp 349 - 354
46) Sage, S.O., and Rink, T.J. (1987) The kinetics of changes in intracellular calcium concentration in Fura-2-loaded human platelets. J. Biol. Chem. 262, 16364 - 16369
47) Rink, T.J., and Sage, S.O. (1990) Calcium signaling in human platelets. Annu. Rev. Physiol. 52, 431 - 449
48) Feinstein, M.B., Zavoico, G.B., and Halenda, S.P. (1985) 'Calcium and cyclic AMP: antagonistic modulators of platelet function' in G.L. Longenecker (ed.) The platelets: physiology and pharmacology. Academic Press, New York, pp 237 - 269
49) Sellers, J.R., and Adelstein, R.S. (1987) 'Regulation of contractile activity' in P.D. Boyer, E.G. Krebs (eds.) The enzymes, third edition, Vol. 17, Academic Press, New York, pp 381 - 418
50) Lamb, N.J.C., Fernandez, A., Conti, M.A., Adelstein, R., Glass, D.B., Welch, W.J., and Feramisco, J.R. (1988) Regulation of actin microfilament integrity in living non-muscle cells by the cAMP-dependent protein kinase and the myosin light chain kinase. J. Cell Biol. 106, 1955 - 1971
51) Haslam, R.J. (1987) 'Signal transduction in platelet activation' in M. Verstraete, J. Vermylen, R. Lijnen, J. Arnout (eds.) Thrombosis and haemostasis 1987. Leuven University Press, Leuven, pp 147-174
52) FOX, J.E.B. (1987) 'The platelet cytoskeleton' in M. Verstraete, J. Vermylen, R. Lijnen, J. Arnout (eds.) Thrombosis and haemostasis 1987, Leuven University Press, Leuven, pp 175 - 225

53) Mendelsohn, M.E., O'Neill, S., George, D., and Loscalzo, J. (1990) Inhibition of fibrinogen binding to human platelets by S-nitro-N-acetylcyteine. J. Biol. Chem. 265, 19028 - 19034

54) van Willigen, G., and Akkerman, J.-W.N. (1991) Protein kinase C and cyclic AMP regulate reversible exposure of binding sites for fibrinogen on the glycoprotein IIb-IIIA complex of human platelets. Biochem. J. 273, 115 - 120

55) Olashaw, N.E., Rhee, S.G., and Pledger, W.J. (1990) Cyclic AMP agonists induce the phosphorylation of phospholipase C-γ and of a 76 kDa protein coprecipated by anti-(phospholipase C-γ) monoclonal antibodies in BALB/ c-3T3 cells. Biochem. J. 272, 297 - 303

56) Siess, W., and Lapetina, E.G. (1990) Functional relationship between cyclic AMP-dependent protein phosphorylation and platelet inhibition. Biochem. J. 271, 815 - 819

57) Darnanville, A., Bredoux, R., Clemetson, K.J., Kiefer, N., Bourdeau, N., Levy-Toledano, S., Caen, J.P., and Enouf, J. (1991) The phosphoprotein that regulates platelet Ca^{++}-transport is located on the plasma membrane, controls membrane-associated Ca^{++}-ATPase and is not glycoprotein Ib ß-subunit. Biochem. J. 273, 429 - 434

58) Levin, R.I., Weksler, B.B., and Jaffe, E.A. (1982) The interaction of sodium nitroprusside with human endothelial cells and platelets: nitroprusside and prostacyclin synergistically inhibit platelet function. Circulation 66, 1299 - 1307

59) Radomski, M.W., Palmer, R.M.J., and Moncada, S. (1987) The antiaggregating properties of vascular endothelium: interactions between prostacyclin and nitric oxide. Br. J. Pharmacol. 92, 639 - 646

60) Lidbury, P.S., Antunes, E., de Nucci, G., and Vane, J.R. (1989) Interactions of iloprost and sodium nitroprusside on vascular smooth muscle and platelet aggregation. Br. J. Pharmacol. 98, 1275 - 1280

61) Willis, A.L., Smith, D.L., Loveday, M., Fulks, J., Lee, C.H., Hedley, L., and van Antwerp, D. (1989) Selective antiplatelet aggregation synergism between a prostacyclin mimetic, RS93427, and the nitrodilators sodium nitroprusside and glyceryl trinitrate. Br. J. Pharmacol. 98, 1296 - 1302

62) Rouzer, C.A., Ford-Hutchinson, A.W., Morton, H.E., and Gillard, J.W. (1990) MK886, a potent and specific leukotriene biosynthesis inhibitor blocks and reverses the membrane association of 5-lipoxygenase in ionophore challenged leukocytes. J. Biol. Chem. 265, 1436 - 1442

PHARMACOLOGICAL MODIFICATION OF PLATELET-DERIVED CYCLOOXYGENASE PRODUCT FORMATION AND ITS CONSEQUENCES FOR PLATELET-VESSEL WALL INTERACTIONS

K. Schrör

Abstract

Platelet-derived cyclooxygenase products are intimately involved in two types of local platelet-vessel wall interactions: Regulation of hemostasis and control of vessel tone. This paper reviews the possible theoretical and clinical benefits of selective pharmacological interference with platelet-derived cyclooxygenase products by thromboxane synthase inhibitors, blockers of PGH_2/TXA_2 receptors and combined-mode compounds in comparison with acetylsalicylic acid (aspirin). It is concluded that low-dose aspirin is safe and effective to reduce the thromboembolic risk in high-risk cardiovascular patients. However, the low selectivity of the compound for different cyclooxygenases and the high sensitivity of the platelet enzyme might result in suppressed vascular PGI_2 formation. Agents, interfering more selectively with thromboxane formation and/or action, do not suppress vascular PGI_2 generation but usually are reversible-type antagonists with limited clinical experience. Fresh insights into transcellular precursor exchange and the regulation and function of thromboxane receptors might result in the development of new promising compounds in the future.

Introduction

Platelet activation is the primary reaction in arterial thrombus formation and is characterized by a unique series of events: Adherence of platelets to exposed subendothelium, "spreading", coherence of additional platelets to the already existent platelet monolayer (aggregation) and secretion of storage products. This finally results in the formation of a platelet-fibrin hemostatic plug at the site of vessel disruption. Fixation of the platelet thrombus to the injured vessel surface, i.e. the interaction between adhering platelets and the vascular subendothelium, requires vasoconstriction to prevent further blood loss and washout of the plug. Both events are controlled by the

A. G. Herman (ed.), Antithrombotics, 139–158.
© 1991 *Kluwer Academic Publishers. Printed in the Netherlands.*

generation of platelet-derived, platelet activating vasoconstrictor mediators, including peroxidation products of arachidonic acid, i.e. prostaglandin endoperoxides (PGEP) and thromboxane A_2 (TXA_2).

Excessive thrombus growth beyond the area of vessel injury is prevented by a complex interaction between platelets, other components of the hemostatic and fibrinolytic system and the vascular endothelium. Thus, in response to aggregating platelets, platelet inhibitory factors are generated in the endothelium, including "EDRF" (8, 44, 100) and PGI_2 (61). Thus, neither systemic thrombosis nor generalized bleeding occur.

This situation changes considerably in atherosclerosis and other kinds of endothelial injury. Increased sensitivity of platelets to aggregating stimuli, enhanced platelet aggregate formation and elevation of circulating platelet secretion products are frequently found in patients with hypercholesterolemia (80, 95), ischemic heart disease (19), unstable angina pectoris (88) and myocardial infarction (62). There is also a disturbed arachidonic acid metabolism in platelets. Patients with unstable angina and acute myocardial infarction exhibit an increased TXA_2 production (24, 41) and a reduced platelet sensitivity to prostacyclin (62). There is also enhanced platelet-derived thromboxane formation after thrombolysis (22). and a considerable increase in urinary thromboxane excretion during the first days after acute myocardial infarction (29, 41). These data demonstrate that thromboxane-dependent platelet activation plays an important role in the dynamic process of coronary thrombosis in unstable angina, myocardial infarction and reocclusion after successful lysis.

This paper reviews some biochemical, physiological and clinical consequences of pharmacological interference with cyclooxygenase product formation in platelets and the possible consequences for platelet vessel wall interactions. Several recent reviews on this issue are available (36, 78, 82, 90).

Cyclooxygenase Metabolites in Platelets

Biosynthesis of cyclooxygenase products

Platelet activation is initiated by binding of a stimulatory agonist to its specific receptor on the platelet surface. This generates a signal for activation of membrane-bound phospholipases, resulting in formation of phospholipid-derived messenger molecules, such as IP_3, diacylglycerol and arachidonic acid (39). In human platelets, arachidonic acid is metabolized into three major products: The lipoxygenase metabolite 12-hydroxy-eicosatetraenoic acid (12-HETE) and the two cyclooxygenase metabolites 12-OH-heptadecatrienoic acid (HHT) + malondialdehyde (MDA) and thromboxane A_2 (TXA_2). TXA_2 is synthezised via prostaglandin (PG) endoperoxides (EP) by the thromboxane synthase and represents the vast majority ($\geq$ 95%) of the cyclooxygenase metabolites. There is no enzymatic degradation of TXA_2 by platelets. The action of locally released TXA_2 is terminated by dilution with the bloodstream and spontaneous or enzymatic degradation. A significant generation of other metabolites of PGEP is only detected after inhibition of the thromboxane synthase. The profile of these metabolites depends upon the available "converting" enzymes, including PGD_2 isomerase activity of plasma albumin and PGI_2-synthase of the vessel wall.

FUNCTION OF PLATELET-DERIVED CYCLOOXYGENASE PRODUCTS

Platelets. PGEP and TXA_2 stimulate all aspects of platelet function, including aggregation, secretion and release of arachidonic acid. These effects are receptor-mediated. The threshold concentrations for PGEP and TXA_2 amount to about 2 and 40 nM, respectively (59). PGEP and TXA_2 have a central role in mediating platelet secretion since their formation is always associated with dense and α-granule secretion and blockade of their formation by specific inhibitors antagonizes the release reaction. Thus, PGEP/TXA_2 (in addition to ADP) form a most important positive feed-back loop (39). Although some vessels and white cells are also capable of TXA_2 formation, the vast majority of TX-(metabolites), generated during platelet-vessel wall interaction is of platelet origin.

Vessel Tone. The action of platelet-derived cyclooxygenase products, i.e. TXA_2 and PGH_2, on the vessel wall is more complex. TXA_2 contracts isolated vessels in vitro (18, 91). The threshold concentrations are $\geq$ 100-200 nM (91) and depend on the type of vessel studied. For example, bovine cerebral arteries are considerably more sensitive to TXA_2 than coronary arteries of this species (18). If platelets are used as source of TXA_2, the long-lasting vasoconstrictor response in isolated coronary (98) and cerebral vessels (4) is caused by TXA_2-induced 5-HT secretion. However, the coronary microcirculation with an intact endothelium does not respond with vasoconstriction to endogenous TXA_2 at concentrations large enough to cause a profound contraction of a rabbit aorta, superfused with the coronary effluent (79). Studies in dogs were also unable to demonstrate any larger constrictor effect of TXA_2 on the coronary microcirculation (50).

Studies with synthetic TXA_2 clearly demonstrated an increase in coronary vascular resistance after injection into coronary arteries of anesthetized dogs. However, threshold concentrations varied greatly between dogs, ranging from 0.125 to 2 μg/kg, and involved platelet aggregate formation. Both blood flow reduction and decrease in platelet count were transient responses and reversible within 70-80 sec (43). Thus, the vasoconstrictor action of TXA_2 in intact circulations is variable and modulated by endothelium-derived vasoactive mediators. This is also in line with the general concept that eicosanoids are local mediators of vessel tone and are rapidly inactivated by metabolic degradation or dilution by the blood-stream.

A different situation exists if endogenous TXA_2 is generated at an area of endothelial injury or turbulent blood flow, caused for example by critical narrowing of a large coronary artery. This results in cyclic reductions in blood flow, caused by the release of vasoactive mediators from platelet aggregates at the site of vessel obstruction. Formation of platelet aggregates and vasoactive mediator release in this species can be prevented by treatment with aspirin (28), inhibition of thromboxane synthase or blockade of thromboxane receptors (2, 7). These data suggest that (i) endogenous, platelet-derived TXA_2 and/or PGEP are involved in intracoronary thrombus formation and coronary vasoconstriction at the site of platelet adhesion and (ii) that this process is limited to the site of formation by antagonistic, i.e. vasodilator and platelet inhibitory mediators, released from healthy endothelium in the vicinity.

Thromboxane A_2/PGH_2-Receptors. The actions of TXA_2 and PGH_2 on platelets and vascular smooth muscle may involve different types of receptors (37). In human platelets, PGH_2 is more potent than TXA_2 and binds to the same receptor (59). Thus, PGH_2, accumulating for example after inhibition of its conversion into TXA_2 by inhibitors of the thromboxane synthase, might replace this ligand at its binding site. This may result in maintained platelet aggregation (69) and/or desensitization of the thromboxane receptor (9).

More recently, two different types of PGH_2/TXA_2 receptors have been identified in human platelets. These receptors are probably coupled to different effector systems to mediate separately platelet shape change and the aggregation/secretion response (16, 92). Importantly, there is evidence for noncompetive inhibition of platelet aggregation by some of the more recent PGH_2/TXA_2 receptor antagonists, such as GR 32191 (92) and Bay u 3405 (71). Following incubation of human platelets with GR 32191 and subsequent washout, there was no formation of IP_3 or stimulation of protein kinase C by a thromboxane mimetic (U 46.619). Platelet aggregation and secretion were abolished, indicating an irreversible blockade of a PGH_2/TXA_2 receptor by this compound. In contrast, platelet shape change and increase in $[Ca^{++}_i]$ following administration of U 46.619 were maintained but could be blocked by SQ 29,548, a reversible type PGH_2/TXA_2 receptor antagonist (92). Patscheke (71) demonstrated a pseudo-irreversible inhibition of platelet aggregation using Bay u 3405, due to a slow-dissociation of the antagonists after occupation of the receptors.

The extent of platelet aggregation after addition of a thromboxane mimetic is also determined by the number of PGH_2/TXA_2 receptors, coupled to the intracellular signal-transducing pathways. There is evidence for cyclic variations of the TXA_2/PGH_2-receptor number on human platelets (15). If platelets in vitro are exposed to subthreshold concentrations of a thromboxane mimetic, subsequent addition of this agonist results in a reduced aggregation. This inhibition is time-dependent, complete at about 5 min and probably due to a reduced number of available PGH_2/TXA_2 receptors (71). Another fascinating aspect of agonist-induced thromboxane receptor desensitization is the sensitization of the platelet adenylate cyclase, i.e. an enhanced cAMP generation in response to receptor-dependent (iloprost) and -independent (forskolin) stimulation of the enzyme (64). Both the reversible (SQ 29,548) and irreversible (GR 32191) PGH_2/TXA_2 receptor antagonists were equieffective inhibitors of the U 46.619-induced adenylate cyclase sensitization (64).

In addition to these in vitro investigations, several recent in vivo studies also indicated that the number of thromboxane receptors may vary under conditions of altered endogenous thromboxane generation. In acute myocardial infarction, the number of thromboxane receptors was increased (17) while the number of PGI_2 receptors tended to be reduced (48-49). More information about receptor regulation is doubtless necessary for an improved design of TX-directed drugs.

PLATELET-VESSEL WALL PRECURSOR EXCHANGE

Eicosanoids are mediators of intercellular signal transfer. Therefore, contacts between platelets and vascular endothelium or subendothelial smooth muscle cells might involve transcellular precursor exchange. Several lines of evidence suggest that vascular endothelium may use platelet-derived endoperoxides to enhance local PGI_2 generation (58, 66). A similar precursor exchange may also take place between platelets and vascular smooth muscle cells.

The possible use of platelet-derived PGEP by the vessel wall to enhance PGI_2 production (Figure 1) was one of the strategic concepts to introduce selective thromboxane synthase inhibitors (see below). Another compound that stimulates endothelial PGI_2 production by a platelet-dependent mechanism is defibrotide (55). Defibrotide enhances cardiocoronary PGI_2 production in acute myocardial ischemia (42) and reduces infarct size (77). Eventually, these effects are due to the stimulation of platelet function (77). In other terms, platelet hyperreactivity, e.g. in severe atherosclerosis (26) and unstable angina (24) may represent a compensatory mechanism to increase local PGI_2 generation by improved supply of the vessel wall with PGEP. Consequently, inhibition of platelet cyclooxygenase by aspirin may result in reduced vascular PGI_2 formation rather by its antiplatelet effect than by direct inhibition of the vascular enzyme. Interestingly, the amount of prostacyclin synthase is not different between vascular endothelial and vascular smooth muscle cells while the amount of cyclooxygenase is about 8-fold lower in endothelial cells (13). Thus, provision of PGH_2 by adhering platelets could be quite effective in stimulating local PGI_2 generation.

Another important issue is of whether or not local PGI_2 generation is sufficient to inhibit platelet function. It had been shown that the maximal plasma concentrations of PGI_2, 3-4 pg/ml, were about 10-fold lower than the concentrations necessary to alter platelet function. In healthy volunteers, Nowak and FitzGerald (66) have recently demonstrated that a peak concentration of 305 pg/ml PGI_2 can be expected after local vascular damage. Administration of the thromboxane synthase inhibitor CGS 13.080 resulted in a 3-5-fold increase of PGI_2, PGD_2 and PGE_2 and there was also enhanced (up to 2.5-fold) urinary excretion of PGI_2 metabolites (25) after single administration to man.

These data clearly demonstrate biologically relevant transcellular metabolism of platelet-derived PGEP by the vessel wall in man.

PHARMACOLOGICAL MODIFICATION OF PLATELET FUNCTION VIA CYCLOOXYGENASE PRODUCT FORMATION

There are several possibilities to interfere with the platelet thromboxane formation. For example, if platelets are hyperreactive all sucessful means to reduce hyperreactivity may also result in reduced stimulation of arachidonic acid release and will not be discussed here. The same is true for endothelium-derived inhibitors of platelet function, including "EDRF" (8) which will be covered in separate sections of this book. The present paper is focussed entirely upon pharmacological interventions that are directly related to the platelet cyclooxygenase pathway: (i) cyclooxygenase inhibitors (aspirin-type agents), (ii) TX-synthase inhibitors, (iii) TX-receptor antagonists, (iv) combined TX-synthase inhibitors/receptor antagonists (Figure 1). The clinical significance of these mechanisms (as far as known) will be exemplified with the two most important thrombembolic complications of atherosclerosis: myocardial infarction and ischemic stroke.

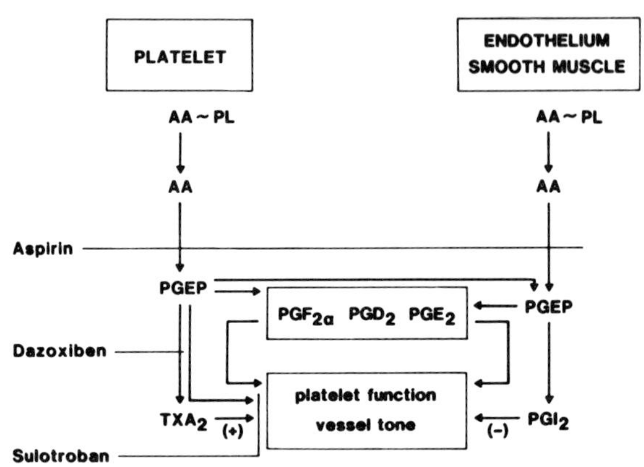

Figure 1: Arachidonic acid metabolism by platelets and the vessel wall and its modification by drugs. (+) stimulation; (-) inhibition.

Acetylsalicylic Acid (Aspirin)

Pharmacology. The systematic pharmacology on antiplatelet effects of acetylsalicylic acid (aspirin) started with the detection by Smith and Willis (87) that aspirin inhibits prostaglandin formation in platelets. The underlying mechanism is an irreversible inhibition of the platelet cyclooxygenase, caused by acetylation of an amino acid that results in steric prevention of access of the enzyme to its substrate

(14). This results in permanent inhibition of TXA_2 formation in the platelet and antagonism of the secretion response, including 5-HT release. The action is not selective for the platelet but may also result in impaired formation of PGI_2 by the vessel wall (68). In contrast to platelets, endothelial cyclooxygenase and subsequent PGI_2 generation may recover within several hours (40). As aspirin undergoes a high first-pass metabolism in the liver, a relative selectivity for the platelets may be acchieved by oral administration of low doses (e.g. 40-50 mg) (56, 68), allowing for presystemic inhibition of the platelet cyclooxygenase without greater reductions in systemic PGI_2 formation (27, 51).

Clinics. The first report on successful use of aspirin as an antithrombotic was published more than 40 years ago (10). In this study, it was found that 10-30 grains of aspirin per day to male patients aged 40-65 years was sufficient to completely prevent coronary thrombosis: None of the 400 patients investigated suffered a coronary thrombosis or myocardial infarction during a 2 years' observation period. About 20 years later, a platelet study was conducted in healthy volunteers (67). According to the results, 175 mg aspirin were recommended as daily antithrombotic dose. It is interesting to note that current research on antithrombotics is now again approaching similar doses, i.e. $\leq$ 160 mg/die (32) after having the experience of 20 more years of research on aspirin and related compounds.

Aspirin is the reference standard antiplatelet drug. The compound is effective in patients at high vascular risk (33, 90). Two recent, placebo-controlled studies have demonstrated the efficacy of 100 mg/day aspirin vs. placebo and 1,000 mg aspirin for prevention of the reinfarction in patients at high risk (45, 99). A significant reduction of reinfarction rate but not of infarct related death or infarct size was observed in one of these investigations (99). Another placebo-controlled trial, using 75 mg aspirin, was conducted in patients with unstable angina or non-Q-wave infarction. There was a 50% reduction in the risk of myocardial infarction over a 3 months observation period (75). The usefulness of aspirin to prevent cerebral ischemia and ischemic stroke is also well established (38, 97). In young patients with brain infarction, aspirin (100 mg/day for 7-10 days) normalized the reduced arachidonic acid content of platelets suggesting enhanced generation of arachidonic acid-derived platelet metabolites in untreated patients (54). According to the UK-TIA study group (97), doses of 300 mg per day are as effective as 1,200 mg/day but less toxic.

Potential negative effects of aspirin involve the relatively low selectivity of the compound for the platelet cyclooxygenase. The possible clinical consequences of simultaneous inhibition of vascular PGI_2 production are currently unknown. Despite of some positive initial results in the U.S. Physicans' Health Study (89), more recent data from this trial suggested that aspirin (325 mg on alternate days) did not reduce the incidence of angina pectoris after an average duration of treatment for 5 years (57). Although available data on secondary prevention of myocardial infarction and preservation of coronary bypass patency suggest the usefulness of a low-dose, i.e. around 100 mg/day, the possibility always exists that additional aspirin may be taken by the patient without knowing it, e.g. by taking combined-drug pain-relievers. Thus, the theoretical benefit to preserve endothelial PGI_2 production by reducing the aspirin dosage may not always work in general practice. Aspirin inhibits fibrinolysis, eventually by reducing vascular PGI_2 formation (3). Aspirin does not prolong the reduced platelet survival in atherosclerosis and, as has to be expected, does not increase the exercise tolerance in patients with stable angina (30). The compound does also only partially antagonize the release of platelet-derived vasoconstrictors in vitro (100) and one might speculate that some of the 50% of patients with unstable angina in the Veterans Administration Study who did not respond to aspirin (see in [90]) might represent those patients with insufficient inhibition of platelet-derived vasoconstrictor release by aspirin alone. In this context, the synergistic action between several types of platelet stimulating factors, in particular thrombin, adrenaline (53) and PGH_2/TXA_2 should also be considered.

Thromboxane Synthase Inhibitors

Pharmacology. These compounds block selectively thromboxane A_2 biosynthesis without inhibiting vascular PGI_2 formation. This results in reduced TXA_2 generation and redirection of the prostaglandin endoperoxide (PGEP) metabolism towards primary prostaglandins (PGE_2, PGD_2) and PGI_2 (12). In a combined system, consisting of human vessels bathed in clotting blood, addition of a thromboxane synthase inhibitor resulted in conversion of the accumulating PGEP mainly to primary prostaglandins (PGE_2) as well as to some PGI_2 (1). The same inhibitor also caused significant generation of PGE_2, PGD_2 and PGI_2 in blood ex vivo, collected from a vascular injury in man (66). However, possible long-term effects of enhanced prostaglandin formation, e.g. PGE_2, are unknown.

Experimental Studies. A number of thromboxane synthase inhibitors have been investigated in animal studies on myocardial and cerebral ischemia. Beneficial effects were reported for most of them (see [82]). It should be noted that these experiments were carried out in healthy animals, i.e. animals with an intact endothelium. Thus, the question arises whether the beneficial effects observed were due to the prevention of deleterious product formation, i.e. TXA_2, or due to the stimulation of protective PGEP metabolites, i.e. PGI_2. Mullane and Fornabaio (63) have shown that cardioprotection from ischemic injury in dogs by two different thromboxane synthase inhibitors was antagonized by platelet antiserum and aspirin pretreatment. This suggests that thromboxane synthase inhibition operates via an aspirin-sensitive, platelet-dependent pathway and that it is not the inhibition of thromboxane formation *per se* which explains the beneficial effects of the compounds. Enhanced PGI_2 biosynthesis might also contribute to improved regional blood supply to the jeopardized myocardium after administration of dazoxiben (23).

Clinics. Clinical trials with thromboxane synthase inhibitors in patients with vasospastic angina, unstable angina or acute myocardial infarction in general did not provide encouraging results (see [82]). In two reports, a significant reduction of transcardiac thromboxane gradients in pacing induced angina, inhibition of lactate release and a significantly increased pacing level were found (46, 93). The clinical position of thromboxane synthase inhibitors in treatment of cerebral ischemia is also largely unknown (31).

There is a number of possible explanations for this clinical failure of thromboxane synthase inhibitors. As mentioned above, PGEP themselves are agonists at the platelet thromboxane receptor with a molar potency comparable to TXA_2 and thus may substitute for TXA_2 at its binding sites to blood platelets. A virtually complete blockade of serum TX must be obtained before TX-dependent platelet activation is influenced in vivo (73). Additionally, platelet-derived prostaglandin endoperoxides might both enzymatically and spontaneously be converted to $PGF_{2\alpha}$, PGE_2 and PGD_2. All of these compounds are constrictors of human cerebral and coronary vessels.

There is also evidence from human studies that the biological actions of thromboxane synthase inhibitors are determined by conversion of PGEP into antiplatelet prostaglandins and elevated platelet cAMP levels rather than by prevention of TXA_2 generation (35, 85). Consequently, addition of an phosphodiesterase inhibitor enhanced the platelet cAMP (53) and amplified the effectivity of thromboxane synthase inhibition (85).

In contrast to aspirin, available thromboxane synthase inhibitors are reversible inhibitors of the platelet enzyme. The duration of action (50% inhibition of serum thromboxane) after single oral administration of compounds that have also been studied in man, i.e. dazoxiben (96), dazmegrel (21) and ozagrel (47, 84) is in the range of 4-6 h. However, repeated administration of some of the compounds, including dazmegrel (21) and OKY 1581 (47) may result in more permanent inhibition of thromboxane formation. Any aspirin-type blockade of TXA_2 formation, lasting for several days after one single tablet (68) is not obtained. Furthermore, an at least 90% suppression of thromboxane-generating capacity is required to prevent thromboxane- dependent platelet activation (73).

Thromboxane Receptor Antagonists

Pharmacology. Thromboxane receptor antagonists differ principally from synthase inhibitors because they do not interfere with thromboxane synthesizing pathways. Consequently, there is no accumulation of thromboxane precursors. These compounds inhibit both TXA_2/PGEP-mediated platelet secretion, including antagonism of TXA_2-mediated granule secretion, i.e. serotonin release and vasoconstriction of coronary (98) and cerebral arteries (4). Like synthase inhibitors, receptor antagonists do also not inhibit endothelial PGI_2 generation.

Experimental Studies. Thromboxane receptor antagonists, such as sulotroban, daltroban, GR 32.191 and Bay u 3405 are potent antithrombotic and antiischemic compounds in animal experiments (60). These compounds acted beneficially in experimental myocardial ischemia at antiplatelet doses (6, 20, 34, 86, 94) and prevented stenosis-induced platelet activation (2). Although thromboxane receptor antagonists have been shown to suppress experimental coronary thrombus formation even more efficiently than aspirin, it is not known whether this is the only or even the major effect to explain their cardioprotective properties. For example, daltroban was found in experimental studies to inhibit ischemia-induced neutrophil activation as well (86, 94).

Clinics. There are only limited and controversial data on the use of thromboxane receptor antagonists as antithrombotics in man (see [60]). Short-term trials and theoretical considerations suggest these compounds as being useful for prevention of streptokinase-induced platelet activation during fibrinolytic treatment of acute myocardial infarction (22), prevention of acute coronary restenoses after PTCA (74) and prevention of platelet deposition to vascular prostheses (52). The newer compounds GR 32.191 (76) and Bay u 3405 (72) exhibit significant inhibition of platelet function still 8 and 12 hours after single oral dosing of 50 and 80 mg, respectively. This long-lasting effect is explained by the non-competitive type of inhibition of the platelet thromboxane receptor(s) (see above).

The problem of longer lasting inhibition of platelet function might be solved by improved knowledge about the nature of platelet thromboxane receptors. Similar to thromboxane synthase inhibitors, thromboxane action has to be suppressed by more than 85% to obtain a significant antithrombotic effect by a thromboxane receptor antagonist (83).

Combined receptor antagonist/synthase inhibitors and future aspects

Pharmacology. These compounds are active at the two important sites of thromboxane generation and action. Pinane-thromboxane A_2 was probably the first compound, exhibiting both TX-receptor blocking and synthase inhibitory activities at 10-50-fold higher concentrations (65). A similar combined action in the opposite direction, i.e. about 100-fold higher concentrations for blockade of the TX-receptor than for inhibition of synthase was described for ridogrel (11). Potent dual inhibitors have been recently also found among 1,3-dioxane derivatives (5).

Experimental studies. Pinane thromboxane A_2 was a potent cardioprotective agent in myocardial ischemia (81). Alternatively, thromboxane synthase inhibitors and receptor antagonists may be used in combination (23, 71) and has been found to exert supraadditive beneficial effects in experimental coronary thrombosis (71, 73). In addition, agents that stimulate platelet cAMP, e.g. inhibitors of the platelet phosphodiesterase (36) may also be added.

Ridogrel was found to be active in man (11). It will be interesting to know whether this new approach will also provide clinical benefit in patients with ischemic heart disease.

In conclusion, new concepts on thromboxane-related antithrombotics may be generated in the future if more detailed information on structure and function of PGH_2/TXA_2-receptors is available. From a teleological point of view, it appears to be more logical to take advantage from locally enhanced, platelet-derived PG-endoperoxide formation by appropriate redirection of their metabolism instead of non-selective prevention of their generation.

Acknowledgements

The competent secretarial assistance of Erika Lohmann is gratefully acknowledged.

References

1. Asai, F. and Schrör, K. (1987) 'Different effects of thromboxane synthetase inhibition on PGI_2 and PGE_2 synthesis in human vascular tissue bathed in clotting blood', in H. Sinzinger and K. Schrör (eds.), Prostaglandins in Clinical Research, Alan R. Liss Inc., New York, pp. 259-264.

2. Ashton, J., Schmitz, J., Campbell, W., Ogletree, M., Raheja, S., Taylor, A., FitzGerald, C., Buja, L., and Willerson, J.T. (1986) 'Inhibition of cyclic flow variations in stenosed canine coronary arteries by thromboxane A_2/prostaglandin H_2 receptor antagonists', Circ. Res. 59, 568-578.

3. Bertele, G., Mussoni, V., Pintucci, G., del Rosso, G., Romano, C., de Gaetano, G., and Libretti, A. (1989) 'The inhibitory effect of aspirin on fibrinolysis is reversed by iloprost, a prostacyclin-analogue', Thromb. Haemostasis 61, 286-288.

4. Braun, M. and Schrör, K. (1990) 'Bay U 3405 inhibits cerebral vasospasm induced by authentic thromboxane A_2', Stroke 21 (Suppl IV), 152-154.

5. Brewster, A. G., Braun, G. R., Jessup, R., Smithers, M. N. J., and Stocker, A. (1990) '1,3-dioxane derivatives possessing potent thromboxane A_2 receptor antagonism and thromboxane A_2 synthase inhibition', Proc. 7th Intern. Conf. Prostagl., p.178

6. Brezinski, M. E., Yanagisawa, A., Darius, H., and Lefer, A. M. (1985) 'Anti-ischemic actions of a new thromboxane receptor antagonist during acute myocardial ischemia in cats', Am. Heart. J. 110, 1161-1167.

7. Bush, L. R. and Smith III, E. F. (1987) 'Comparative and combined effects of U-63557A, a TxA_2 synthetase inhibitor, and BM 13.177, a TxA_2 receptor antagonist, on cyclic flow reductions in stenosed canine coronary arteries', Fed. Proc. 46, 1316.

8. Busse, R., Lückhoff, A., and Bassenge, E. (1987) 'Endothelium-derived relaxant factor inhibits platelet activation', Naunyn-Schmiedeberg's Arch. Pharmacol. 336, 566-571.

9. Carmo, L. G., Hatmi, M., Rotilio, D., and Vargaftig, B. B. (1985) 'Platelet desensitization induced by arachidonic acid is not due to cyclooxygenase inactivation and involves the endoperoxide receptor', Br. J. Pharmacol. 85, 849-859.

10. Craven, L. L. (1950) 'Acetylsalicylic acid, possible prevention of coronary thrombosis', Ann. West Med. Surg. 4, 95-99.

11. De Clerck, F., Beetens, J., de Chaffoy de Courcelles, D., Freyne, E., and Janssen, P. A. J. (1989) 'R 68070: Thromboxane A_2 synthetase inhibition and thromboxane A_2/prostaglandin endoperoxide receptor blockade combined in one molecule - I. Biochemical profile in vitro', Thrombosis Haemostasis 61, 35-42.

12. Defreyn, G., Deckmyn, H. and Vermylen, J. (1982) 'A thromboxane synthetase inhibitor reorients endoperoxide metabolism in whole blood towards prostacyclin and prostaglandin E_2', Thromb. Res. 26, 389-400.

13. DeWitt, D. L., Day, J. S., Sonnenburg, W. K., and Smith, W. L. (1983) 'Concentrations of prostaglandin endoperoxide synthase and prostaglandin I_2 synthase in the endothelium and smooth muscle of bovine aorta', J. Clin. Invest. 72, 1882-1888.

14. DeWitt, D. L., El-Harith, E. A., Kraemer, S. A., Andrews, M. J., Yao, E. F., Armstrong, R. L., and Smith, W. L. (1990) 'The aspirin- and heme-binding sites of bovine and murine prostaglandin endoperoxide synthases', J. Biol. Chem. 265, 5192-5198.

15. Dorn II, G. W. (1990) 'Cyclic oxidation-reduction reactions regulate thromboxane A_2/prostaglandin H_2 receptor number and affinity in human platelet membranes', J. Biol. Chem. 265, 4240-4246.

16. Dorn II, G. W. and de Jesus, A. (1991) 'Human platelet aggregation and shape change are coupled to separate thromboxane A_2-prostaglandin H_2 receptors', Am. J. Physiol. 260, H327-H334.

17. Dorn II, G. W., Liel, N., Trask, J. L., Mais, D. E., Assey, M. E., and Halushka, P. V. (1990) 'Increased platelet thromboxane

A_2/prostaglandin H_2 receptors in patients with acute myocardial infarction', Circulation 81, 212-218.

18. Ellis, E. F., Oelz, O., Roberts II, L. J., Payne, N. A., Sweetman, B. J., Nies A. S., and Oates, J. A. (1976) 'Coronary arterial smooth muscle contraction by a substance released from platelets: Evidence that it is thromboxane A_2', Science 193, 1135-1137.

19. Elwood, P. C., Renaud, S., Sharp, D. S., Beswick, A. D., O'Brien, J. R., and Yarnell, J. W. G. (1991) 'Ischemic heart disease and platelet aggregation', Circulation 83, 38-44.

20. Fiedler, V. B., Perzborn, E., Seuter, F., Rosentreter, U., and Böshagen, H. (1989) 'Reduction of in vivo coronary artery thrombosis by the novel thromboxane antagonist (3R)-3-(-4-fluorophenylsulfonamido)-1,2,3,4-tetrahydro-9-carbazole-propanoic acid', ArzneimittelForsch. 39, 1527-1530.

21. Fischer, S., Struppler, M., Böhlig, B., Bernutz, Ch., Wober, W., and Weber, P. C. (1983) 'The influence of selective thromboxane synthetase inhibition with a novel imidazole derivative, UK-38,485, on prostanoid formation in man', Circulation 68, 821-826.

22. FitzGerald, D. J., Catella, F., Roy, L., and FitzGerald, G. A. (1988) 'Marked platelet activation in vivo after intravenous streptokinase in patients with acute myocardial infarction', Circulation 77, 142-150.

23. FitzGerald, D. J., Fragetta, J., and FitzGerald, G. A. (1988) 'Prostaglandin endoperoxides modulate the response to thromboxane synthase inhibition during coronary thrombosis', J. Clin. Invest. 82, 1708-1713.

24. FitzGerald, D. J., Roy, L., and FitzGerald, G. A. (1985) 'Enhanced prostacyclin and thromboxane A_2 synthesis in vivo in ischemic heart disease: noninvasive evidence of sporadic platelet activation in unstable angina', Circulation 72 (Suppl 3), III-113.

25. FitzGerald, G. A., Fisher, D. M., Doran, J., and Oates, J. A. (1985) 'Pharmacological modulation of arachidonic acid metabolism in platelet-vascular interactions', in J. A. Oates, J. Hawiger and R. Ross (eds.), Interactions of the platelets with the vessel wall, Am. Physiol. Soc., Bethesda, pp. 103-110.

26. FitzGerald, G. A., Smith, B., Pedersen, A. K., and Brash, A. R. (1984) 'Prostacyclin biosynthesis is increased in patients with severe atherosclerosis and platelet activation', New Engl. J. Med. 310, 1065-1068.

27. FitzGerald, G. A., Oates, J. A., Hawiger, J. A., Maas, R. L., Roberts II, L. J., Lawson, J. A., and Brash, A. R. (1983) 'Endogenous biosynthesis of prostacyclin and thromboxane and platelet function during chronic administration of aspirin in man', J. Clin. Invest. 71, 676-688.

28. Folts, J. D., Crowell, E. D., and Rowe, G. G. (1976) 'Platelet aggregation in partially obstructed vessels and its elimination with aspirin', Circulation 54, 365-370.

29. Friedrich, T., Lichey, J., Nigam, S., Priesnitz, M., and Wegscheider, K. (1985) 'Follow-up of prostaglandin plasma levels after acute myocardial infarction', Am. Heart J. 109, 218-222.

30. Frishman, W. H., Christodoulou, J., Weksler, B. B., Smithen, C., Killip, T., and Scheidt, S. (1976) 'Aspirin therapy in angina pectoris: effects on platelet aggregation, exercise tolerance, and echocardiographic manifestations of ischemia', Am. Heart J. 92, 3-10.

31. Fukumori, T., Tani, E., Maeda, Y., and Sukenaga, A. (1984) 'Effect of selective inhibitor of thromboxane A_2 synthetase on experimental cerebral vasospasm', Stroke 15, 306-311.

32. Fuster, V., Cohen, M., and Halperin, J. (1989) 'Aspirin in the prevention of coronary disease', New Engl. J. Med. 321, 183-185.

33. Fuster, V., Stein, B., Halperin, J. L., and Chesebro, J. H. (1990) 'Antithrombotic therapy in cardiac disease: An approach based on pathogenesis and risk stratification', Am. J. Cardiol. 65, 38C-44C.

34. Giessen van der, W. J., Zijlstra, F. J., Berk, L., and Verdouw, P. D. (1988) 'The effect of the thromboxane receptor antagonist BM 13.177 on experimentally induced coronary thrombosis in the pig', Eur. J. Pharmacol. 147, 241-248.

35. Gresele, P., Blockmans, D., Deckmyn, H., and Vermylen, J. (1988) 'Adenylate cyclase activation determines the effect of thromboxane synthase inhibitors on platelet aggregation in vitro. Comparison of platelets from responders and nonresponders', J. Pharmacol. Exp. Ther. 246, 301-307.

36. Gresele, P., Deckmyn, H., Nenci, G.G., and Vermylen, J. (1991) 'Thromboxane synthase inhibitors, thromboxane receptor antagonists and dual blockers in thrombotic disorders', TiPS 12, 158-163.

37. Halushka, P. V., Mais, S. E., and Saussy Jr., D. L. (1987) 'Platelet and vascular smooth muscle thrombaxane A_2/prostaglandin H_2 receptors', Fed. Proc. 46, 149-153.

38. Hass, W. K., Easton, J. D., Adams Jr., H. P., Pryse-Phillips, W., Molony, B. A., Anderson, S., and Kamm, B. (1989) 'A randomized trial comparing ticlopidine hydrochloride with aspirin for the prevention of stroke in high-risk patients', New Engl. J. Med. 321, 501-507.

39. Hawiger, J. (1989) 'Methods in Enzymology. Platelets: Receptors, Adhesion, Secretion' Part A, Vol 169, Academic Press, San Diego.

40. Heavey, D. J., Barrow, S. E., Hickling, N. E., and Ritter, J. M. (1985) 'Aspirin causes short-lived inhibition of bradykinin-stimulated prostacyclin production in man', Nature 318, 186-188.

41. Henriksson, P., Wennmalm, A., Edhag, O., Vesterqvist, O., and Green, K. (1986) 'In vivo production of prostacyclin and thromboxane in patients with acute myocardial infarction', Br. Heart J. 55, 543-548.

42. Hohlfeld, Th., Strobach, H., and Schrör, K. (1991) 'Stimulation of prostacyclin synthesis by defibrotide: improved contractile recovery from myocardial stunning', J. Cardiovasc. Pharmacol. 17, 108-115.

43. Holzgrefe, H. H., Buchanan, L. V., and Bunting, S. (1987) 'In vivo characterization of synthetic thromboxane A_2 in canine myocardium', Circ. Res. 60, 290-296.

44. Houston, D. S., Sheperd, J. T., and Vanhoutte, P. M. (1986) 'Aggregating human platelets cause direct contraction and endothelium-dependent relaxation of isolated coronary arteries. Role of serotonin, thromboxane A_2 and adenine nucleotides', J. Clin. Invest. 78, 539-544.

45. Husted, S. E., Kraemmer-Nielsen, H., Krusell, L. R., and Faergeman, O. (1989) 'Acetylsalicylic acid 100 mg and 1000 mg daily in acute myocardial infarction suspects: a placebo-controlled trial', J. Int. Med. 226, 303-310.

46. Hutton, I., Tweddel, A. C., Rankin, A. C., Walker, I. D., and Davidson, J. F. (1983) 'Effects of dazoxiben on transcardiac thromboxane levels and haemodynamics in coronary heart disease', Br. J. Clin. Pharmacol. 15, 79S-82S.

47. Ito, T., Ogawa, K., Watanabe, J., Chen, L. S., Shikano, M., Shibata, T., Ito, Y., Miyazaki, Y., and Satake, T. (1984) 'Selective thromboxane inhibitor and ischemic heart disease', Biomed. Biochim. Acta 43, S125-S132.

48. Jaschonek, K., Karsch, K. R., Weisenberger, H., Tidow, S., Faul, C., and Renn, W. (1986) 'Platelet prostacyclin binding in coronary artery disease', J. Am. Coll. Cardiol. 8, 259-266.

49. Kahn, N. N., Mueller, H. S., and Sinha, A. K. (1990) 'Impaired prostaglandin E_1/I_2 receptor activity of human blood platelets in acute ischemic heart disease', Circ. Res. 66, 932-940.

50. Kaley, G., Messina, E. J., Hintze, T. H., Roberts, A. M., Martin, E. G., and Slomiany, B. L. (1977) 'Effects of the metabolites of arachidonic acid on coronary blood flow', Prostaglandins 13, 1011.

51. Knapp, H. R., Healy, C., Lawson, J., and FitzGerald, G. A. (1988) 'Effects of low-dose aspirin on endogenous eicosanoid formation in normal and atherosclerotic men', Thromb. Res. 50, 377-386.

52. Lane, I. F., Lumley, P., Michael, M. F., Peters, A. M., and McCollum, C. N. (1990) 'A specific thromboxane receptor blocking drug, AH 23848, reduces platelet deposition on vascular grafts in man', Thromb. Haemost. 64, 369-373.

53. Lanza, F., Berettz, A., Stierle, A., Hanau, D., Kubina, M., and Cazenave, J.-P. (1988) 'Epinephrine potentiates human platelet activation but is not an aggregating agent' Am. J. Physiol. 255, H1276-H1288.

54. Lee, T. K., Chen, Y. C., Lien, I. N., Liu, M. C., and Huang, Z. S. (1988) 'Inhibitory effect of acetylsalicylic acid on platelet function in patients with completed stroke or reversible ischemic neurologic deficit', Stroke 19, 566-570.

55. Löbel, P. and Schrör, K. (1985) 'Selective stimulation of coronary vascular PGI_2 but not of platelet thromboxane formation by defibrotide in the platelet perfused heart', Naunyn-Schmiedeberg's Arch. Pharmacol. 331, 125-130.

56. Lorenz, R. L., Boehlig, B., Uedelhoven, W. M., and Weber, P. C. (1989) 'Superior antiplatelet action of alternate day pulsed dosing versus split dose administration of aspirin', Am. J. Cardiol. 64, 1185-1188.

57. Manson, J. E., Grobbee, D. E., Stampfer, M. J., Taylor, J. O., Goldhaber, S. Z., Gaziano, J. M., Ridker, P. M., Buring, J. E., and Hennekens, C. H. (1990) 'Aspirin in the primary prevention of angina pectoris in a randomized trial of United States physicians', Am. J. Med. 89, 772-776.

58. Marcus, A. J., Weksler, B. B., Jaffe, E. A., and Broekman, M. J. (1980) 'Synthesis of prostacyclin from platelet-derived

endoperoxides by cultured human endothelial cells', J. Clin. Invest. 66, 979-986.

59. Mayeux, P. R., Morton, H. E., Gillard, J., Lord, A., Morinelli, T. A., Boehm, A., Mais, D. E., and Halushka, P. V. (1988) 'The affinities of prostaglandins H_2 and thromboxane A_2 for their receptors are similar in washed human platelets', Biochem. Biophys. Res. Comm. 157, 733-739.

60. Mehta, J. L. and Nichols, W. W. (1990) 'The potential role of thromboxane inhibitors in preventing myocardial ischaemic injury', Drugs 40, 657-665.

61. Moncada, S., Palmer, R. M. J., and Higgs, E. A. (1987) 'Prostacyclin and endothelium-derived relaxing factor: biological interactions and significance', in M. Verstraete, J. Vermylen, H. R. Lijnen, and J. Arnout (eds.), Thrombosis and Hemostasis, Leuven University Press, pp. 597-618.

62. Mueller, H. S., Rao, P. S., Greenberg, M. A., Buttrick, P. M., Sussman I. I., Levite, H. A., Grose, R. M., Perez-Davila, V., Strain, J. E., and Spaet, T. H. (1985) 'Systemic and transcardiac platelet activity in acute myocardial infarction in man: resistance to prostacyclin', Circulation 72, 1336-1345.

63. Mullane, K. M. and Fornabaio, D. (1988) 'Thromboxane synthetase inhibitors reduce infarct size by a platelet-dependent, aspirin sensitive pathway', Circ. Res. 62, 668-678.

64. Murray, R., Shipp, E., and FitzGerald, G. A. (1990) 'Prostaglandin endoperoxide thromboxane A_2 receptor desensitization - Cross talk with adenylate cyclase in human platelets', J. Biol. Chem. 265, 21670-21675.

65. Nicolaou, K. C., Magolda, R. L., Smith, J. B., Aharony, D., Smith, E. F., and Lefer, A. M. (1979) 'Synthesis and biological properties of pinane-thromboxane A_2, a selective inhibitor of coronary artery constriction, platelet aggregation and thromboxane formation', Proc. Natl. Acad. Sci. 76, 2566-2570.

66. Nowak, J. and FitzGerald, G. A. (1989) 'Redirection of prostaglandin endoperoxide metabolism at the platelet-vascular interface in man', J. Clin. Invest. 3, 380-385.

67. O'Brien, J. R. (1969) 'Effects of salicylates on human platelets', Lancet I, 779-783.

68. Patrono, C. (1989) 'Aspirin and human platelets: from clinical trials to acetylation of cyclooxygenase and back', TiPS 10, 453-458.

69. Patscheke, H. (1985) 'Thromboxane synthase inhibition potentiates washed platelet activation by endogenous and exogenous arachidonic acid', Biochem. Pharmacol. 34, 1151-1156.

70. Patscheke, H., Staiger, C., Neugebauer, G., Kaufmann, B., Strein, K., Endele, R., and Stegmeier, K. (1986) 'The pharmacokinetic and pharmacodynamic profiles of the thromboxane A_2-receptor blocker BM 13.177', Clin. Pharmacol. Ther. 39, 145-150.

71. Patscheke, H. (1990) 'Thromboxane A_2/Prostaglandin H_2 receptor antagonists. A new therapeutic principle', Stroke (Suppl IV), 139-142.

72. Perzborn, E., Fiedler, V. B., Seuter, F., Stasch, J. P., Weber, H., Sander, E., Böshagen, H., and Rosentreter, U. (1990) 'Characterization of Bay U 3405, a novel thromboxane A_2/endoperoxide receptor antagonist', Stroke 21 (Suppl IV), 143-151.

73. Reilly, I. A. and FitzGerald, G. A. (1987) 'Inhibition of thromboxane formation in vivo and ex vivo: implications for therapy with platelet inhibitory drugs', Blood 69, 180-186.

74. Riess, H., Höfling, B., v. Arnim, T., and Hiller, E. (1986) 'Thromboxane receptor blockade versus cyclooxigenase inhibition: antiplatelet effects in patients', Thromb. Res. 42, 235-245.

75. RISC-Group (1990) 'Risk of myocardial infarction and death during treatment with low-dose aspirin and intravenous heparin in man with unstable coronary artery disease', Lancet 336: 827-830.

76. Ritter, J. M., Doktor, H. S., Benjamin, N., Barrow, S. E., and Stewart-Long, P. (1990) 'On the mechanism of the prolonged action in man of GR 32191, a thromboxane receptor antagonist', Adv. Prostaglandin Thromboxane Leukotriene Res. 21, 351-354.

77. Schrör, K., Ackermann, G., Hohlfeld, Th., Löbel, P., Ney, P., Schröder, H., and Strobach, H. (1989) 'Endothelial protection by defibrotide - a new strategy for treatment of myocardial infarction?', Z. Kardiol. 6, 35-41.

78. Schrör, K. and Braun, M. (1990) 'Platelets as a source of vasoactive mediators', Stroke 21 (Suppl IV), 32-35.

79. Schrör, K., Köhler, P., Müller, M., Peskar, B. A., and Rösen, P. (1981) 'Prostacyclin-thromboxane interactions in the platelet-perfused in vitro heart', Am. J. Physiol. 241, H18-H25.

80. Schrör, K. (1990) 'Platelet reactivity and arachidonic acid metabolism in type II hyperlipoproteinaemia and its modification by cholesterol-lowering agents, Eicosanoids 3, 67-73.

81. Schrör, K., Smith III, E. F., Bickerton, M., Smith, J. B., Nicolaou, K. C., Magolda, R., and Lefer, A. M. (1980) 'Preservation of the ischemic myocardium by pinane thromboxane A_2', Am. J. Physiol. 238, H87-H92.

82. Schrör, K. (1990) 'Thromboxane A_2 and platelets as mediators of coronary arterial vasoconstriction in myocardial ischaemia', Eur. Heart J. 11 (Suppl B), 27-34.

83. Schumacher, W. A., Heran, C. L., Goldenberg, H. J., Harris, D. N., and Ogletree, M. L. (1989) 'Magnitude of thromboxane receptor antagonism necessary for antithrombotic activity in monkeys', Am. J. Physiol. 256, H726-H734.

84. Shikano, M., Ito, T., Ogawa, K., and Satake, T. (1987) 'Effects of a selective thromboxane synthetase inhibitor (OKY-046) in patients with coronary artery disease during exercise', Jap. Heart J. 28, 663-674.

85. Sills, T. and Heptinstall, S. (1986) 'Effects of a thromboxane synthetase inhibitor and a cAMP phosphodiesterase inhibitor, singly and in combination, on platelet behaviour', Thromb. Haemostasis 55, 305-308.

86. Smith III, E. F., Griswold, D. E., Egan, J. W., Hillegass, L. M., and DiMartino, M. J. (1989) 'Reduction of myocardial damage and polymorphonuclear leukocyte accumulation following coronary artery occlusion and reperfusion by the thromboxane receptor antagonist BM 13.505', J. Cardiovasc. Pharmacol. 13, 715-722.

87. Smith, J. B. and Willis, A. L. (1971) 'Aspirin selectively inhibits prostaglandin production in human platelets', Nature New Biol. 231, 235-237.

88. Sobel, M., Salzman, E. W., Davies, G. C., Handin, R. I., Sweeney, J., Ploetz, J., and Kurland, G. (1981) 'Circulating platelet products in unstable angina pectoris', Circulation 63, 300-306.

89. Steering Committee of the physician's health study research group (1989) 'Final report on the aspirin component of the ongoing physician's health study', New Engl. J. Med. 321, 129-135.

90. Stein, B., Fuster, V., Israel, D. H., Cohen, M., Badimon, L., Badimon, J.J., and Chesebro, J. H. (1989) 'Platelet inhibitor agents in cardiovascular disease: an update', J. Am. Coll. Cardiol. 14, 813-836.

91. Svensson, J. and Hamberg, M. (1976) 'Thromboxane A_2 and prostaglandin H_2: potent stimulators of the swine coronary artery', Prostaglandins 12, 943-950.

92. Takahara, K., Murray, R., FitzGerald, G. A., and FitzGerald, D. J. (1990) 'The response to thromboxane A_2 analogues in human platelets. Discrimination of two binding sites linked to distinct effector systems', J. Biol. Chem. 265, 6836-6844.

93. Thaulow, E., Dale, J., and Myhre, E. (1984) 'Effects of selective thromboxane sythetase inhibitor, dazoxiben and of acetyl salicylic acid on myocardial ischemia in patients with coronary artery disease', Am. J. Cardiol. 53, 1255.

94. Thiemermann, C., Ney, P., and Schrör, K. (1988) 'The thromboxane receptor antagonist, daltroban, protects the myocardium from ischaemic injury resulting in suppression of leukocytosis', Eur. J. Pharmacol. 155, 57-67.

95. Tremoli, E., Maderna, P., Colli, S., Morazzoni, G., Sirtori, M., and Sirtori, C. R. (1984) 'Increased platelet sensitivity and thromboxane B_2 formation in type II hyperlipoproteinaemic patients', Eur. J. Clin. Invest. 14, 329-333.

96. Tyler, H. M., Saxton, C. A. P. D., Parry, M. J. (1981) 'Administration to man of UK-37,248-01, a selective inhibitor of thromboxane synthetase', Lancet 1, 629-632.

97. UK-TIA Study Group (1988) 'United kingdom transient ischaemic attack trial: interim results', Br. Med. J. [Clin. Res.] 296, 316-320.

98. Verheggen, R. and Schrör, K. (1986) 'The modification of platelet-induced vasoconstriction by a thromboxane receptor antagonist', J. Cardiovasc. Pharmacol. 8, 483-490.

99. Verheugt, F. W. A., van der Laarse, A., Funke-Küpper, A. J., Sterkman, L. G. W., Galema, T. W., and Roos, J. P. (1990) 'Effects of early intervention with low-dose aspirin (100 mg) on infarct size, reinfarction and mortality in anterior wall acute myocardial infarction', Am. J. Cardiol. 66, 267-270.

100. Yang, Z., Stulz, P., v. Segesser, L., Bauer, E., Turina, M., and Lüscher, T. F. (1991) 'Different interactions of platelets with arterial and venous coronary bypass vessels', Lancet 337, 938-943.

ANTITHROMBOTICS AND THE LIPOXYGENASE PATHWAY

M.R. Buchanan and S.J. Brister

ABSTRACT

The current strategy used to achieve an antithrombotic effect in the prevention and treatment of vascular disease or following vascular injury, is based upon the concept that platelet activation and coagulation are the principle factors responsible for thrombogenesis. There has been a major focus on understanding platelet pathophysiology the activation of the coagulation cascade, and identifying those "antiplatelet" and "anticoagulant" agents which most effectively alter these processes. While it is clear that many of these agents provide some clinical benefit, it is also clear that they are not optimal and are associated with many untoward side-effects. Since the injured vessel wall acts as a potent stimulus for platelet activation and coagulation, it is suggested that an alternative strategy to achieve an antithrombotic effect is, to alter the thrombogenic properties of the vessel wall, thereby ameliorating the response to the stimulus by platelets and/or procoagulants. In this chapter, we will discuss this latter approach,. paying particular attention to the relative benefits and/or shortcomings of modulating the lipoxygenase pathway in platelets and the vessel wall.

1. INTRODUCTION

The rationale for using "antiplatelet" drugs as a strategy to prevent or to ameliorate a thrombotic event, is based upon the concept that activated platelets secrete constituents which facilitate thrombogenesis. Under homeostatic conditions, platelets circulate as discoid-shaped, inert cell bodies which do not interact either with other circulating blood cells or with the vascular endothelium (1,2). However, when blood vessel walls are injured, their luminal surface properties are altered, such as in response to injury, inflammation or the release of procoagulants and cytokines generated elsewhere. Platelets become activated and adhere to the damaged vascular endothelium or exposed basement membrane underlying the endothelium, and secrete a number of other procoagulants, proaggregatory agents and

A. G. Herman (ed.), Antithrombotics, 159–179.
© 1991 *Kluwer Academic Publishers. Printed in the Netherlands.*

mitogenic factors which are normally stored in their intercellular granules (3-6). These factors, in turn, facilitate haemostasis and vessel wall repair. Unfortunately, if these platelet-associated responses are not regulated, further vessel wall damage and thrombus formation occur. The degree of platelet activation and subsequent adhesion to the injured vessel wall surface is, in part, influenced by the extent and depth of the vessel wall injury (7-9); the greater the thrombogenic response, the greater the platelet activation, coagulation and subsequent vessel wall occlusion.

2. PROTHROMBOTIC BEHAVIOUR OF PLATELETS

Platelets secrete a number of clotting factors which facilitate thrombin generation (10-13). Platelets provide a site on their activated membranes for activation of factor X, and the assembly of the prothrombinase complex, which, in turn, enhance coagulation (14-16). It is not surprising therefore, that the use of anticoagulants such as heparin or coumadin which may down-regulate or counter-balance the procoagulant effects mediated by the activated blood cells, are included in the strategy to prevent thrombus formation.

Other agents released from activated platelets include adenosine diphosphate (ADP), and thromboxane A_2 (TxA_2), the prostanoid generated from arachidonic acid by the cyclooxygenase pathway (4,5). These facilitate the recruitment of more platelets into the thrombotic process. ADP is released from the platelet dense granule in response to a variety of stimuli (4). Once released, ADP binds to a specific platelet receptor site, causing secondary and irreversible platelet aggregation. TxA_2 also induces platelet aggregation (5). Free arachidonic acid liberated from the membrane phospholipids following stimulation, is oxidized into unstable endoperoxides, PGG_2 and PGH_2 by a reaction that utilizes molecular oxygen and that is catalysed by the enzyme, cyclooxygenase (5). In the platelet, these unstable endoperoxides are rapidly converted predominantly into TxA_2, which in turn, promotes platelet aggregation and acts synergistically with ADP and other stimuli (eg: thrombin and collagen), to augment further the platelet release reaction (4). In addition, the unstable endoperoxides (PGG_2 and PGH_2) have also been shown to induce platelet aggregation (17).

Finally, platelets release two constituents which influence smooth muscle cell proliferation, platelet factor (PF4) and platelet-derived growth factor (PDGF). PF4 neutralizes heparin (3) thereby preventing the antiproliferation effect of heparin (18). PDGF facilitates smooth muscle cell proliferation (6). The combined effects of PF4 and PDGF are likely to enhance thrombogenesis by facilitating hyperplasia and subsequent vessel wall narrowing.

3. ANTITHROMBOTIC STRATEGY

Consequently, the concept that utilization of agents which antagonize or inhibit the production of these metabolites or compete with their receptors, has evolved as a reasonable strategy to prevent and treat thrombosis. For example, aspirin and sulphinpyrazone have been shown to inhibit cyclooxygenase (19,20), thereby preventing the metabolism of arachidonic acid into TxA_2. As a consequence, platelet aggregation in response to some thrombogenic stimuli, is impaired. Alternatively, a variety of TxA_2 competitors or TxA_2 receptor inhibitors are also thought to be useful (21). Finally, agents such as persantine (dipyridamole) have been used to render platelets hyporesponsive. The underlying mechanism of the persantine effect is not clear, but has been attributed to effects on the platelet metabolic pool, adenosine metabolism and PGI_2 synthesis (22-24). However, when used clinically, these agents have not been as promising as initially anticipated. For example, all of the drugs have had a modest, albeit significant, beneficial effect (25-29). The Anturan Reinfarction trial (27) and the randomized control trials using aspirin (acetylsalicylic acid) to prevent mortality due to stroke or secondary myocardial infarction, all show an improved benefit with therapy (25,28,29). However, many patients receiving treatment still suffered a recurrent myocardial infarction. Is it possible that the drug treatment itself actually facilitated thrombosis in some of those patients who suffered a recurrent myocardial infarction? This possibility has not been considered previously nor has it been excluded. Evidence to support this possibility is discussed later as an unwanted side-effect in addition to the well-known bleeding side-effect associated with many "antiplatelet" agents.

In summary, there are a number of constituents released from platelets which contribute to further platelet aggregation, the activation of the coagulation system and promote vessel wall hyperplasia, such as those illustrated in Figure 1. This has lead to the adoption of a strategy which utilizes agents which can effectively block the synthesis and/or secretion of these constituents in the platelet, and hence reduce the thrombotic response.

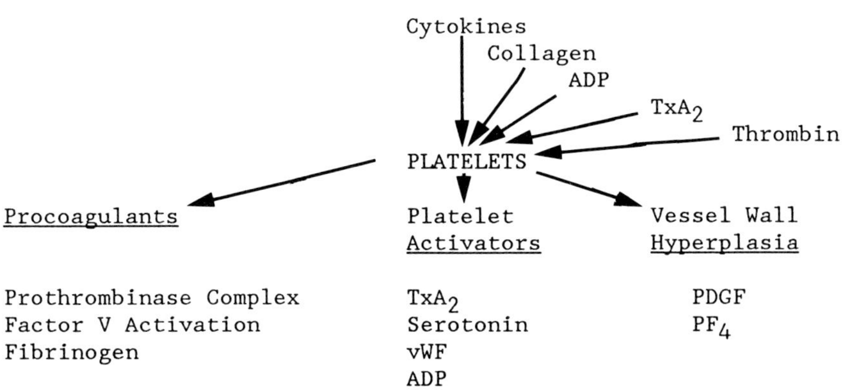

Figure 1. Constituents secreted by or expressed on activated platelets which facilitate thrombogenesis.

4. LIMITATIONS OF ANTIPLATELET THERAPY

There are, however, a number of aspects to this approach which may merit further consideration when using a strategy which employs "antiplatelet drugs" to achieve an antithrombotic effect. The first is well-documented and obvious to most; namely, that inhibition of platelet function by any "antiplatelet" agent, which does not destroy the platelets, necessitating their removal from the circulation, renders the platelets haemostatically defective, thereby contributing to a prolonged cutaneous bleeding time. What is not so obvious, but what may be fundamental to our rationale of using "antiplatelet" drugs is, that the haemostatic defect of platelets can be overcome, simply by increasing the stimulus for platelet activation. This is illustrated in Figure 2, using platelets obtained from rabbits treated with 0, 3 or 100 mg/kg of aspirin 2 hours beforehand. First, platelet aggregation is increased in a concentration-dependent manner when increasing amounts of thrombin are added to platelets harvested from untreated (0 mg/kg) rabbits (Figure 2A-2C). When the platelets are obtained from rabbits which had received 3 mg/kg of aspirin 2 hours beforehand, platelet aggregation induced by the lowest concentrations of thrombin (0.013 U) is inhibited by ≈ 50%. When the platelets are obtained from rabbits receiving the higher dose aspirin, (100 mg/kg), platelet aggregation is abolished (Figure 2A). However, simply by increasing the thrombin concentration, the inhibitory effects of both aspirin doses seen in Figure 2A, are overcome (see Figure 2B and C).

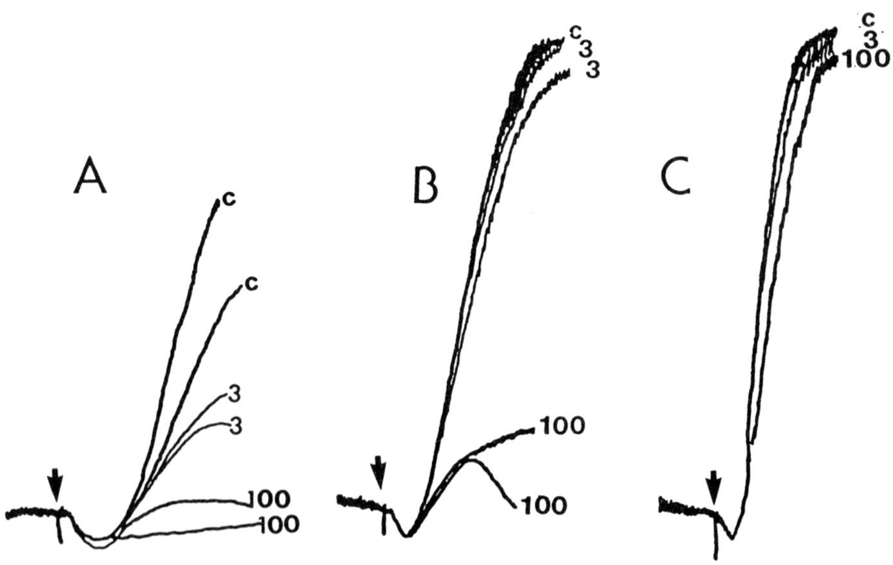

Figure 2. Thrombin-induced aggregation of platelets obtained from rabbits receiving 0 (Control, C), 3 or 100 mg/kg aspirin 2 hr beforehand. A,B and C = 0.013, 0.025 and 0.05 U/ml thrombin, resp.

These results may be interpreted to indicate that the inhibitory effect of "antiplatelet" agents in vivo may be easily overcome, simply by increasing the extent of platelet activation, i.e. dependent upon the strength of the stimulus, despite any apparent impression that platelet function has been abolished, as assessed either in vitro or ex vivo. If this is truly the case, it is very likely that "antiplatelet" drugs will be relatively weak in preventing thrombogenesis in patients with severe vascular disease or vessel wall injury, such as is the case, in fact, with peripheral vascular disease.

The second aspect of "antithrombotic" therapy which has received little attention, concerns the role of the lipoxygenase pathway in platelet function and the potential prothrombotic effects of "antiplatelet drugs" on this pathway. When platelets are stimulated and arachidonic acid is liberated from the phospholipid stores, the arachidonic acid is metabolized not only by cyclooxygenase into TxA_2, but also by lipoxygenase into the monohydroxide fatty acid, 12-hydroxyeicosatetraenoic acid (12-HETE) (Figure 3). The amounts of 12-HETE produced are at least 10-fold greater than the amounts of TxA_2 produced by the platelets (31-32). It should also be noted that in the presence of albumin, platelet arachidonic acid metabolism is redirected from cyclooxygenase towards lipoxygenase. Consequently, 12-HETE synthesis is increased even further (32). Little attention has been given to the importance of this metabolite when developing "antiplatelet" drugs for antithrombotic therapy. This is surprising, particularly since 12-HETE is produced in far greater amounts than TxA_2. The possible roles that platelet 12-HETE play in platelet function and thrombogenesis are discussed below.

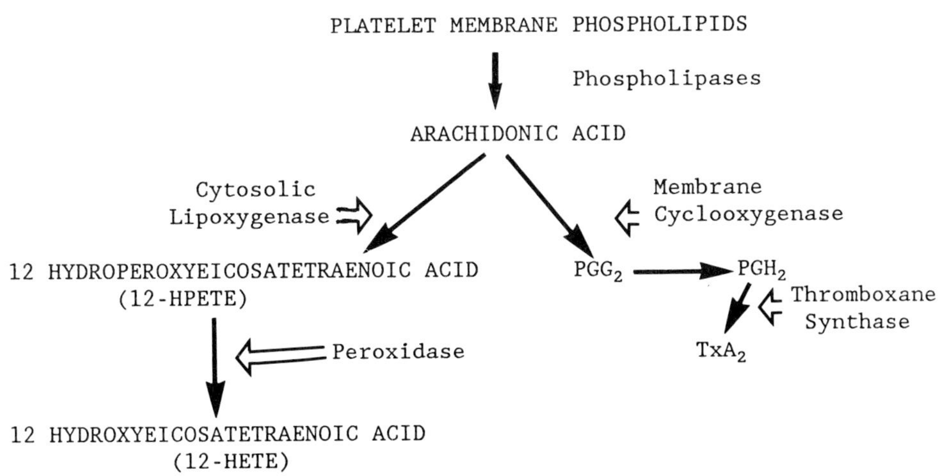

Figure 3. Metabolism of arachidonic acid by cyclo- and lipoxygenase.

A number of in vitro studies suggest that 12-HETE and/or its precursor, 12-HPETE facilitate or are necessary for platelet function (31, 33-36). Platelets obtained from patients with myeloproliferative disease, have a lipoxygenase deficiency; the greater the deficiency, the greater the tendency for bleeding, i.e. the less the ability of the platelets to synthesize 12-HETE, the less haemostatically effective the platelets (34,37). Morita (35) found that the precursor of 12-HETE, 12-HPETE, increases arachidonic acid-induced platelet aggregation. He suggested that 12-HETE alters platelet membrane permeability, thereby making more arachidonic acid available for metabolism. In the presence of albumin, this would appear to take place mainly via the lipoxygenase pathway (32). Early studies by us and others suggest that irreversible platelet aggregation is dependant in part, upon the generation of 12-HETE (31,38). Furthermore, we demonstrated that by selectively inhibiting the 12-lipoxygenase pathway in platelets, platelet adhesion is also impaired, independent of any effect on platelet aggregation (31,38). More importantly, inhibition of 12-HETE synthesis and subsequent platelet adhesion are associated with increased TxA_2 synthesis and increased collagen-induced platelet aggregation. In contrast, when platelets are treated with low dose aspirin and are unable to aggregate to the collagen stimulus, they had an **increased ability** to adhere to a collagen-coated surface (31). This ability is associated with enhanced 12-HETE synthesis. These latter results suggest that low dose aspirin can enhance thrombogenesis in some settings, which, in fact, has been confirmed experimentally. We found that the low dose aspirin which enhances platelet adhesivity in vitro, also increases thrombus formation in vivo (39). It is also interesting to note that platelet 12-HETE has been shown to stimulate procoagulant tissue factor activity in monocytes (40).

Thus, a number of clinical and experimental studies in vitro, ex vivo and in vivo provide evidence that 12-HETE facilitates platelet adhesion, independent of aggregation. If these observations are relevant to man, they suggest that agents which block platelet aggregation per se may increase the capacity of the platelets to adhere, for example, to an injured vessel wall. Thus, while aspirin may be an effective antithrombotic agent in some patients suffering transient ischemic attacks by preventing "platelet aggregation" (25,28,29), the possibility remains that low dose aspirin may facilitate a thrombogenic event eg. myocardial infarction, in other patients receiving the same treatment. This possibility cannot be excluded without first demonstrating that platelet adhesion and 12-HETE synthesis are not increased in these patients.

5. ANTITHROMBOTICS DERIVED FROM THE VESSEL WALL

The rationale for developing drugs to inhibit the interaction of platelets (as well as other blood cells) with the vessel wall, neglects to take into consideration using agents that would alter the thrombogenic properties of the vessel wall. Since the development of endothelial cell culture systems, a wealth of information has been generated concerning the antithrombotic properties of the vascular endothelium under both homeostatic and pathologic conditions. From this perspective, we have focussed our attention on the role of fatty acid metabolites generated from the endothelium under basal and stimulated conditions, and how these metabolites influence platelet/vessel wall interactions. As a consequence of these studies, a possible new strategy of achieving an antithrombotic effect emerges, namely, the strategy of manipulating vessel wall thrombogenecity and reducing the strength of the stimulus initiating thrombogenesis. It is from this perspective that we will focus the rest of this chapter.

While it is clear that the damaged vessel is highly thrombogenic (7,9,41,42), it is equally clear that constituents synthesized and/or secreted by the stimulated endothelium of the vasculature, regulate thrombus formation, growth and its dissolution. Thus, endothelial cells metabolize arachidonic acid into the prostanoid, PGI_2 which in turn, acts synergistically with endothelial cell-derived relaxant factor (EDRF) and endothelin to down-regulate platelet responses (43-45). Endothelial cells synthesize and secrete tissue plasminogen activator (tPA) and its inhibitor (PAI) which regulate thrombolysis (46,47). Our understanding of the potent antithrombotic effects of many of these endothelial cell-derived constituents such as tPA and PGI_2 have expanded our strategy of utilizing these constituents to block or impair platelet activation and/or coagulation during or following thrombosis. Lysis of a coronary thrombus following myocardial infarction can be achieved successfully with a rapid infusion of tPA (48,49). It is important to note however, that despite the rapid resolution of the formed thrombus by this lytic treatment, rapid reocclusion of the vessel wall will occur unless an adjunct therapy of heparin and/or antiplatelet drugs are included (for review, see 50). Furthermore, maintenance of vessel wall patency can only be achieved by continuous adjunct therapy of anticoagulants or antiplatelet drugs. However, it should also be recognized that with such long term therapy, while reducing recurrent myocardial infarction and general mortality, it is fraught with an increased risk of haemorrhagic events, particularly in stroke (51).

Thus, similar to the strategy using "antiplatelet" agents, the use of components derived from the vessel wall after injury, while achieving short-term benefit in treating and preventing thrombosis, are not without significant rethrombosis or bleeding side-effects (50,51).

6. VESSEL WALL THROMBOGENECITY

One possible explanation for this limited "antithrombotic effect" is that none of these agents alter the thrombogenic properties of the stimulus, namely, the thrombogenic properties of the damaged vessel wall. It is possible that thrombosis will continue unless vessel wall thrombogenecity is decreased. If so, it raises the possibility that an alternative approach to antithrombotic treatment is to reduce vessel wall thrombogenecity.

It has been suggested that many of these antithrombotic constituents synthesized and/or secreted by the vessel wall, in particular, by the endothelium, not only regulate thrombogenesis following vessel wall injury, but also maintain vessel wall biocompatibility under basal conditions. We would argue against the latter possibility since it is apparent that synthesis and secretion of tPA, PGI_2, endothelin, and other antithrombotic agents derived from the endothelium, all require **endothelial cell stimulation** (43-47). There is little evidence to indicate that under basal conditions, endothelial cells synthesize any of these components. What then, is the component(s) of the healthy, intact endothelium which render(s) the healthy vessel wall non-thrombogenic? For a number of years, our laboratory has addressed this question from the perspective of fatty acid metabolism.

7. LINOLEIC ACID AND THE LIPOXYGENASE PATHWAY

Endothelial cells are metabolically active under basal conditions. Denning et al (52) and others have demonstrated that triglycerides are continuously turned over in unstimulated endothelial cells (53). Linoleic acid is continuously released from this cytosolic triglyceride pool and metabolised intracellularly by the endothelial cell enzyme, 15-lipoxygenase, into the monohydroxide, 13-hydroxyoctadecadienoic acid or 13-HODE, see Figure 4 (53-55). 13-HODE is retained in vesicles inside endothelial cells and is not released from the endothelial cells into the ambient surroundings.

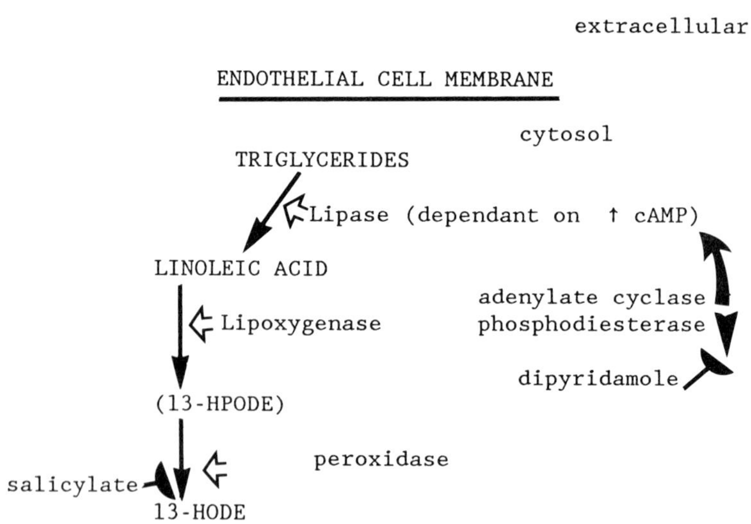

Figure 4. Linoleic acid is only metabolized by the lipoxygenase enzyme in endothelial cells, since linoleic acid has only 2 double bonds and therefore, is a poor substrate for the cyclooxygenase enzyme. And, triglyceride turnover and linoleic acid release are cAMP dependant. This latter point is important for the discussion below.

When endothelial cells are stimulated, 13-HODE synthesis rapidly decreases, such as in response to thrombin, endotoxin, Interleukin 1, or other cytokines (53-56). In contrast, the level of intracellular 13-HODE can be elevated by increasing the intracellular levels of cAMP, both in vitro and in vivo (53,56). Increased synthesis of 13-HODE associated with increased cAMP levels, appears to be due to an increased availability of free linoleic acid released from the triglyceride pool (53). In early studies, we observed that the amount of 13-HODE synthesized in the resting endothelial cell is inversely correlated with the thrombogenecity of the endothelial cell surface. When 13-HODE synthesis is increased, less platelets, tumour cells and other circulating cells adhere to the endothelium (53-56). On the other hand, when 13-HODE synthesis is decreased, the endothelial cell surface becomes more reactive to circulating blood cells.

These observations suggested to us that 13-HODE acts as an intracellular regulator of vessel wall adhesivity. Thus, we explored the possibility that the expression of adhesion molecules on the endothelial cell surface are regulated by 13-HODE, thereby influencing platelet endothelial cell adhesion. We found that Interleukin 1-stimulated endothelial cells synthesize and express the vitronectin receptor on the endothelial cell surface (57). [The vitronectin receptor is a two chain glycoprotein belonging to the integrin family (58)]. In unstimulated endothelial cells, the vitronectin receptor appears to be retained in vesicles lying immediately below the plasma membrane (59). Upon stimulation, this receptor appears to re-locate at the apical surface, unfolding its RGD recognizing binding site, thereby rendering the endothelial cell surface more adhesive. We also demonstrated that 13-HODE and the vitronectin receptor are co-localized within the same vesicles of non-adhesive endothelial cells (59-60). When the endothelial cells are stimulated, the vitronectin receptor and 13-HODE dissociate, and the vitronectin receptor is detected on the apical surface of the cells, at a time when the endothelial cells are more adhesive to platelets (59).

These observations suggest to us that 13-HODE interacts with the lipophilic site of the alpha chain of the vitronectin receptor, down-regulating its expression on the endothelial cell surface. Consistent with the possibility that fatty acid metabolites can alter the ability of integrins to recognize their specific ligands, and hence alter their adhesivity, Conforti et al (61) demonstrated that the ability of the vitronectin receptor to recognize its specific ligands could be altered by varying the fatty acid environment in which it was located. Other investigators have also suggested a similar relationship between the linoleic and arachidonic acid-derived lipoxygenase metabolites and glycoprotein IIb/IIIa dependent adhesion among tumour cells, platelets and endothelial cells (56,62,64).

Thus, a battery of evidence provides support to the idea that adhesion molecule expression necessary for cell adhesion, be it to endothelial cells, platelets or to other circulating blood cells, can be manipulated by altering the fatty acid milieu, in particular, by altering the relative amounts of lipoxygenase products derived from linoleic and arachidonic acids. The linoleic acid metabolite, 13-HODE, is associated with down-regulating the expression of adhesion molecules while the arachidonic acid metabolites (12-HETE in platelets, 15-HETE in tumour cells), appears to up-regulate the expression of these adhesion molecules.

We also found that when the vessel wall is de-endothelialized by selectively removing the endothelium, the exposed subendothelium is not reactive to circulating blood cells, but is, in fact, as thromboresistant as the healthy intact endothelium itself (9,65). These results, at first glance, appeared to be in marked contrast to many studies in which the injured vessel wall is reported to be highly thrombogenic (1,2,7,8). To further explore this apparent contradiction, experiments were performed to determine whether 13-HODE is released abluminally from endothelial cells, and if so, whether its presence in the basement membrane influences basement membrane thrombogenecity. We found that the thrombogenecity of the exposed basement membrane surface is dependent, in part, upon the amount of 13-HODE associated with it (64). The initial observation of this relationship using *in vitro* cell culture systems has been confirmed *in vivo* both in animal and human tissue (9,66-68). These observations therefore, lend credence to the concept that 13-HODE binds not only to the adhesion molecules on the luminal surface of the endothelium but also is secreted to the abluminal basement membrane, rendering the adhesion molecules in a conformational presentation which prevents them from recognizing their adhesive ligands, and hence, reducing basement membrane thrombogenecity.

....

In summary, a number of studies, using intact cell preparation *in vitro* and live animal studies *in vivo*, suggest that lipoxygenase metabolites regulate cell/cell adhesion by up- or down-regulating blood cell and vessel wall integrin expression.

8. ALTERNATIVE ANTITHROMBOTIC STRATEGIES: Altering Vessel Wall Thrombogenecity

The concept of achieving an antithrombotic effect by impairing or blocking adhesion molecule expression is not new. Many studies have adopted a strategy of blocking these adhesion molecule on platelets, such as with the use of the glycoprotein IIb/IIIa antibodies (69,70). Not surprisingly however, this approach has been fraught with bleeding side-effects similar to those seen with other antiplatelet agents (71). The recognition that adhesion molecules are also expressed on the vessel wall however, suggests an alternative approach, to alter vessel wall thrombogenecity without impairing platelet function, namely to selectively alter vessel wall adhesion molecule expression and decrease vessel wall thrombogenecity.

A number of experimental studies performed both in animals and humans suggest that manipulating vessel wall 13-HODE synthesis may contribute to this approach. Our first approach was based upon the earlier *in vitro* observations that increasing cAMP increases endothelial cell triglyceride turnover and 13-HODE production. If relevant to the *in vivo* situation, we argued that increasing vessel wall cAMP should lead to increased availability of linoleic acid, increased 13-HODE synthesis, and as a result, decreased adhesivity of both the intact and the injured vessel wall. As a consequence, fewer platelets should adhere to the injured vessel wall surface, and thrombogenesis should be ameliorated. We also argued that if the lipoxygenase pathway was impaired, 13-HODE synthesis should decrease, and platelet adhesion to the injured vessel wall should increase.

Rabbits were treated with drugs which we had reason to believe, would influence the lipoxygenase pathway, either by reducing 13-HODE synthesis or by elevating cAMP. Salicylate was used as an inhibitor of the peroxidation of the unstable precursor, 13-HPODE to 13-HODE, see Figure 4 (54,55,72). Dipyridamole was used to inhibit phosphodiesterase, permitting increased vessel wall cAMP, see Figure 4 (24,53,56,64). After one week of oral treatment with either salicylate, dipyridamole or the appropriate control, both carotid arteries of each animal were isolated. The endothelium was removed using a selective injury technique (9), and three hours later, the animals were injected with radiolabelled platelets. The number of ^{3}H-platelets adherent to the injured area of the vessel wall was determined one hour later, as a measure of vessel wall thrombogenecity. Other vessel wall segments (proximal or distal to the injury site) were removed for the analysis of vessel wall 13-HODE and cAMP.

Adhesion of platelets to the injured carotid arteries increased two-fold in the salicylate-treated animals as compared to platelet adhesion to injured carotid arteries in untreated rabbits. This increase in platelet adhesion was associated with a 67 % decrease in vessel wall 13-HODE, Table 1, (66). In contrast platelet adhesion to the injured vessel walls in the dipyridamole-treated animals was decreased by half, relative to the control animals. This was associated with an increase in 13-HODE synthesis. 13-HODE synthesis in the dipyridamole-treated animals correlated significantly with both the dipyridamole plasma level and the vessel wall cAMP level, $p < 0.001$. It should be noted that neither the dipyridamole nor the salicylate treatment impaired platelet function assessed ex vivo (66). Thus, these observations provide direct

Table 1 **RELATIONSHIP BETWEEN VESSEL WALL THROMBOGENECITY *IN VIVO* AND VESSEL WALL 13HODE LEVELS IN SALICYLATE AND DIPYRIDAMOLE TREATED ANIMALS**

TREATMENT	PLT ADH	13-HODE
Salicylate	+ 205 ± 25%*	33 ± 4%*
Dipyridamole	- 54 ± 6%*	141 ± 5%*

Data are expressed as, % of Control, mean ± SEM, n = 8* $p < 0.001$.

in vivo evidence that 13-HODE synthesis in the vessel wall correlates with vessel wall thromboresistance. These observations also suggest that manipulating vessel wall thromboresistance per se, is just as effective an approach to prevent platelet vessel wall interactions in vivo following vessel wall injury as inhibiting platelet function.

Our second approach was to alter vessel wall thrombogenecity by diet. The rationale was based in part upon i) our in vitro observations that increasing the availability of linoleic acid results in increased 13-HODE synthesis (53), and ii) epidemiological studies which suggest that cardiovascular disease is significantly lower in populations which ingest diets rich in linoleic acid (73,74). Rabbits were fed a semi-purified synthetic diet rich either in linoleic acid, linoleic acid and γ-linoleic acid, or eicosapentaenoic acid (EPA). After 4 weeks of feeding, injured carotid artery thrombogenecity was measured in the rabbits as described earlier.

When the animals were fed a diet rich in linoleic acid ± gamma linolenic acid, there was an increased synthesis of 13-HODE and a decrease in vessel wall thrombogenecity. Platelet adhesion and platelet aggregation were not significantly impaired. In contrast, EPA had a minimal effect on vessel wall thrombogenecity despite significantly impairing platelet adhesion. The latter effect was associated with a marked decrease in platelet 12-HETE production. These dietary effects on platelet and vessel wall adhesivity were due to selective uptake of these fatty acids from the plasma. EPA was selectively incorporated by the platelet, decreasing platelet 12-HETE synthesis and impairing platelet adhesivity as measured ex vivo. In contrast, the blood vessel wall selectively incorporated linoleic acid, facilitating a marked increase in 13-HODE synthesis (66).

In summary, we demonstrated that vessel wall thrombogenecity can be selectively altered in vivo both by drugs and diet without rendering platelets dysfunctional. Whether rendering the vessel wall less thrombogenic acutely results in decreased thrombogenesis and vessel wall reocclusion chronically, is at present, not known. Experimental studies to test this possibility are presently ongoing. Nonetheless, some clinical data are suggestive of this possibility. Recently, Harker et al (75) examined the effects of [aspirin plus persantine] in preventing hyperplasia in patients following carotid endarectomies. They concluded that the "antiplatelet" treatment regime was ineffective since chronic vessel wall hyperplasia and restenosis were not inhibited. In that study, persantine was given 2 hours pre-operative, and [aspirin plus persantine] was given for 12 months post-operative. In another study, Chesebro (76) examined the effects of [aspirin + persantine] in preventing hyperplasia in patients undergoing elective coronary artery bypass grafting. He found that [aspirin plus persantine] decreased significantly saphenous vein graft hyperplasia. In this study, the patients were given persantine for 48 hours before the surgery and [aspirin plus persantine] 12 months post-operative. Albeit the two clinical situations are considerably different, but the end-points measured were similar, ie, vessel wall hyperplasia. How is it possible that with an apparent minor difference in pre-surgery treatment regime, there was such a marked difference on the end-point? Is it possible that in the Chesebro study, the two day pre-treatment with persantine increased vessel wall cAMP levels, resulting in increased 13-HODE synthesis and decreased vessel wall thrombogenecity? If so, is it possible that the decreased platelet/vessel wall interaction immediately post-surgery, was reduced sufficiently to minimize platelet PF4 and PDGF secretion and subsequent vessel wall hyperplasia? It is interesting that in our animal study, we had to pretreated our rabbits for one week to ensure a consistent effect of dipyridamole (persantine) on vessel wall cAMP and 13-HODE levels, since earlier studies indicated that this dipyridamole effect required at least 24-48 hours (53,56).

Recent evidence demonstrates that human blood vessels also synthesize 13-HODE and that this activity correlates with vessel wall thrombogenecity. Segments of internal mammary arteries and saphenous veins obtained from patients undergoing elective coronary artery bypass surgery, produce significant amounts of 13-HODE. The arteries produce 6-fold more 13-HODE than the veins. More interestingly however, 13-HODE synthesis in both the arteries and the veins decreases with age. This decrease in 13-HODE synthesis is parallelled by a significant increase in vessel wall thrombogenecity (77). Studies presently ongoing in our laboratory in this patient population, will determine whether increasing 13-HODE synthesis pre-operatively is associated with a corresponding decrease in vessel wall thrombogenecity at the time of surgery.

9. CONCLUSIONS AND IMPLICATIONS

The concept of repairing the vessel wall as a strategy to decrease thrombogenesis has been limited primarily to cardiologic and surgical intervention, such as angioplasty and coronary artery bypass grafting. These treatments also require adjunct antiplatelet and anticoagulant therapy (75-79). However, the experimental data reviewed above, suggest an alternative strategy, namely altering vessel wall thrombogenecity. A number of earlier studies have proposed rendering the vessel wall less thrombogenic after injury by targeting specific thrombin inhibitors at thrombin bound to fibrin or the injured vessel wall (80-83). Others have suggested seeding genetically altered endothelial cells on artificial grafts or damaged vessel walls (84-85). We propose an alternative strategy which would change the inherent thrombogenic properties of the vessel wall, rather than attempt to counter the thrombogenic components already expressed on the vessel wall surface. Part of this strategy includes manipulating 13-HODE in an attempt to regulate adhesion molecule expression not only on the apical surface of the endothelium, but also on the subendothelial surface which is exposed following injury. Interestingly, a number of studies suggest a possible vehicle with which to deliver such agents to potential thrombogenic sites in the vessel wall. Mizushima et al (86,87) reported that certain lipid microspheres containing PGE_1 (lipo-PGE_1) are selectively incorporated in areas of vascular damage in the spontaneous hypertensive rat and the atherosclerotic rabbit, suggesting that a specific effect could be targetted in a cardiovascular system. It is interesting to note that in these latter studies, the lipid microspheres carrying PGE_1, were 55% linoleic acid. Bertomeu et al (67) have demonstrated that linoleic acid is selectively incorporated by the vessel wall. These latter experimental data provide evidence therefore, to suggest that not only manipulating vessel wall thrombogenecity is an alternative approach to achieve an antithrombotic effect, but also that the technology to target specific delivery of agents to thrombogenic sites of the vessel wall to achieve this effect, is possible. Further studies exploring this alternative approach of antithrombotic therapy therefore, merits further investigation.

ACKNOWLEDGEMENTS

The studies performed by us and referred to in this manuscript have been supported, in part, by the Ontario Heart and Stroke Foundation of Canada and the Medical Research Council of Canada.

REFERENCES

1. Ross, R. (1986). The pathogenesis of atherosclerosis - an update. *N. Engl. J. Med.* 314:488-500.

2. Packham, M.A., Mustard, J.F. (1986). The role of platelets in the development and complications of atherosclerosis. *Semin. Hematol.* 23:8-26.

3. Moore, S., Pepper, D.S., Cash, J.D. (1975). The isolation and characterisation of platelet factor 4 release from thrombin-aggregated washed human platelets and its dissociation into subunits and the isolation of membrane-bound antiheparin activity. *Biochim. Biophys. Acta.* 379:370-384.

4. Mustard, J.F., Perry, D.W., Kinlough-Rathbone, R.L., Packham, M.A. (1975). Factors responsible for ADP-induced release reaction of human platelets. *Am. J. Physiol.* 228(6):1757-1768.

5. Hamberg, M., Svensson, J., Samuelsson, B. (1974). Prostaglandin endoperoxides. A new concept concerning the mode of action and release of prostaglandins. *Proc. Natl. Acad. Sci. USA* 71:3824-3828.

6. Ross, R. (1987). Platelet derived growth factor. *Ann. Rev. Med.* 38:71-79.

7. Stemerman, M.B., Spaet, T.H. (1972). The subendothelium and thrombogenesis. *Bull. N.Y. Acad. Med.* 48:289-301.

8. Mustard, J.F., Packham, M.A., Kinlough-Rathbone, R. (1978). Platelets, thrombosis and atherosclerosis. *Adv. Exp. Med. Biol.* 104:127-144.

9. Buchanan, M.R., Richardson, M., Haas, T., Hirsh, J., Madri, J. (1987). The basement membrane underlying the vascular endothelium is not thrombogenic. *Thromb. Haemost.* 58:698-704.

10. Keenan, J.P., Solum, N.O. (1972). Quantitative studies on the release of platelet fibrinogen by thrombin. *Br. J. Haematol.* 23:461-466.

11. Lajmanovich, A., Hudry-Clergeon, G., Freyssinet, J.M., Marguerie, G. (1981). Human factor VIII procoagulant activity and phospholipid interaction. *Biochim. Biophys. Acta.* 678:132-136.

12. Lipscomb, M.S., Walsh, P.N. Human platelet factor XI. (1979). Localization in platelet membranes of factor XI-like activity and its function distinction from plasma factor XI. *J. Clin. Invest.* 63:1006-1014.

13. Tuszynski, G.P., Bevacona, S.J., Schmaier, A.H., CoLman, R.W., Walsh, P.N. (1982). Factor XI antigen and activity in platelets. *Blood* 59:1148-

14. Ozge-Anwar, A.H., Ofosu, F.A., Blajchman, M.A. (1985). Evidence that intact human platelets provide factor VII-like activity for the activation of factor X by the extrinsic coagulation pathway. *Thromb. Haemost.* 54:176/P1042.

15. Nesheim, M.E., Eid, S., Mann, K.G. (1981). Assembly of the prothrombinase complex in the absence of prothrombin. *J. Biol. Chem.* 256:9874-9882.

16. Stenflo, J., Dahlback, B. (1980). Activation of prothrombin by factor Xa on the surface of platelets. In: *"The Regulation of Coagulation"*. (K.G. Mann, F.B. Taylor (eds.). Elsevier, New York, p. 225.

17. Needleman, P., Turk, J., Jakschik, B.A., Morrison, A.R., Lefkowith, J.B. (1986). Arachidonic acid metabolism. *Ann. Rev. Biochem.* 55:69-102.

18. Castellot, J.J., Jr., Favreau, L.B., Karnovsky, M.J., Rosenberg, R.D. (1982). Inhibition of vascular smooth muscle cell growth by endothelial cell-derived heparin. *J. Biol. Chem.* 257, 19:11256-11260.

19. Al-Mondhiry, H., Marcus, A.J., Spaet, T.H. (1970). On the mechanism of platelet function inhibition by acetylsalicylic acid. *Proc. Soc. Exp. Dial. Med.* 133:632-636.

20. Ali, M., McDonald, J.W.D. (1977). Effects of sulfinpyrazone on platelet prostaglandin synthesis and platelet release of serotonin. *J. Lab. Clin. Med.* 89:868-875.

21. Willerson, J.T., Golino, P., McNatt, J. Eidt, J., Yao, S-K., Buja, L.M. (1991). Role of new antiplatelet agents as adjunctive therapies in thrombolysis. *Am. J. Cardiol.* 67:12A-18A.

22. German, D.C., Kredich, N.M., Bjornsson, T.D. (1989). Oral dipyridamole increases plasma adenosine levels in human beings. *Clin. Pharmacol. Ther.* 45:80-84.

23. Smith, J.B., Mills, D.C.B. (1970). Inhibition of adenosine 3':5'-cyclic monophosphate phosphodiesterase. *Biochem. J.* 120: 20P.

24. Moncada, S., Korburt, R. (1978). Dipyridamole and other phosphodiesterase inhibitors act as antithrombotic agents by potentiating endogenous prostacyclin. *Lancet* 1:1286- 1289.

25. Hennekens, C.H., Buring, J.E., Sandercock, P., Collins, R., Peto, R. (1989). Aspirin and other antiplatelet agents in the secondary and primary prevention of cardiovascular disease. *Circ.* 80:749-756.

26. Harker, L.A., Slichter, S.J. (1972). Platelet and fibrinogen consumption in man. *N. Engl. J. Med.* 287:999-1005.

27. The Anturane Reinfarction Trial Research Group. (1980). Sulfinpyrazone in the prevention of sudden death after myocardial infarction. *N. Engl. J. Med.* 302:250-256.

28. Canadian Cooperative Study Group. (1978). A randomized trial of aspirin and sulfinpyrazone in threatened stroke. *N. Engl. J. Med.* 299:53-59.

29. Cairns, J., Turpie, A.G.G., ISIS-2. (1988). Randomized trial of intravenous streptokinase, oral aspirin, both, or neither among 17, 187 cases of suspected acute myocardial infarction: ISIS-2. *Lancet* 350-360.

30. Marcus, A.J. (1978). The role of lipids in platelet function with particular reference to the arachidonic acid pathway. *J. Lipid Res.* 19:793-826.

31. Buchanan, M.R., Butt, R.W., Hirsh, J., Markham, B.A., Nazir, D.J. (1986). Role of lipoxygenase metabolism in platelet function: effect of aspirin and salicylate. *Prost. Leuk. Med.* 21:157-168.

32. Broekman, M.J., Eiroa, A.M., Marcus, A.J. (1989). Albumin redirects platelet eicosanoid metabolism toward 12(S)-hydroxyeicosatetraenoic acid. *J. Lipid Res.* 30:1925-1932.

33. Dutilh, C.E., Haddeman, E., Don, J.A., Hoor, F.T. (1981). The role of arachidonate lipoxygenase and fatty acids during irreversible blood platelet aggregation in vitro. *Prost. Med.* 6:111-126.

34. Gibson, B.E.S., Buchanan, M.R., Barr, R.D., White J.G. (1987). Primary thrombocythaemia in childhood: Symptomatic episodes and their relationship to thromboxane A2, 6-keto-PGE1 and 12-hydroxyeicosatetraenoic acid production. A case report. *Prost. Leuko. Med.* 26:221-231.

35. Morita, I., Murota S.I. (1987). Role of 12-lipoxygenase products of arachidonic acid on platelet aggregation. *Adv. Prost. Thromb. Leuko. Res.* 17:219-223.

36. Herrman, K.S. (1985). Lipoxygenase Products: Leukotrienes C4, D4, A4s breakdown products and 12-HPETE influence platelet aggregation in vivo. *Prostaglandins* 29, No 3:459-465.

37. Okuma, M., Uchino, H. (1979). Altered arachidonate metabolism by platelets in patients with myeloproliferative disorders. *Blood* 13:1258-1271.

38. Van Ryn-McKenna, J., Buchanan, M.R. (1989). Relative effects of flurbiprofen on platelet 12-hydroxyeicosatetraenoic acid and thromboxane A2 production: Influence on collagen induced platelet aggregation and adhesion. *Prost. Leuko. and Med.* 36:171-174.

39. Buchanan, M.R., Dejana, E., Gent, M. (1981). Enhanced platelet accumulation onto injured carotid arteries in rabbits after aspirin treatment. *J. Clin. Invest.* 67:503-508.

40. Lorenzet, R., Niemetz, J., Marcus, A.J., Broekman, M.J. (1986). Enhancement of mononuclear procoagulant activity by platelet 12-hydroxyeicosatetraenoic acid. *J. Clin. Invest.* 78:418-423.

41. Ross, R. (1981) Atherosclerosis: A problem of the biology of arterial wall cells and their interaction with blood components. *Arteriosclerosis* 1:293-311.

42. Stemerman, M.B. (1982). Relationship to atherosclerosis. In: *Thrombosis and Haemostasis.* Basic principles and usual practice. R.W. Coleman, J. Hirsh, V. Marder, E.W. Salzlman (eds.). JB Lippincott, Philadelphia pp 781-88.

43. Moncada, S., Gryglewski, R., Bunting, S., Vane, J.R. (1976). An enzyme isolated form arteries transforms prostaglandin endoperoxides to an unstable substance that inhibits platelets aggregation. *Nature* 263:663-665.

44. Doni, M.G., Whittle, B.J.R., Palmer, R.M.J., Moncada, S. (1988). Actions of nitric oxide on the release of prostacyclin from bovine endothelial cells in culture. *Eur. J. Pharm.* 151:19-25.

45. Lopez, J.A., Armstrong, M.L. Piegors, D.J., Heistad, D.D. (1990). Vascular responses to endothelin-1 in atherosclerotic primates. *Arteriosclerosis* 10:1113-1118.

46. Levin, E.G., Marzec, U., Anderson, J., Harker, L.A. (1984). Thrombin stimulates tissue plasminogen activator release from cultured human endothelial cells. *J. Clin. Invest. 74:1988-1995.*

47. *Hekman, C.M., Loskutoff, D.J. (1985). Endothelial cells produce a latent inhibitor of plasminogen activators that can be activated by denaturants.* J. Biol. Chem. 260, No 21:11581-11587.

48. Hsia, J., Hamilton, W.P., Kleiman, N., Roberts, R., Ghaitman, B.R., Ross, A.M. (1990). A comparison between heparin and low-dose aspirin as adjunctive therapy with tissue plasminogen activator for acute myocardial infarction. *N. Engl. J. Med.* 323:1433-1437.

49. Collen, D., Topol, E.J., Tiefenbrunn, A.J. et al. (1984). Coronary thrombolysis with recombinant human tissue-type plasminogen activator: a prospective, randomized-placebo controlled trial. *Circ.* 70:1012-1017.

50. Prins, M.H., Hirsh J. (1991). Heparin as an adjunctive treatment after thrombolytic therapy for acute myocardial infarction. *Am. J. Cardiol.* 67:3A-11A.

51. Lotto, A., Colombo, A., Talarico, G., Fratianne, G., Lettino, M. (1990). Heparin and secondary prevention of acute myocardial infarction. *Haemostasis* 20:132-141.

52. Denning, G.M., Figard, P.H., Kaduce, T.L., Spector, A. (1983). Role of triglycerides in endothelial cell arachidonic acid metabolism. *J. Lipid Res.* 24:993-1011.

53. Haas, T.A., Bertomeu, M.C., Bastida, E., Buchanan, M.R. Cyclic AMP regulation of endotheial cell triglyceride turnover, 13-hydroxyoctadecadienoic acid (13-HODE) synthesis and endothelial cell thrombogenecity. *Biochim. Biophys. Acta.* 1031:174-178.

54. Buchanan, M.R., Butt, R.W., Magas, Z., Van Ryn, J., Hirsh, J., Nazir, D.J. (1985). Endothelial cells produce a lipoxygenase derived chemorepellant with influences platelet/endothelial cell interactions: effect of aspirin and salicylate. *Thromb. Haemost.* 53:306-311.

55. Buchanan, M.R., Haas, T.A, Lagarde, M., Guichardant, M. (1985). 13-hydroxyoctadecadienoic acid is the vessel wall chemorepellant factor, LOX. *J. Biol. Chem.* 260:16056-16059.

56. Lauri, D., Bertomeu, M.C., Orr, F.W., Bastida, E., Sauder, D., Buchanan, M.R. (1990). Interleukin-1 increases tumor cell adhesion to endothelial cells through an RGD dependant mechanism: in vitro and in vivo studies. *Clin. Expl. Metastasis* 8:27-32.

57. Lafrenie, R.M., Podor, T.J., Buchanan, M.R., Orr, F.W. (1990). Interleukin 1α induced vitronectin receptor expression and tumor cell endothelial cell adhesion. *FASEB* 4:A1134.

58. Hynes, R.O. (1987). Integrins: a family of cell surface receptors. *Cell* 48:549-554.

59. Buchanan, M.R., Bertomeu, M.C., Haas, T.A., Gallo, S., Eltringham-Smith, L. (1991). Endothelial cell 13-HODE synthesis and tumor cell endothelial cell adhesion. *Adv. Prost.Thromb.Leuko.Res.* 20:909-912.

60. Aznar-Salatti, J., Bastida, E., Buchanan, M.R., Castillo, R., Ordinas, A., Escolar, G. (1990). Differential localization of von Willebrand factor, fibronectin and 13-HODE in human endothelial cell cultures. *Histochemistry* 93:507-514.

61. Conforti, G., Zanetti, A., Pasquali-Ronchetti, I., Quaglino, D. Jr., Neyroz, P., Dejana, E. (1990). Modulation of vitronectin receptor binding by membrane lipid composition. *J. Biol. Chem.* 265:4011-4019.

62. Bastida, E., Bertomeu, M.C., Haas, T.A., Almirall, L., Lauri, D., Orr, F.W., Buchanan, M.R. (1990). Regulation of tumor cell adhesion by intracellular 13-HODE:15-HETE ratio. *J. Lipid Med.* 2:281-293.

63. Grossi, I.M., Fitzgerald, L.A., Umbarger, L.A., Nelson, K.K., Diglio, C.A., Taylor, J.D., Honn, K.V. (1989). Bidirectional control of membrane expression and/or activation of tumor cell IRGpIIb/IIIa receptor and tumor cell adhesion by lipoxygenase products of arachidonic acid and linoleic acid. *Canc. Res.* 49:1029-1037.

64. Buchanan, M.R., Bastida, E. (1988). Endothelium and underlying membrane reactivity with platelets, leukocytes and tumor cells: regulation by the lipoxygenase-derived fatty acid metabolites, 13-HODE and HETE's. *Med. Hypothesis,* 27:317-325.

65. Aznar-Salatti, J., Bastida, E., Haas, T.A., Escolar, G., Ordinas, A., de Groot, P.H.G., Buchanan, M.R. (1991). The reactivity of the extracellular matrix with platelets is dependant upon the method of its preparation. *Arterosclerosis,* 11:In Press.

66. Weber, E., Haas, T.A., Mueller, T.H., Eisert, W.G., Hirsh, J. Richardson, M., Buchanan, M.R. (1990). Relationship between vessel wall 13-HODE synthesis and vessel wall thrombogenecity following injury. Influence of salicylate and dipyridamole treatment. *Thromb. Res.* 57:383-392.

67. Bertomeu,M.C.,Crozier,G.L.,Haas,T.A.,Fleith,M.,Buchanan, M.R.(1990). Selective effects of dietary fats on vascular 13-HODE synthesis and platelet/vessel wall interactions. *Thromb. Res.* 59:819-830.

68. Simon, T.C., Makheja, A.N., Bailey, J.M. (1989). The induced lipoxygenase in atherosclerotic aorta converts linoleic acid to the platelet chemorepellant factor 13-HODE. *Thromb. Res.* 55:171-178.

69. Roth, G.J. (1991). Developing relationships: arterial platelet adhesion, glycoprotein 1b, and leucine-rich glycoproteins. *Blood* 77:5-19.

70. Coller, B.S., Folts, J.D., Smith, S.R., Scudder, L.E., Jordan, R. (1989). Abolition of in vivo platelet thrombus formation in primates with monoclonal antibodies to the platelet GPIIb/IIIa receptor:correlation with bleeding time, platelet aggregation, and blockade of GPIIb/IIIa receptors. *Circ.* 80:1766-1774.

71. FitzGerald, D.J. (1989). Platelet inhibition with an antibody to glycoprotein IIb/IIIa. *Circ.* 80:1918-1919.

72. Siegel, M.I., McConnell, R.T., Cuatrecasas, P. (1979). Aspirin-like drugs interfere with arachidonate metabolism by inhibition of the 12-hydroperoxy-5,8,10,14-eicosatetraenoic acid peroxidase activity of the lipoxygenase pathway. *Biochemistry* 76:3774-3778.

73. Wood, D.A., Riemeisma, R.A., Butler, S., Thomson, M., MacIntyre, C., Elton, R.D., Oliver, M.F. (1987). Linoleic and eicosatetraenoic acids in adipose tissue and platelets and risk of coronary heart disease. *Lancet* 1:177-183.

74. Oliver, M.F., Riemeisma, R.A., Thomson, M., Fulton, M., Abraham, R.A., Wood, D.A. (1989). Linoleic acid and coronary heart disease. *Br. J. Hosp. Med.* 42:298-300.

75. Harker, L., Bernstein, E., Scala, T. (1990). Effect of aspirin/dipyridamole on restenosis after carotid endarterectomy: randomized placebo controlled clinical trial. *Circulation* 80:III-5.(Abstr.)

76. Chesebro, J.H. (1990). Effect of dipyridamole and aspirin on vein graft patency after coronary bypass operations. *Thromb. Res.* XII:5-10.

77. Brister, S.J., Haas, T.A., Bertomeu, M.C., Austin, J., Buchanan, M.R. (1990). 13-HODE synthesis in internal mammary arteries and saphenous veins: Implications in cardiovascular surgery. In: *Adv. Prost. Thromb. Leuko. Res.* 21:667-670.

78. Dehmer, G.J., Popma, J.J., Van Den Berg, M.D., Eichhorn, E.J., Prewitt, J.B., Campbell, W.B., Jennings, L., Willerson, J.T., Schmitz, J.M. (1988). Reduction in the rate of early restenosis after coronary angioplasty by a diet supplemented with n-3 fatty acids. *N. Engl. J. Med.* 319:733-740.

79. GISSI-2. (1990). A factorial randomised trial of alteplase versus streptokinase and heparin versus no heparin among 12,490 patients with acute myocardial infarction. *Lancet* 336:65-71.

80. Jang, I-K., Gold, H.K., Ziskind, A.A., Leinbach, R.C., Fallon, J.T., Collen, D. (1990). Prevention of platelet-rich arterial thrombosis by selective thrombin inhibition. *Circ.* 81:219-225.

81. Eisenberg, P.R. (1991). Role of new anticoagulants as adjunctive therapy during thrombolysis. *Am. J. Cardiol.* 67:19A-24A.

82. Marzec, U.M., Kelly, A.B., Hanson, S.R., Lasslo, A., Harker, L.A. (1990). Inhibition of thrombus formation in vivo by novel antiplatelet agent. *Arteriosclerosis* 10:367-371.

83. Okwusidi, J., Falcone, M., Van Ryn-McKenna, J., Hirsh, J., Ofosu, F.A., Buchanan, M.R. (1990). In vivo catalysis of thrombin inhibition by antithrombin III and heparin co-factor II and antithrombotic effect: Differential effects of dermatan sulfate and unfractioned heparin. *Thromb. & Haemorrh. Dis.* 1/2:77-80.

84. Johnson, R.C., Augustin-Voss, H.G., Zhu, D., Pauli, B.U. (1991). Endothelial cell membrane vesicles in the study of organ preference of metastasis. Canc. Res. 51:394-399.

85. Dichek, D.D., Neville, R.F., Zwiebel, J.A., Freeman, S.M., Leon, M.B., Anderson, W.F. (1989). Seeding of intravascular stents with genetically engineered endothelial cells. *Circ.* 80:1347-1353.

86. Mizushima, Y. (1991). Lipo-prostaglandin preparations. *Prost. Leuko. Essent. Fatty Acids* 42:1-6.

87. Mizushima, T., Hamano, T., Haramoto, S. Kiyokawa, S., Yanagawa, A., Nakura, K., Shintome, M., Watanabe, M. (1990). Distribution of lipid microspheres incorporating prostaglandin E1 to vascular lesions. *Prost. Leuko. Essent. Fatty Acids* 41:269-272.

PATHOLOGICAL EXPRESSIONS OF PLATELET-VESSEL WALL INTERACTIONS: IMPLICATIONS OF SEROTONIN

F. DE CLERCK

ABSTRACT. Platelet-derived serotonin activates vascular smooth muscle cells, endothelial cells and blood platelets, directly and through amplification. Such an activation trigger a) vascular smooth muscle cell mitogenic, and connective tissue synthetic activity; b) vascular smooth muscle cell contraction in particular when endothelial cell-derived relating mechanisms are defective; c) platelet activation resulting in cellular aggregation, and secretion of vasoactive products. By such actions, the platelet-derived mono-amine can contribute to arterial vessel wall proliferation, vasoconstriction and arterial thrombus formation in response to interactions of platelets with a damaged vessel wall, leading to ischemia in particular when normal counterbalance systems are disturbed by underlying pathologies such as hypertension or atherosclerosis. Molecules directed specifically against the receptors by which serotonin elicits these actions on target cells thus may offer possibilities for the treatment of human ischemic heart disease.

1. Introduction

On the list of autocoids, suspected to be involved in cardiovascular pathology, serotonin is an "old-timer" (De Clerck *et al.*, 1984; De Clerck and Vanhoutte, 1982; Page, 1958; Vanhoutte, 1985).

In a series of papers, published between 1940-1950, Page and colleagues (Page, 1958), reported the isolation of the substance responsible for the vasoconstricitve properties of blood serum and called it "*serotonin*" - due to its presence in serum and its tonic action on vascular smooth muscle cells. Soon thereafter, they identified it chemically as being *5-hydroxytryptamine*. In the same period, Erspamer and colleagues (1954), extracted a substance from the enterochromaffin cells, called it "*enteramine*" and chemically characterized it as being identical to 5-hydroxytryptamine. The compound has since been found widely distributed in vegetal and animal organisms.

In mammals, serotonin is produced enzymatically from dietary tryptophan by enterochromaffin cells of the gut, central and peripheral nerve cells, mast cells and renal tissue. The monoamine, produced by the enterochromaffin cells in the intestine, is released into the veno-portal blood and destroyed to a large extent in the liver and the lungs by monoamine oxidases, except for that fraction which is taken up by the platelets, stored in their dense granules in a super-complex with adenine nucleotides and calcium and thus carried throughout the cardiovascular system (De Clerck and Vanhoutte, 1982; Vanhoutte, 1985). When, in the course of their 7-10 days life span in the human

A. G. Herman (ed.), Antithrombotics, 181–194.
© 1991 *Kluwer Academic Publishers. Printed in the Netherlands.*

circulation, blood platelets are activated as, for example, by a contact with a lesion of the vessel wall, they secrete prostaglandins derived from arachidonic acid, as well as products stored in their granules, including serotonin; these mediators act locally on vascular tissue and on blood cells (De Clerck and De Chaffoy de Courcelles, 1989).

Despite the early recognition of its impact on vascular smooth muscle cells, endothelial cells, blood platelets (De Clerck and Vanhoutte, 1982; Vanhoutte, 1985), interest in serotonin soon lingered off and its potential contribution to vascular pathologies as hypertension or arterial thrombosis remained underestimated for several decades after its discovery.

Interactions between blood cells and the arterial wall have been suggested as early events in atherogenesis (Ross *et al.*, 1985) and thrombogenesis (Bertele and Salzman, 1985), leading to a variety of cardiovascular pathologies in which platelets are major participants (Harker and Ritchie, 1980).

Indeed, platelets activated at the site of a vessel wall injury accelerate the local formation of thrombin by catalyzing the conversion of prothrombin and release a multitude of endogenous products including prostaglandin endoperoxides and thromboxane A_2 (TXA_2), serotonin, adenosine diphosphate, and platelet derived growth factor (Vermylen *et al.*, 1986). These autocoids can contribute to vascular abnormalities in several ways. They may stimulate vascular smooth muscle cell and fibroblast proliferation, contributing to a local thickening of the arterial intima and a progressive reduction of the arterial lumen (Ross *et al.*, 1985; Nemecek *et al.*, 1986); they can cause vasoconstriction in areas of defective endothelial cell-dependent relaxation mechanisms

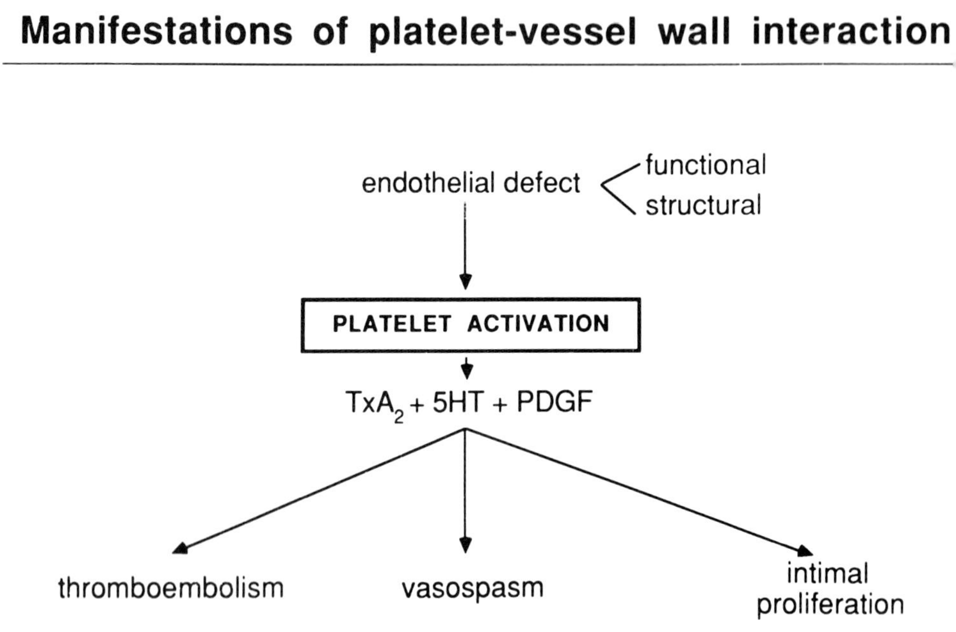

FIGURE 1. Manifestations of platelet-vessel wall interactions in which serotonin (5-HT) can play a role.

(Vanhoutte *et al.*, 1990); and they may facilitate platelet aggregation and fibrin formation to produce an acute thrombotic occlusion of the damaged artery with consequent ischaemic repercussions on organ function (Bevers *et al.*, 1987; De Clerck and de Chaffoy de Courcelles, 1989).

Various data suggest that platelet-derived serotonin plays a central role in such pathological repercussions of platelet-vessel wall interactions (Fig. 1).

Extensive reviews and details on serotonergic mechanisms in platelet endothelial cell function and vascular smooth muscle cell behaviour are available to the interested reader elsewhere (De Clerck *et al.*, 1984; Vanhoutte, 1985; De Clerck and Janssen, 1990; Hillis and Lange, 1991).

1.1. VASCULAR PROLIFERATION

Via activation of 5-HT_2 serotonergic receptors (Nemecek *et al.*, 1986), serotonin stimulates the mitogenesis of bovine aortic smooth muscle cells in culture (Fig. 2). Such an effect is induced by low concentrations of the mono-amine ($1x10^{-8}$ to $1x10^{-6}$ M),

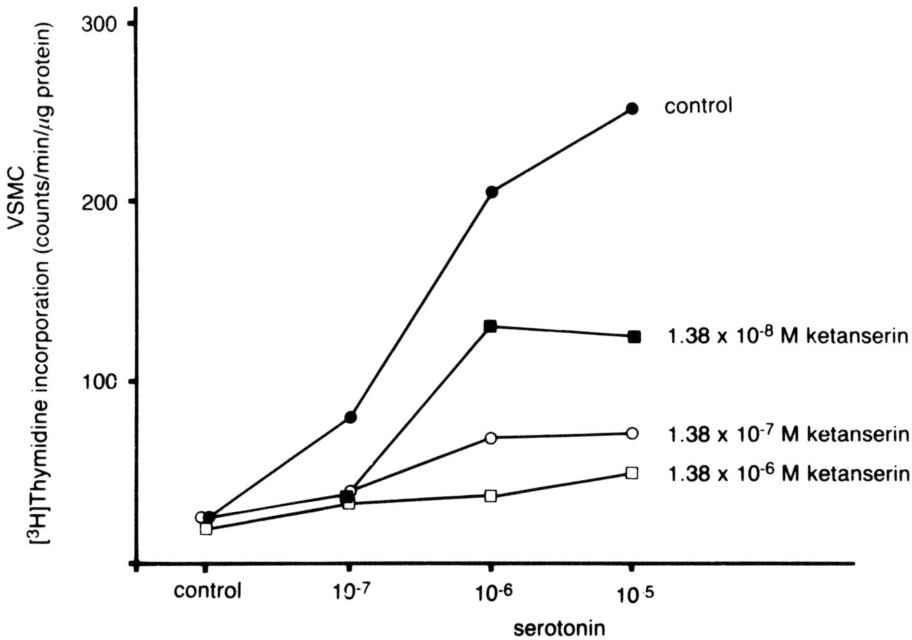

FIGURE 2. Mitogenic effect of serotonin on cultured vascular smooth muscle cells (VSMC) is mediated via 5-HT_2 serotonergic receptors. Isolated VSMC derived from bovine aorta incubated with serotonin (10^{-7} to 10^{-5} M). Mitogenic effect, quantified by measuring [^{3}H]thymidine incorporation, is attenuated by ketanserin, a 5-HT_2 serotonergic receptor antagonist (derived from De Clerck and Janssen, 1990).

readily liberated locally by platelets interacting with a vessel wall lesion (Ashton *et al.*, 1986). Although less potent in this respect than platelet-derived growth factor, a strong mediator released from platelets adhering to exposed subendothelial connective tissue, serotonin substantially enhances the mitogenic response to platelet derived growth factor (Ross *et al.*, 1985; Nemecek *et al.*, 1986). Via stimulation of 5-HT_{1b} receptors, the mono-amine enhances the proliferation of cultured fibroblasts (Boucek and Alvarez, 1970; Bazin *et al.*, 1973; Boucek and Alvarez, 1971; Mann, 1967; Seuwen and Pouysségur, 1990) and promotes the production of collagen by such cells *in vitro* (Aalto and Kulonen, 1972; Boucek *et al.*, 1972). The development of fibroelastosis, intimal hyperplasia, cellular infiltration of the vascular wall and deposits of mucopolysaccharides in subendothelial layers resembling atherosclerosis upon chronic administration of serotonin to experimental animals *in vivo* (Rossi and Zamboni, 1958; Ahmed and Harrison, 1964; Kokot, 1959) may result from such serotonergic effects. These observations create the possibility that platelet-derived serotonin contributes to the initiation and/or progression of myointimal arterial lesions, characteristic e.g. for atherosclerosis and late vascular restenosis after angioplasty (Ross *et al.*, 1985; Chesebro *et al.*, 1986).

1.2. VASCULAR TONE

Low concentrations of platelet-derived serotonin cause constriction of isolated large blood vessels via the activation of 5-HT_2 receptors receptors respectively on vascular smooth muscle cells; additionally, the monoamine potentiates such a reaction triggered by ineffective concentrations of various other agonists such as catecholamines, or angiotensin II (Van Nueten *et al.*, 1987). Vasoconstriction by serotonin occurs in particular when counterregulation of vasorelaxation by normal endothelial cells is defective (Fig. 3) (Vanhoutte and Houston, 1985; Vanhoutte *et al.*, 1990).

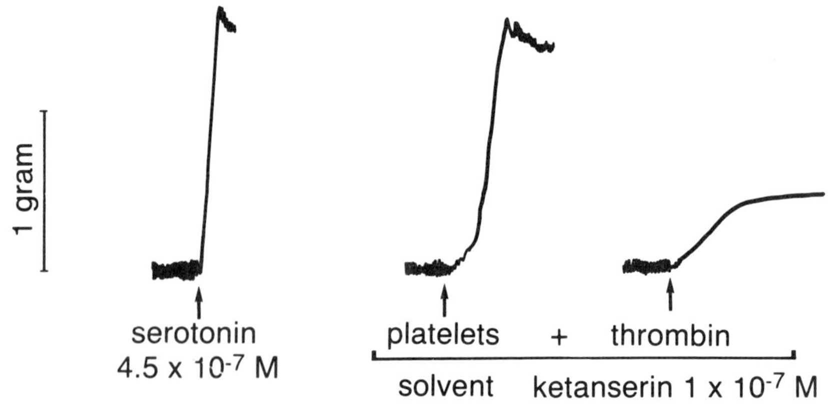

FIGURE 3. Contraction of de-endothelialized artery strips by serotonin and by thrombin-activated platelets is mediated via 5-HT_2 serotonergic receptors. Isolated rat caudal artery strips are constricted by exogenous serotonin and by washed rat platelets

(2.5×10^{10} cells/l) stimualted with thrombin (200 U/l). Platelet-mediated constriction is attenuated by ketanserin, a 5-HT_2 serotonergic receptor antagonist (derived from De Clerck and Janssen, 1990).

Such an endothelial cell dysfunction results in an oversensitivity specifically to the monoamine, delivered either exogenously or released by platelets. This peculiar oversensitivity occurs in isolated vessel segments taken from animals with established, dietary-induced atherosclerosis (Heistad *et al.*, 1984; Verbeuren, 1990), but also in vessels with early stages of vascular disease as occurring in spontaneously hypertensive rats (Heistad *et al.*, 1990) or after regeneration of endothelium in mechanically denuded porcine coronary arteries (Shimokawa *et al.*, 1987). Such a vasospastic overreactivity to serotonin also occurs *in vivo* during the recruitment phase of collateral vessels subsequent to a ligation of a major artery in experimental animals such as rats, cats and rabbits (Verheyen *et al.*, 1988; De Clerck *et al.*, 1986; Hollenberg, 1988; Verheyen *et al.*, 1991) (Fig. 4).

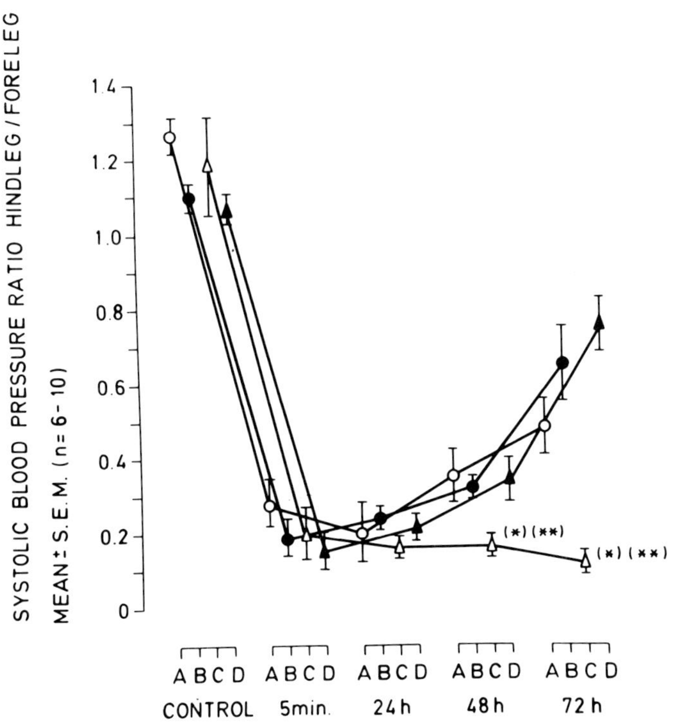

FIGURE 4. Correction by 5-HT_2 serotonergic receptor antagonism of the platelet-mediated reduction of peripheral collateral circulation, reflected by the systolic blood pressure ratio hind leg/foreleg in cats as a function of time after aortic occlusion. Mean ± S.E.M. of values obtained after aortic ligation alone (A, n = 6), ligation plus ketanserin 1.25 mg/kg i.p. daily (B, n = 7), aortic ligation with an intra-aortic stasis thrombus alone (C, n = 10), or additionally treated with ketanserin (D, n = 8). * $P < 0.05$ versus ligation plus ketanserin, 48 h; ** $P < 0.05$ versus ligation plus ketanserin, 72 h (derived from De Clerck *et al.*, 1986).

Of crucial importance are the findings that in patients with normal coronary arteries, intracoronary infusion of serotonin increase cross-sertional area and blood flow, an effect enhanced by 5-HT_2 serotonergic receptor blockade with ketanserin (Golino *et al.*, 1991).

However, in those with coronary atherosclerosis such a delivery of the mono-amine constructs coronary vessels and reduces blood flow markedly (Golino *et al.*, 1991; McFadden *et al.*, 1991), coronary artery constriction in patients with coronary atheroslerosis being attenuated by ketanserin (Golino *et al.*, 1991) (Fig. 5).

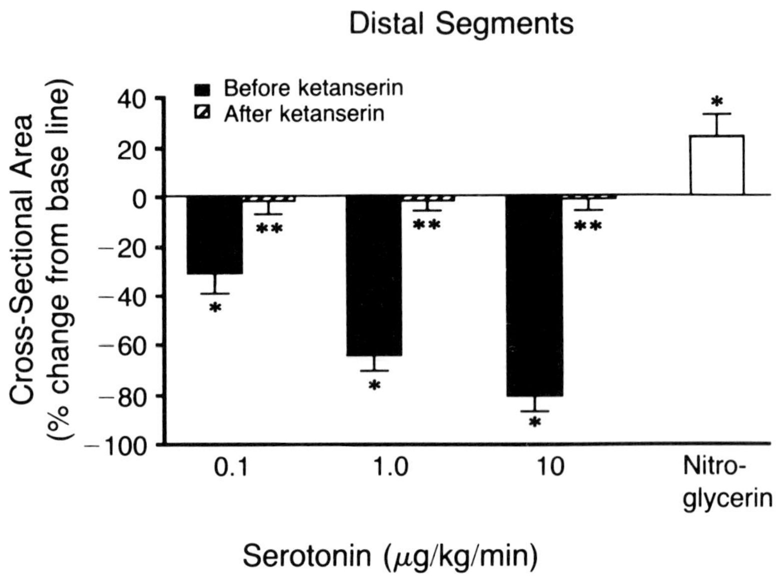

FIGURE 5. Reduction of coronary cross-sertional area by intracoronary serotonin in patients (n = 7) with coronary atheroslerosis is inhibited by ketanserin, a 5-HT_2 serotonergic receptor antagonist (0.25 mg/kg i.v.). * $P < 0.001$ versus baseline; ** $P < 0.01$ versus before ketanserin (adapted from information appearing in NEJM, Golino *et al.*, 1991).

This vascular hypersensitivity in pathologically modified arteries creates the possibility that serotonin released by those platelets initially activated at the site of a vessel wall injury before an occluding blood clot is formed can already induce localized vasospasms via 5-HT_2 serotonergic receptors. Such vasospasms are bound to jeopardize the magnitude and regularity of blood flow and can crack open an adjacent atheroslerotic plaque, thus favouring the build-up of an, occluding arterial thrombus (Mustard *et al.*, 1981).

1.3. PLATELET REACTIONS

Serotonin activates platelets functionally through 5-HT_2 serotonergic receptors, resembling the ones labeled with [^{3}H]spiperone or [^{3}H]ketanserin in cerebral membrane preparations and involved in vascular smooth muscle contractions. As for some other agonists, such an agonist-receptor interaction enhances the turnover of polyphosphoinositides, eventually resulting in an activation of the enzyme protein kinase

C and in an increase of cytoplasmic levels of Ca^{2+}-ions; these changes then mediate the platelet functional response.

In blood obtained from normal men, the functional response of platelets, exposed to serotonin as a single agonist, is a weak one: a shape change and a modest, transient aggregation reaction, the intensity of which does not suggest any physiological or pathological relevance (De Clerck and Vanhoutte, 1982; De Clerck *et al.*, 1984; De Clerck and de Chaffoy de Courcelles, 1989).

However, the mono-amine markedly amplifies platelet reactions to a variety of other agonists including TXA_2, catecholamines, adenosine diphosphate and thrombin via activation of 5-HT_2 serotonergic receptors on platelets. In that way, it enhances the extent of platelet aggregation, release of intragranular products and of arachidonic acid metabolites in response to otherwise ineffective agonist concentrations of other agonists (De Clerck and de Chaffoy de Courcelles, 1989) (Fig. 6). Such an amplification operates at low concentrations of serotonin, as seeping out of platelets subjected to

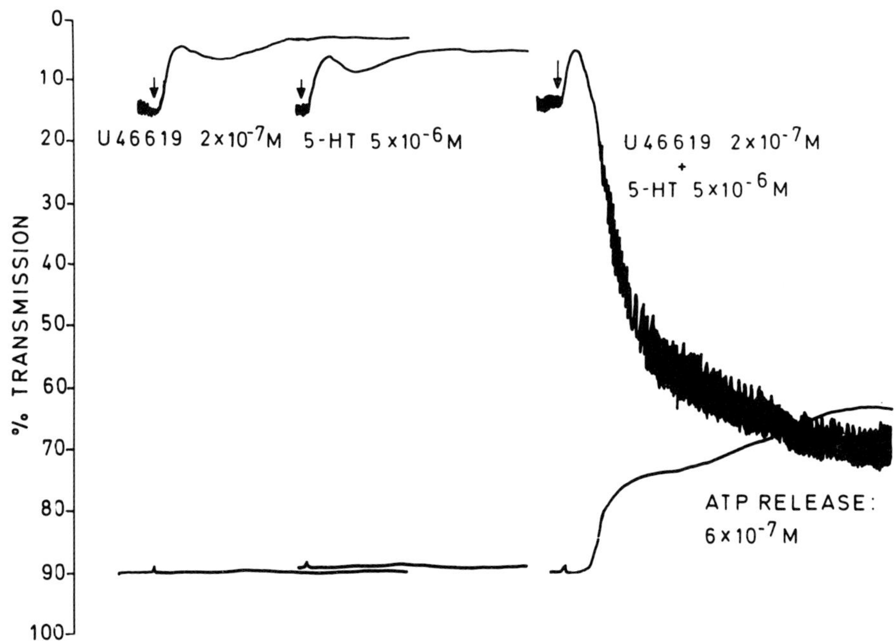

FIGURE 6. Amplification of human platelet activation by simultaneous activation of 5-HT_2 serotonergic receptors and of TXA_2/prostaglandin endoperoxide receptors. Combined challenge with separately ineffective concentrations of U46619 (left curve) and serotonin (5-HT; middle curve) results in an amplified response (right curve) in terms of platelet aggregation and release of intragranular products (ATP) (derived from De Clerck and Janssen, 1990).

shear stresses in physiological blood flow conditions *in vivo* (Osim and Wyllie, 1982) or released on the spot where platelets interact with an arterial wall lesion (Ashton *et al.*, 1986). Thereby, platelet-derived serotonin can play a substantial role in the progression of an initially modest mural thrombus, covering the vessel wall lesion, into a thrombus occluding the artery, causing cessation of blood flow. For example, cyclic cessations of blood flow caused by platelet aggregation/dislodgement at the locus of discrete endothelial cell injury in critically stenosed canine coronaries are eliminated by either TXA_2 synthase inhibition, TXA_2/prostaglandin endoperoxide receptor antagonism, or cyclo-oxygenase inhibition (Table 1) (Aiken, 1985), but also by 5-HT_2 serotonergic receptor blockade (Bush *et al.*, 1984; Golino *et al.*, 1988; De Clerck and Janssen, 1990) (Fig. 7).

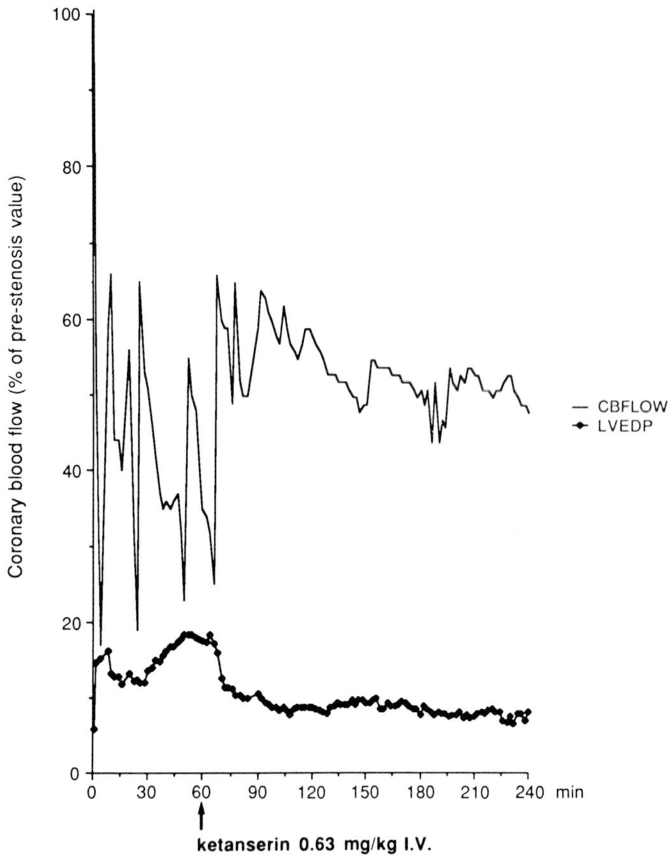

FIGURE 7. Cyclic blood flow reductions (CB-FLOW) in critically stenosed canine coronary arteries are caused by platelet deposition and subsequent dislodgement at the site of endothelial cell injury. Elimination by 5-HT_2 serotonergic receptor blockade with ketanserin points to a major contribution of platelet-derived serotonin in the coronary thrombotic process (LVEDP: left ventricular end diastolic pressure) (derived from De Clerck and Janssen, 1990).

TABLE 1. Involvement of serotonin and thromboxane A_2/prostaglandin endoperoxides in platelet aggregation/dislodgement causing cyclic reductions of blood flow in critically stenosed canine coronaries at sites of endothelial cell damage.

Antagonist	Efficacy*
- $5HT_2$ receptor antagonism (e.g. ketanserin)	> 90%
- TXA_2 synthase inhibition (e.g. OKY 1581, ridogrel)	> 90%
- TXA_2/PGH_2 receptor antagonism (e.g. SQ28668, ridogrel)	≥ 80 %
- Cyclo-oxygenase inhibition (e.g. aspirin)	50 %
- α_2-adrenoceptor antagonism (e.g. yohimbine)	50 %
- Heparin, dipyridamole	0 %

* Elimination of cyclic flow reductions in stated % of experiments. Based upon Aiken, 1985; Bush *et al.*, 1984; Golino *et al.*, 1988; Ashton *et al.*, 1986; Vandeplassche *et al.*, 1989.

In settings of extensive activation, platelet-dependent thrombus formation often escapes single pharmacological control. In such cases, a blockade of the serotonergic pathway of platelet activation substantially enhances the anti-platelet effect of other pharmacological interventions: extensive platelet aggregation produced by intra-aortic infusions of collagen in cats is only modestly influenced by single 5-HT_2 serotonergic receptor blockade with ketanserin; by contrast, it is strongly reduced or eliminated when ketanserin is combined with aspirin for cyclo-oxygenase inhibition or with ridogrel for dual TXA_2 synthase inhibition-TXA_2/prostaglandin endoperoxide receptor antagonism respectively (Fig. 8). This demonstrates the relevance for arterial thrombogenesis of synergistic interactions between the serotonin-dependent pathways of platelet activation with other platelet activating pathways (De Clerck *et al.*, 1990)

Apart from a contribution to occlusive thrombus formation in damaged arteries, platelet-derived serotonin also is involved in platelet-dependent reocclusion of coronary arteries subsequent to successful thrombolysis.

The simultaneous administration of thromboxane A_2/prostaglandin endoperoxide - (SQ29548) and 5-HT_2 serotonergic receptor (ketanserin, LY 53857) antagonists enhances the speed of thrombolysis and prevents or delays reocclusion after rt-PA in a canine, heparinised model in comparison with the effects of the single drugs (Golino *et al.*, 1988; Golino *et al.*, 1989). These observations suggest that the interaction of platelet-derived serotonin and thromboxane A_2 may compromise the efficacy of thrombolytic therapy by supporting further activation of platelets and their incorporation into the thrombus already during initial lysis of the thrombus.

To some extent, clinical data obtained so far with the 5-HT_2 serotonergic receptor antagonist ketanserin in man support the concept that platelet-derived serotonin contributes to the pathological expressions of platelet-vessel wall interactions, in particular those caused by arterial thrombus formation and blood flow reduction.

Indeed, a first controlled trial of percutaneous coronary angioplasty compared the effects of ketanserin 0.1 mg/min intravenously for 24 h, in addition to standard therapy comprising aspirin and heparin, in 21 patients, with those in control group of 22 patients given only standard therapy. Early restenosis at 24 h, due to platelet-dependent thrombus formation (Chesebro *et al.*, 1986), was significantly less in patients given ketanserin (Klein *et al.*, 1988).

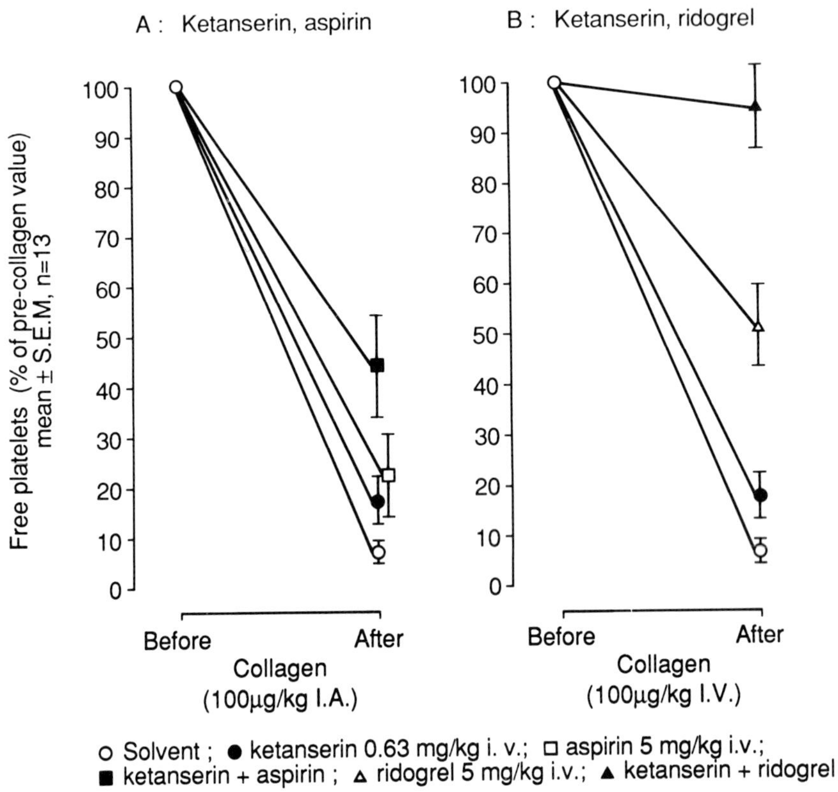

FIGURE 8. Extensive platelet aggregation, reflected by a drop in free circulating platelets, induced by intra-aortic infusion of collagen in cats is markedly reduced by combined treatment with ketanserin and aspirin (A) and with ketanserin and ridogrel (B). $P < 0.05$ for ketanserin, aspirin, ridogrel versus controls; $P < 0.05$ for ketanserin + aspirin and for ketanserin + ridogrel versus single compounds. This demonstrates synergistic interactions between serotonin-dependent and arachidonic-acid-dependent pathways of platelet activation (derived from De Clerck *et al.*, 1990).

Another trial in 62 patients with critical coronary stenosis again suggests a potential protective effect of ketanserin against platelet-related pathology: over a period of 2 years, 6 of 30 patients treated with aspirin (300 mg orally/day) developed myocardial infarction, compared with none of 32 given ketanserin (40 mg orally three times daily) (Noble and Drake-Holland, 1989).

A large double-blind, placebo-controlled study of the possible protective effects of ketanserin against thrombus formation or inadequate tissue perfusion was conducted in 3,899 patients with intermittent claudication. Primary events were vascular death, major stroke, myocardial infarction, leg amputation or excision of ischaemic viscera (PACK,

1989a; PACK, 1989b). Ketanserin, at the dose used in this trial (40 mg orally three times daily) can cause prolongation of the QT interval on the ECG and, probably because of this, a harmful interaction occurred when the active drug was given with potassium-wasting diuretics. This adverse effect did not occur when ketanserin was given alone or when prescribed with a potassium-conserving agent, whether or not a potassium-wasting agent was also given.

Overall "intention-to-treat" analysis was neutral: 136 study end-points were seen in the 1,930 patients treated with ketanserin, compared with 132 in the 1,969 given placebo. However, the number of patients undergoing amputation was significantly reduced (17 with ketanserin versus 32 with placebo; $P < 0.05$) (PACK, 1989b). This overall analysis was clouded by the adverse interaction between ketanserin and potassium-wasting diuretics. A secondary analysis, after exclusion of patients taking potassium-losing diuretics of anti-arrhythmic agents, showed 65 end-points in 1,514 patients taking ketanserin compared to 87 in 1,557 taking placebo, a 23 % reduction on ketanserin.

In a later and detailed evaluation of the trial, it was pointed out that after removal of the diuretic-treated patients the study lacked power and thus the trends in favour of ketanserin were not significant. Nevertheless, it was considered that, placed in context, they are sufficiently impressive to warrant other controlled trials to elucidate the possible value of 5-HT_2 receptor blockade with ketanserin (Chalmers and Murray, 1989; Doyle, 1990).

In conclusion, serotonin seems to be causally involved in platelet-vessel wall interactions leading to vascular smooth muscle cell proliferation, vasospasms, arterial thrombosis and its ischaemic repercussions on the myocardium. Therefore, compounds directed specifically against this autocoid may offer possibilities for treating human ischaemic heart disease.

2. References

Aalto, M. and Kulonen, E. (1972) 'Effects of serotonin, indomethacin and other antirheumatic drugs on the synthesis of collagen and other proteins in granulation tissue slices', Biochem. Pharmacol. 21, 2835-2840.

Ahmed, F.S. and Harrison, C.V. (1964) 'Morphological effects of serotonin on pulmonary arteries: an experimental study in rabbits', J. Path. Bact. 87, 325.

Aiken, J.W. (1985) 'Pharmacological analysis of factors influencing platelet aggregation in stenosed coronary arteries of dogs', Ann. N.Y. Acad. Sci. 454, 131-134

Ashton, J.H., Benedict, C.R., Fitzgerald, C., Raheja, S., Taylor, A., Campbell, W.B., Buja, L.M. and Willerson, J.T. (1986) 'Serotonin as a mediator of cyclic flow variations in stenosed canine coronary arteries', Circulation 73, 572-578.

Bazin, S., Pelletier, M. and Delaunay, A. (1973) 'The influence of chemical mediators of acute inflammation on the cells of a subacute inflammation', Agents Actions 3, 317-322.

Bertele, B. and Salzman, E.W. (1985) 'Anti-thrombotic therapy in coronary artery disease', Arteriosclerosis 5, 119-134.

Bevers, E.M., Rosing, J. and Zwaal, R.F.N. (1987) 'Platelets and coagulation', in: D.E. Mac Intyre, J.L. Gordon (eds.), Platelets in Biology and Pathology III, Amsterdam, Elsevier, pp. 127-1607.

Boucek, R.J. and Alvarez, T.R. (1970) '5-Hydroxytryptamine: a cytospecific growth stimulator of cultured fibroblasts', Science 167, 898-899.

Boucek, R.J. and Alvarez, T.R. (1971) 'Increase in survival of subcultured fibroblasts mediated by serotonin', Nature 229, 61-62.

Boucek, R.J., Speropoulos, A.J. and Noble, N.L. (1972) 'Serotonin and ribonucleic acid and collagen metabolism of fibroblasts *in vitro*', Proc. Soc. Exp. Biol. Med. 140, 599-603.

Bush, L., Campbell, W.B., Kenn, K., Tilton, G.P., Apprill, P., Ashton, J., Schmitz, J., Buja, L.M. and Willerson, J.T. (1984) 'The effects of alpha$_2$-adrenergic and serotonergic receptor antagonists on cyclic blood flow alterations in stenosed canine coronary arteries', Circ. Res. 55, 642-652.

Chalmers, T.C. and Murray, G.D. (1989) 'Retrospective analyses for hypothesis generation: a commentary on the PACK Trial (Prevention of Atherosclerotic Complications with Ketanserin), Clin. Exp. Hypertens. A11, 1117-1136.

Chesebro, J.H., Lam, J.Y.T. and Fuster, V. (1986) 'The pathogenesis and prevention of aortacoronary vein bypass graft occlusion and restenosis after arterial angioplasty: role of vascular injury and platelet thrombus deposition", J. Am. Coll. Cardiol. 8, 57B-66B.

De Clerck, F. and de Chaffoy de Courcelles, D. (1989) 'Amplification mechanisms in platelet activation', in P. Marche and P. Meyer (eds.), Blood Cells and Arteries in Hypertension and Atheroslerosis, Raven Press, New York, pp. 115-140.

De Clerck, F. and Janssen, P.A.J. (1990) '5-Hydroxytryptamine and thromboxane-A$_2$ in ischaemic heart disease', Blood Coagulation and Fibrinolysis 1, 201-210.

De Clerck, F. and Vanhoutte, P.M. (1982) '5-Hydroxytryptamine in peripheral reactions', Raven Press, New York, pp. 1-230.

De Clerck, F., Loots, W., Jageneau, A. and Nevelsteen, A. (1986) 'Correction by ketanserin of the platelet-mediated inhibition of peripheral collateral circulation in the cat: measurement of blood flow with radioactive microspheres', Drug Dev. Res. 8, 149-158.

De Clerck, F., Loots, W., Somers, Y., Beetens, J., Wijnants, J., Wouters, L. and Janssen, P.A.J. (1990) 5-Hydroxytryptamine and arachidonic acid metabolites modulate extensive platelet activation induced by collagen in cats *in vivo*', Br. J. Pharmacol. 99, 631-636.

De Clerck, F., Van Nueten, J.M. and Reneman, R.S. (1984) 'Platelet-vessel wall interactions: implication of 5-hydroxytryptamine', a review, Agents Actions 15, 611-616.

Doyle, A.E. (1990) 'Serotonin antagonists and vascular protection', Cardiovasc. Drugs Ther. 4, 11-16.

Erspamer, V. (1954) 'Pharmacology of indolealkylamines', Pharmacol. Rev. 6, 425-487.

Golino, P., Ashton, J.H., Glas-Greenwalt, P., McNatt, J., Buja, L.M. and Willerson, J.T. (1988) 'Medation of reocclusion by thromboxane A$_2$ and serotonin after thrombolysis with tissue-type plasminogen activator in a canine preparation of coronary thrombosis', Circulation 77, 678-684.

Golino, P., Ashton, J.H., McNatt, J., Glas-Greenwald, P., Sheng-Kun, Y., O'Brien, R.A., Buja, L.M. and Willerson, J.T. (1989) 'Simultaneous administration of thromboxane A$_2$- and serotonin S$_2$-receptor antagonists markedly enhances thrombolysis and prevents or delays reocclusion after tissue-type plasminogen activator in a canine model of coronary thrombosis', Circulation 79, 911-919.

Golino, P., Buja, L.M., Ashton, J.H., Kulkanni, P., Taylor, A. and Willerson, J.T. (1988) 'Effect of thromboxane and serotonin receptor antagonists on intracoronary platelet deposition in dogs with experimentally stenosed coronary arteries', Circulation 78, 701-711.

Golino, P., Piscione, F., Willerson, J.T., Cappelli-Bigazzi, M., Focaccio, A., Villari, B., Indolfi, C., Russolillo, F., Condorelli, M. and Chiariello, M. (1991) 'Divergent effects of serotonin on coronary artery dimensions and blood flow in patients with coronary atherosclerosis and control patients', N. Engl. J. Med. 324, 641-648.

Harker, L.A. and Ritchie, J.L. (1980) 'The role of platelets in acute vascular events', Circulation 62 (Suppl. V), V13-V18.

Heistad, D.D., Armstrong, M.L., Marcus, M.L., Peigors, D.J. and Mark, A.L. (1984) 'Augmented responses to vasoconstriction stimuli in hypercholesteremic and atherosclerotic monkeys', Circ. Res. 54, 711-718.

Heistad, D.D., Lopez, J.A.G. and Mayhan, W.G. (1990) 'Responses to serotonin in atheroslerotic and hypertensive blood vessels', in: R. Paoletti, P.M. Vanhoutte, N. Brunello, F.M. Maggi (eds.), Serotonin. From cell biology to pharmacology and therapeutics, Dordrecht: Kluwer Academic Publishers, pp. 137-40.

Hillis, L.D. and Lange, R.A. (1991) 'Serotonin and acute ischemic heart disease', N. Engl. J. Med. 324, 688-690.

Hollenberg, N. (1988) 'Serotonin, atherosclerosis and collateral vessel spasms', Am. J. Hypertens. 1, 312S-316S.

Klein, W., Brandt, D., Eber, B. and Dusleag, J. (1988) 'Prävention der frühen Restenosierung nach Perkutaner transluminaler Koronarangioplastie mit Serotonin-Antagonisten', Cor. Vasa. 2, 234-237.

Kokot, F. (1959) 'The role of serotonin in experimental atherosclerosis', Bull. Pol. Med. Hist. Sci. 2, 9-14.

Mann, P.R. (1967) 'Effects of various substances on DNA synthesis in guinea-pig skin *in vitro*', Nature 216, 715-716.

McFadden, E.P., Clarke, J.G., Davies, G.J., Kaski, J.C., Haider, A.W. and Maseri, A. (1991) 'Effect of intracoronary serotonin on coronary vessels in patients with stable angina and patients with variant angina', N. Engl. J. Med. 324, 648-654.

Mustard, J.F., Packham, M.A. and Kinlough-Rathbone, R.L. (1981) 'Mechanisms in thrombosis', in: A.C. Bloom, D.P. Thomas (eds.), Haemostasis and Thrombosis, Edinburgh, Churchill Livingstone, pp. 503-526.

Nemecek, G.M., Coughlin, S.R., Handley, D.A. and Moskowitz, M.A. (1986) 'Stimulation of aortic smooth muscle cell mitogenesis by serotonin', Prod. Natl. Acord. Sci. U.S.A. 83, 674-678.

Noble, M.I.M. and Drake-Holland, A. (1989) 'Prevention of atherosclerotic complications with ketanserin', Br. Med. J. 298, 752.

Osim, E.E. and Wyllie, J.H. (1982) 'Evidence for loss of 5-hydroxytryptamine from circulating platelets', J. Physiol. 325, 25P-26P.

PACK Trial Group (1989a) 'Prevention of atherosclerotic complications: Controlled trial of ketanserin', Br. Med. J. 298, 424-430.

PACK Trial Group (1989b) 'Randomized placebo-controlled, double-blind trial of ketanserin in claudicants: changes in claudication distance and ankle systolic pressure', Circulation 80, 1544-1548.

Page, I.H. (1958) 'Cardiovascular actions of serotonin (5-hydroxytryptamine)', in G.P. Lewis (ed.), 5-Hydroxytryptamine, Pergamon Press, London, pp. 93-108.

Ross, R., Bowen-Pope, D.F. and Raines, E.W. (1985) 'Platelets, macrophages, endothelium and growth factors. Their effects upon cells and their possible roles in atherogenesis', Am. N.Y. Acad. Sci. 454, 254-269.

Rossi, P. and Zamboni, L. (1958) 'Pulmonary atherosclerosis due to serotonin', Nature 181, 1216-1217.

Seuwen, K. and Pouysségur, J. (1990) 'Serotonin as a growth factor', Biochem. Pharmacol. 34, 985-990.

Shimokawa, H., Aarho, L.L. and Vanhoutte, P.M. (1987) 'Porcine coronary arteries with regenarated endothelium have a reduced endothelium-dependent responsiveness to aggregating platelets and serotonin', Circ. Res. 61, 256-270.

Van Nueten, J.M., Janssen, P.A.J., Symoens, J., Janssens, W.J., Heykants, J., De Clerck, F., Leysen, J.E., Van Cauteren, H. and Vanhoutte, P.M. (1987) 'Ketanserin', in: A. Scriabine (ed.), New Cardiovascular Drugs, New York, Raven Press, pp. 1-56.

Vandeplassche, L., Hermans, C., Van de Water, A., Xhonneux, R. and De Clerck, F. (1989) 'Differential effect of TXA_2 synthetase inhibition, singly or combined with TXA_2/PGH_2 receptor antagonism (R 68 070) on thrombosis over endothelial cell damage or deep intimal injury in canine coronary arteries', Thromb. Haemost. 62, 170.

Vanhoutte, P.M. (1985) 'Serotonin and the cardiovascular system', Raven Press, New York, pp. 1-288.

Vanhoutte, P.M. and Houston, D.S. (1985) 'Platelets, endothelium and vasospasm', Circulation 72, 728-734.

Vanhoutte, P.M., Van Nueten, J.M. and Janssen, W.J. (1990) 'Vascular serotonin receptors and cardiovascular disease', in: R. Paoletti, P.M. Vanhoutte, N. Brunello, F.M. Maggi, (eds.), Serotonin. From cell biology to pharmacology and therapeutics, Dordrecht, Kluwer Academic Publishers, pp. 81-96.

Verbeuren, T.J. (1990) '5HT, platelets and experimental atherosclerosis', in: R. Paoletti, P.M. Vanhoutte, N. Brunello, F.M. Maggi (eds.), Serotonin. From cell biology to pharmacology and therapeutics, Dordrecht, Kluwer Academic Publishers, pp. 131-36.

Verheyen, A., Lauwers, F., Vlaminck, F., Wouters, L. and De Clerck, F. (1991) 'Oversensitivity to serotonin of the collateralized vascular bed in rat hind quaters: mechanisms of increased vasoconstriction', Eur. J. Pharmacol. 194, 209-216.

Verheyen, A., Lauwers, F., Vlaminckx, E., Wouters, L. and De Clerck, F. (1988) 'Effects of vasoactive agonists on peripheral collateral arteries in *in situ* perfused rat hind quarters. Supersensitivity to serotonin', Int. J. Microcirc. 7, S132.

Vermylen, J., Verstraete, M. and Fuster, V. (1986) 'Role of platelet activation and fibrin formation in thrombogenesis', J. Am. Coll. Candiol. 8, 2B-9B.

THE INVOLVEMENT OF PAF IN THROMBOTIC EVENTS

C.P. Page, C.M. Herd and W. Paul

ABSTRACT. PAF is a potent stimulus of platelet and neutrophil activation both in vivo and in vitro which has an aggregatory profile distinct from other well known platelet agonists. In laboratory animals, PAF has been shown to induce a dose-related accumulation and subsequent retention of ^{111}Indium-labelled platelets into the pulmonary vascular bed. The release of nitric oxide within the pulmonary vascular bed is suggested to be an important regulatory event in limiting platelet aggregation physiologically. However, the pathological relevance of PAF in terms of human thrombotic conditions remains to be elucidated.

PAF is an ether-linked phospholipid, generated by a number of cell types, which was initially described for its ability to aggregate platelets [1]. PAF is an extremely potent platelet stimulus, since concentrations between 1-10nM are sufficient to induce activation **in vitro** of platelets from a range of species including man [2]. **In vitro**, PAF causes shape change and Ca^{2+} -dependent release of granular contents (eg. serotonin and ADP) [3]. Hence, release or generation of PAF **in vivo** will evoke a wide range of responses that are due to the biological activity of platelet activation products.

It is accepted that PAF produces platelet aggregation via a receptor-mediated process. Specific binding sites have been demonstrated on rabbit and human platelets using radioligand binding [4], and more recently a protein has been isolated from human platelets which is thought to be the PAF receptor [5]. A wide range of PAF receptor antagonists have been evaluated on PAF-induced platelet aggregation in a number of species including man [6]. This has led to the development of potent, orally active PAF antagonists for use in man

A. G. Herman (ed.), Antithrombotics, 195–203.
© 1991 *Kluwer Academic Publishers. Printed in the Netherlands.*

which all selectively inhibit **ex vivo** platelet aggregation induced by PAF in normal volunteers [7-9]. However, while none of these drugs has yet been finally tested in patients with thrombotic disease, these PAF antagonists do not produce overt changes in bleeding time [7], suggesting that PAF is not physiologically important in haemostasis of blood vessels. Nonetheless, PAF has been described to have very potent actions on platelets and other blood elements **in vivo** and has been implicated in the pathogenesis of various thrombotic and ischaemic conditions [10].

Numerous experimental systems have been developed to study platelet function **in vivo** [11-25]. The retention of platelets within the pulmonary vasculature induced by various platelet agonists, assessed histologically, has provided a quantitative index of platelet activation **in vivo** [20,26]. In addition, ^{51}Cr-labelled platelets present in organs (eg. lung tissue) and in blood samples following antigen challenge have been assessed using a gamma scintillation counter for the evaluation of aggregatory stimuli and of inhibitors of platelet function **in vitro** [20]. A technique for automating the detection of the rate of accumulation of radiolabelled platelets **in vivo** was subsequently devised [27], a system adapted from the clinical procedure whereby blood elements radiolabelled with gamma-emitting isotopes such as ^{51}Cr, ^{125}I and ^{111}In are externally imaged with gamma camera devices [28-30].

The intravenous administration of a variety of aggregatory stimuli (eg. ADP, collagen, PAF and antigen) has been shown to evoke increases in thoracic radioactive counts in experimental animals preloaded with ^{111}In-labelled platelets. Such increases can be attributed to the retention of platelets within the pulmonary vasculature, as lungs from animals sacrificed when thoracic counts are elevated show extensive evidence of platelet aggregates [20,31]. The intravenous administration of PAF (0.001 1ug/kg) into the anaesthetized rabbit produces a transient, reversible, dose-related accumulation of platelet-associated radioactivity into the thoracic region. The peak of the PAF response in this system is reached within 1-2 minutes following i.v. administration, i.e. similar to that observed with either collagen (100 ug/kg i.v.) or thrombin (32 IU/kg) but more delayed than that observed with ADP (100 ug/kg i.v., 20-30 seconds). The return to pre-administration levels following i.v. PAF occurs within 5-15 minutes, a much more long-lasting effect compared to ADP (less than 2 minutes) but not as protracted as the responses achieved with collagen (10-25 minutes) or thrombin (10-30 minutes). This increase in radioactive counts recorded over the thoracic area most likely reflects trapping of platelet aggregates within the pulmonary vasculature rather than changes in blood flow or blood volume, since comparable changes were not observed when similar experiments were performed with ^{111}Indium-labelled erythrocytes. In other species, similar profiles have been observed with ^{111}In-labelled platelets and histological sections of the lung tissue removed at the time of maximal increase in thoracic radioactivity reveal intravascular platelet aggregates throughout the pulmonary vasculature [31]. The intrathoracic accumulation of ^{111}In-labelled platelets following i.v. PAF in the rabbit is associated with a parallel loss of platelet-associated radioactivity from the hindlimb region. This most likely reflects the loss of platelets from the peripheral circulation (i.e. thrombocytopaenia) rather than changes in blood flow or blood volume since such changes were not observed when ^{111}In-labelled erythrocytes were used. This finding is in accordance with other reports of thrombocytopaenia following i.v. PAF in the rabbit [32,33]. Furthermore, following the intravenous administration of PAF, a concomitant fall in platelet-associated radioactivity in the cranial circulation was observed. Again, this is unlikely to reflect any changes in blood flow or blood volume, since similar changes were not observed when ^{111}In-labelled erythrocytes were used. These observations would suggest that the platelet aggregates transiently formed in the pulmonary vasculature following i.v. PAF consist of platelets recruited from both the peripheral and cranial circulations.

The PAF antagonists SRI 63-441 [34], (1 mg/kg i.v.) and brotizolam, [35] (1 mg/kg i.v.) fully inhibited PAF-induced intrathoracic ^{111}In-labelled platelet accumulation in the rabbit. Inhibition was selective since this dose of SRI 63-441 and brotizolam did not diminish responses of a similar magnitude induced by ADP (100 ug/kg i.v.) or collagen (100 ug/kg i.v.), [36]. The effect of SRI 63-441 was dose-related over the range 0.01- 1 mg/kg. A similar finding has been reported in guinea pigs [29], using a similar **in vivo** technique.

PAF-induced accumulation of ^{111}In-labelled platelets in the rabbit appears to be thromboxane-independent, as dazmegrel (10 mg/kg i.v.), a potent and selective thromboxane synthetase inhibitor [37,38], does not inhibit platelet accumulation induces by PAF [36]. Furthermore, cyclo-oxygenase inhibitors aspirin and indomethacin caused a significant potentiation of the PAF-induced platelet response, possibly due to stimulation of the platelet lipoxygenase pathway as a consequence of the blockade of the enzyme cyclo-oxygenase, leading to the formation of possible platelet-active lipid products [36].

Under physiological conditions the aggregatory response to i.v. PAF and other agonists of platelet function is reversible. The lung vasculature is a considerable source of vascular endothelium and one product of this endothelium, endothelium-derived nitric oxide (NO) is widely believed to play an important role in vascular haemostasis. NO is a potent vasodilator [39], and inhibits both platelet adhesion [40], and platelet/neutrophil aggregation **in vitro** [41,42]. Stimuli of NO release (eg. carbachol, substance P) have been shown to reduce platelet aggregation in intact animals [43-45]. To investigate the role of NO as a possible regulator of platelet aggregation and/or dis-aggregation **in vivo**, studies have been performed using L-N^G-nitro arginine methyl ester (L-NAME) a potent and selective inhibitor of vascular and non-vascular NO biosynthesis [46,47]. L-NAME (10 mg/kg), but not its biologically inert enantiomer D-NAME, significantly enhanced the intrathoracic accumulation of ^{111}Indium-labelled platelets and neutrophils induced by a sub-maximal dose of PAF administered i.v. in the rabbit [48]. These results suggest that endogenously produced NO from the pulmonary vascular bed may play a role in actively limiting platelet and PMN aggregation within the pulmonary vasculature. Such a mechanism could provide a unique protective mechanism to ensure that blood elements entering the systemic circulation from the pulmonary circulation are not activated and thus reduce the incidence of thrombotic events occurring in peripheral arterial vascular beds, eg. the coronary or cerebral circulation. Furthermore, the failure of this important regulatory role of the pulmonary vascular endothelium could result in initial retention of platelet aggregates within the vascular bed, namely pulmonary embolism. It is therefore of interest that the selective PAF antagonist WEB 2086 has been shown to inhibit pulmonary embolism in sheep [49].

In an **in vivo** rabbit model for investigating platelet function recently described ^{111}In-labelled platelet accumulation in the cranium can be induced by the intracarotid (i.c.) administration of thrombin (100 IU/kg) [30]. Initially, thrombin administration via the carotid artery elicited a similar pattern to that observed following the administration of thrombin via the i.v. route, i.e. accumulation of platelets within the pulmonary vascular bed. However, a pronounced accumulation of ^{111}In-labelled platelets in the cranial vasculature was sustained up to 3 [30], and 6 hours after challenge [48]. This accumulation of platelets is unlikely to be attributable to changes in blood flow or blood volume within the cranial circulation as comparable changes were not observed when ^{111}In-labelled erythrocytes were used [30]. The magnitude of the platelet accumulation within the cranial circulation was approximately 3-fold greater than that seen in the pulmonary circulation with other platelet agonists administered i.v. (i.e. ADP, PAF collagen and thrombin). The precise nature of this platelet-associated radioactivity remains to be determined, but it could represent overt embolisation of platelets within regions of the cranial vasculature or deposition of platelets on damaged vessel walls. Thrombin is certainly known to elicit vascular wall injury [50], and to release a variety of biologically active materials from the vascular endothelium [51]. However, the inability of PAF to mimic the effect of thrombin in this respect suggests that, while thrombin can release PAF from endothelial cells [52], this phospholipid is unlikely to contribute to platelet accumulation observed following intracarotid administration of thrombin. This conclusion is supported by experiments demonstrating that pretreatment of rabbits with the PAF antagonist BN 52021 (10 mg/kg i.v.) 5 minutes prior to the i.c. administration of thrombin (100 IU/kg) had no significant effect on the accumulation of radiolabelled platelets in the cranial vasculature. However, this same dose of BN 52021 abolished the thoracic response to i.v. PAF, but failed to inhibit the response to i.v. ADP [48]. Such results suggest that PAF may not be involved in the initial thrombotic events within the cranial circulation following activation of thrombin. However, there is considerable evidence suggesting the involvement of PAF in central nervous system functions and ischaemic diseases [6]. A potential role for PAF in the CNS was suggested by the finding that triazolobenzodiazepines (alprazolam or triazolam) and some benzodiazepines exert PAF antagonism. Evidence based on the beneficial effects of various PAF antagonists now exists demonstrating the involvement of PAF in animal models of cerebral ischaemia [53, 54]. PAF is known as a highly potent mediator of injury responses in a variety of tissues including gastric intestinal and cardiac ischaemia [6]. It therefore remains to be established whether or not PAF contributes to the ischaemic injury resulting from occlusion of the cranial vasculature in man.

References

1. Benveniste J, Henson PM, Cochrane CG. (1972) Leucocyte dependent histamine release from rabbit platelets: the role of IgE, basophils and a platelet activating factor. J Exp Med 136, 1356-1377.
2. Chignard M, Le Couedic JP, Vargaftig BB, Benveniste J. (1979) The role of platelet activating factor in platelet aggregation. Nature 279, 799-800.
3. Henson PM. (1976) Activation of rabbit platelets by platelet activating factor derived from IgE-sensitised basophils: I. Characteristics of the secretory

response. J Exp Med 143, 937-952.
4. Hwang SB, Lee CSC, Cheah MJ, Shen TY. (1983) Specific receptor sites for 1-O-alkyl-2-O-acetyl-sn-glycero-3-phosphorylcholine (platelet activating factor) on rabbit platelet and guinea pig smooth muscle membranes. Biochemistry 22, 4756-4763.
5. Valone FH. (1984) Isolation of a platelet membrane protein which binds the platelet-activating factor 1-O-hexadecyl-2-acetyl-sn-glycero-3-phosphocholine. Immunology 52, 169-174.
6. Braquet P, Touqui L, Shen TY, Vargaftig BB. (1987) Perspectives in platelet activating factor research. Pharmacol Rev 39, 97-145.
7. Adamus WS, Huer H, Meade CJ, Frey G, Brecht HM (1988) Inhibitory effect of oral WEB 2086, a novel selective PAF-acether antagonist, on **ex vivo** platelet aggregation, Eur J Clin Pharmacol 35, 237-240.
8. Chung KF, Dent G, McCusker M, Guinot Ph, Page CP, Barnes CP. (1987). Effects of a specific antagonist of platelet activating factor (BN 52063). Lancet i, 248-251.
9. Heuer HO, Casals-Stenzel J, Muacevic G, Weber KH. (1990) Pharmacologic activity of bepafant (WEB 2170), a new and selective hetrazepinoic antagonist of platelet activating factor. J Pharmacol Exp Ther 255, 962-968.
10. Bourgain RH, Vargaftig BB. (1990) PAF and blood cells - pathophysiological correlates. In: Barnes PJ, Page CP, Henson PM eds. PAF and human disease. Oxford: Blackwell Scientific Publications, 220-230.
11. Born GVR, Cross MJ. (1963) Effect of adenosine diphosphate on the concentration of platelets in circulating blood. Nature 197, 974-976.
12. Hornstra G. (1970) A method for the determination of thrombocyte aggregation in circulating rat blood. Experientia 26, 111-112.
13. Smith GM, Freuler F. (1973) The measurement of intravascular aggregation by continuous platelet counting. Bibl Anat 12, 229-234.
14. Bourgain RH, Six F. (1974) A continuous registration method in experimental arterial thrombosis in the rat. Thromb Res 4, 599-607.
15. Wu KK, Hoak JC (1974) A new method for the quantitative detection of platelet aggregates in patients with arterial insufficiency. Lancet ii, 924-926.
16. Baumgartner HR, Muggli R, Tschopp TB, Turitto VT. (1976) Platelet adhesion, release and aggregation in flowing blood: effects of surface properties and platelet function. Thrombos Haemostas 35, 124-138.
17. Kohler C, Wooding W, Ellenbogen L. (1976) Intravenous arachidonate in the mouse: a model for the evaluation

of antithrombotic drugs. Thromb Res 9, 67-80.

18. Buchanan MR, Hirsch J. (1978) A comparison of the effects of aspirin and dipyridamole on platelet aggregation **in vivo** and **ex vivo**. Thromb Res 13, 517-529.
19. Gryglewski RJ, Korbut R, Ocetkiewicz A, Spawinski J, Wojtaszek B, Swies J. (1978) Lungs as a generator of prostacyclin - hypothesis on physiological significance. Arch Pharmacol 304, 45-50.
20. Butler KD, Walls RB, White AM. (1979) A study of the relationship between **ex vivo** and **in vivo** effects of sulphinpyrazone in the guinea pig. Haemostasis 9, 353-360.
21. Shishido M, Katori M. (1981) A quantitative method using continuous recording of platelet thrombus size in hamster cheeck pouch. Microvasc Res 22, 199-209.
22. Garcia-Rafanell J, Forn J. (1982) Intravenous arachidonate-induced respiratory distress: comparative study of three **in vivo** models for the measurement of antithrombotic activity. J Pharmacol Meth 7, 231-238.
23. Badimon L, Fuster V, Chesebro JH, Dewanjee MK. (1983) New **ex vivo** radioisotopic method of quantitation of platelet deposition studies in four animal species. Thromb Haemostas 50, 639-644.
24. Pinon JF. (1984) **In vivo** study of platelet aggregation in rats. J Pharmacol Meth 12, 79-84.
25. Del Zoppo GJ, Copeland BR, Harker LA, Waltz TA, Zyroff J, Hanson SR, Battenberg E. (1986) Experimental acute thrombotic stroke in baboons. Stroke 17, 1254-1265.
26. Pinckard RN, Halonen M, Palmer JD, Butler C, Shaw JO , Henson PM. (1977) Intravascular aggregation and pulmonary sequestration of platelets during IgE induced systemic anaphylaxis in the rabbit: abrogation of lethal anaphylactic shock by platelet depletion. J Immunol 119, 2185-2193.
27. Davies OJ, Morley J, Page CP,Paul W. (1981) **In vivo** aggregation of guinea-pig platelets. J Physiol 320, 3-4P.
28. Page CP, Paul W, Morley J. (1982) An **in vivo** model for studying platelet aggregation and disaggregation. Thromb Haemostas 47, 210-213.
29. Smith D, Sanjar S, Herd C, Morley J. (1989) **In vivo** method for the assessment of platelet accumulation. J Pharmacol Med 21, 45-59.
30. May GR, Herd CM, Butler KD, Page CP. (1990) A radioisotopic model for investigating thromboembolism in the rabbit. J Pharmacol Meth 24, 19-35.
31. Dewar A, Archer CB, Paul W, Page CP, Macdonald DM , Morley J. (1984) Cutaneous and pulmonary histopathological responses to platelet activating factor (Paf-acether) in the guinea pig. J Pathol 144,

25-34.

32. Honey AC, Lad N, Tuffin DP. (1986) Effect of indomethacin and dazoxiben on intravascular platelet aggregation in the anaesthetized rabbit. Thromb Haemostas 56, 80-85.
33. McManus LM. (1987) Acute lung injury induced by intravascular platelet activating factor. In: Winslow CM, Lee ML eds. New horizons in platelet activating factor research. Chichester: John Wiley and Sons, 233-244.
34. Handley DA, Tomesch JC, Saunders RN. (1986) Inhibition of PAF-induced systemic responses in the rat, guinea-pig, dog and primate by the receptor antagonist SRI 63-441. Thromb Haemostas 56, 40-44.
35. Casals-Stenzel J. (1987). The inhibitory activity of brotizolam and related compounds on platelet activating factor (PAF)-induced effects **in vitro** and **in vivo**. In: Winslow CM, Lee ML eds. New horizons in platelet activating factor research. Vol. 29, John Wiley and Sons Ltd, 277-285.
36. Herd CM. (1991) Pharmacological modulation of PAF-induced platelet accumulation in the pulmonary circulation of the rabbit. Brit J Pharmacol 102, 175.
37. Vermylen J, DeFreyn G, Carreras LO, Machin SJ, Van Schaeren J, Verstraete M. (1981) Thromboxane synthetase inhibition as antithrombotic strategy. Lancet i, 1073-1075.
38. Fitzgerald GA, Oates JA. (1984). Selective and nonselective inhibition of thromboxane formation. Clin Pharmacol Ther 35, 633-640.
39. Furchgott RF, Zawadzki JV. (1980) The obligatory role of endothelial cells in the relaxation of arterial smooth muscle by acetylcholine. Nature 288, 373-376.
40. Radomski MW, Palmer RMJ, Moncada S. (1987) Endogenous nitric oxide inhibits human platelet adhesion to vascular endothelium. Lancet ii, 1057-1058.
41. Azuma H, Ishikawa M, Sekizaki S. (1986) Endothelium-dependent inhibition of platelet aggregation. Brit J Pharmacol 88, 411-415.
42. McCall TB, Boughton-Smith NK, Palmer RMJ, Whittle BJR, Moncada S. (1989) Synthesis of nitric oxide from L-arginine by neutrophils: release and interaction with superoxide anion. Biochem J 261, 293-296.
43. Bhardwaj R, Page CP, May GR, Moore PK. (1988). Endothelium derived relaxing factor inhibits platelet aggregation in human whole blood and in the rat **in vivo**. Eur J Pharmacol 157, 83-92.
44. Hogan JC, Lewis MJ, Henderson AH. (1988) **In vivo** EDRF actifity influences platelet function. Brit J Pharmacol 94, 1020-1022.
45. Humphries RG, Tomlinson W, O'Connor SE, Leff P. (1990)

Inhibition of collagen- and ADP-induced platelet aggregation by substance P **in vivo:** involvement of endothelium-derived relaxing factor. J Cardiovasc Pharmacol 16, 292-297.

46. Gibson A, Mirzazadeh S, Hobbs A, Moore PK. (1990) L-N^G-monomethyl arginine and L-N^G-nitro arginine inhibit non-adrenergic, non-cholinergic relaxation of the mouse anococcygeus muscle. Brit J Pharmacol 99, 602-606.
47. Moore PK, Al-Swayeh OA, Chong NWS, Evans RA, Gibson A. (1990) L-N^G-nitro arginine (L-NOARG), a novel L-arginine-reversible inhibitor of endothelium-dependent vasodilation **in vitro.** Brit J Pharmacol 99, 408-412.
48. May GR, Crook P, Moore KP, Page CP. (1991) The role of nitric oxide as an endogenous regulator of platelet and neurophil activation within the pulmonary circulation of the rabbit. Brit J Pharmacol 102, 759-763.
49. Malik AB (1991) Platelets and pulmonary embolism. In: Page CP ed. The platelet in health and disease. Blackwell Scientific Publications, in press.
50. Malik AB. (1983) Pulmonary microembolism. Physiol Rev 63, 1115-1207.
51. Schuman MA. (1986) Thrombin-cellular interactions. Ann NY Acad Sci 485, 228-239.
52. Prescott SM, Zimmerman GA, McIntyre TM. (1984) Human endothelial cells in culture produce platelet activating factor (1-alkyl-2-acetyl-sn-glycero-3-phosphocholine) when stimulated with thrombin. Proc Natl Acad Sci USA 81, 3534-3538. Immunol 119, 2185-2193.
53. Braquet P, Paubert-Braquet M, Koltai M, Bourgain R, Bussolino F, Hosford D. (1989) Is there a case for PAF antagonists in the treatment of ischaemic states? Trends Pharmacol Sci 10, 23-30.
54. Braquet P, Spinnewyn B, Demerle C, Hosford D, Marcheselli V, Rossawska M, Bazan N. (1989) The role of platelet activating factor in cerebral ischaemia and related disorders. In: Barkai V, Bazan NG eds. New York Acadamy of Science, 559, 296-312.

PROSTAGLANDINS AND -ANALOGS IN THE TREATMENT OF PLATELET VESSEL WALL INTERACTION

Helmut SINZINGER

ABSTRACT. Endogenous prostaglandins have been shown to beneficially affect the haemostatic balance. Experimental as well as clinical pharmacological data confirmed this benefit for PGE1, PGI2 and the analogs iloprost and taprostene. Controlled trials are available in the sequence of number and quality for PGE1, iloprost and PGI2. The intermittent, intravenous long-term treatment seems to be the preferable one, especially in the studies conducted more recently. In general, the above mentioned studies show a clear benefit for the patients concerning various endpoints such as painfree walking distance, pain relief, ulcer healing or amputation rate. These results underline the clinical value of this group of substances and the promise in the treatment of peripheral vascular disease.

Introduction

After the discovery and the structural identification of prostaglandin (PG) E1 (Bergström et al., 1963) and later on PGI2 (Moncada et al., 1976), their antiaggregatory capacity attracted central interest. This mechanism was claimed as a rationale for the substitutional treatment in situations such as atherosclerosis which was assumed to be a deficiency stage of endogenous synthesis (Szczeklik et al., 1979). The examination of underlying background mechanisms, however, has almost been neglected at this early time. Initially very enthusiastic reports were follwed by later rather pessimistic views. This resulted in a variety of different therapeutic schemes tested with different success. In the meanwhile a variety of antiatherosclerotic actions for both PGE1 and PGI2 as well as synthetic analogs has been demonstrated. In parallel, a significant benefit has been documented in the sequence of the amount of data available for PGE1, iloprost and PGI2. However, due to their extremely varying design a comparison concerning qualitative and quantitative profile is very difficult.

A. G. Herman (ed.), Antithrombotics, 205–220.
© 1991 *Kluwer Academic Publishers. Printed in the Netherlands.*

Mechanisms

The prostaglandins mentioned are beneficially interfering with all the 3 major pathogenetic mechanisms of atherosclerosis, i.e. a. (parietal) thrombus formation (Rokitansky, 1852), b. cellular proliferation (Virchow, 1856) and c. lipid metabolism (Anitschkow, 1913; for overview see table 1). As a matter of fact, due to the interspecies differences, the wide variety of test models and in experimental animals and the differences in study designs actual comparisons are difficult.

a. Thrombus formation: PGE1, PGI2 and analogs have been shown to inhibit platelet activity via specific receptors and an elevation of intracellular cAMP in vitro. The antiplatelet-activity for PGE1 ex-vivo is much less pronounced as for the I-family compounds. All the substances show the synergism with nitric oxide (NO; Radomski et al., 1987a), one of the acting compounds of the endothelium derived relaxing factor (EDRF; Radomski et al., 1987b). EDRF acts via alterations in cGMP. This synergism has been shown also in-vivo for PGE1 and PGI2 with in-vivo NO-donors (isosorbidedinitrate, molsidomine; Sinzinger et al., 1990, 1991a). A stabilization of vascular surface lining is evidenced also by a decreased number of circulating endothelial cells. Furthermore, all the compounds share the unique property of inducing thromboresistance both in-vitro and in-vivo, keeping cells (not only platelets) apart from the vessel wall (Sinzinger et al., 1983). In this context, the decrease in neutrophil activation exerted especially by PGE1 and probably by taprostene is of particular interest (Hecker et al., 1990). This effect is mediated by cAMP too. PGI2 itself does not seem to possess their property. In-vitro studies further demonstrated an inhibitory effect on the release of various mitogens, in particular the platelet derived growth factor (PDGF; Willis et al., 1986). For PGE1 an increased red blood cell flexibility and a diminished erythrocyte aggregation have been documented. Fibrinolytic activity was shown both in-vitro and in-vivo for PGE1, PGI2 and analogs.

b. Cellular proliferation: All the prostaglandins (I2, E1) inhibit mitotic and proliferative activity of smooth muscle cells (SMC), extracellular matrix synthesis (glycosaminoglycans and collagen) partly studied in vitro or in experimental animals. One study performed in human indicates a similar benefit (Sinzinger et al., 1986a). From these data it becomes evident that the effect on SMC is mediated in part directly and in part by the inhibitory action on the release of mitogens from different cells.

c. Lipid metabolism: Especially for PGE1 (I-series less effective?) a benefit at the vascular wall level was demonstrated. There seems to be a decreased cholesterol esterification, while the degradation is stimulated in parallel, resulting in a net decrease of cholesterol in SMC (Willis et al., 1986). Reduced arterial surface areas of Sudan III-positive staining and a decreased vascular cholesterol content have been measured as well (Sinzinger et al., 1991b). A decreased entry of 125I-LDL into the arterial wall has been documented in rabbits, while a comparable benefit in human was recently confirmed after autologous LDL-labelling with 123I (Sinzinger et al., 1986b). At the liver an increased number of LDL-receptors without a change in binding affinity can be seen (Virgolini et al., 1991), being most likely due to an increase in messenger RNA for receptor protein synthesis. It appears that this effect applies for the E- and I-series as well.

TABLE 1. Mechanisms of action of PGE1, PGI2, (13,14-DH-PGE1)

Mechanisms	PGE1	PGI2	(13,14-DH PGE1)	analogs
White blood cells	+	-	+	+
Red blood cells	+	+	-	?
Mitotic activity	+	+	+	?
SMC-proliferation	+	+	+	?
GAG-synthesis	+	+	+	?
Collagen synthesis	+	+	+	?
Cholesterol synthesis	+	?	+	?
Cholesterol degradation	+	+	+	?
LDL-entry ↓	+	?	+	?
LDL-receptors ↑	+	?	+	?
thromboresistance	+	+	-	+
cytoprotection	+	+	-	+
substrate utilization	+	?	-	?
antiarrhythmic	+	+	-	+

Clinical trials

The number of trials available and the evidence of clinical efficacy of the various substances are highly dependent on the activities of the pharmaceutical companies marketing these compounds. At least for 3 of them (in the sequence of evidence), namely PGE1, iloprost and PGI2 clinical benefit has been proven in certain stages of peripheral arterial disease.

TABLE 2. Continuous i.a. PGE1-infusion

Author	design	n	dosis PGE1	duration	stage of PVD	results s/ns
Carlson et al. (1973)	n.c.	4	1ng/kg min	24-72 h	III/I V	pain gangrain healing
Sakaguchi (1984)	con.	65	0.05ng/kg min	24 d	III/IV	27% UH(s) 82% pain pos. long-term
Gruss et al. (1984)	n.c.	105	0.19ng/kg min	38 d mean	III/IV	Thromb.obl: 71% III/IV>IIb Ath+MOD:30% III/IV>IIb Ath-MOD:47% III/IV>IIb pos. long-term
Biedermann (1984)	n.c.	22	0.09-0.48 ng/kg/min	15 d	III/IV	impr: 12/14
Hirai (1986)	n.c.	12	0.1-03 ng/kg/min	3x1 h	III/IV	change IIb: 9/12

s ... significant, ns ... not significant
con ... controlled; n.c. ... not controlled
UH ... ulcer healing

The greatest number of clinical data is available at present for PGE1 (most of them administering α-cyclodextrin PGE1) allowing to group the studies communicated according to the route (i.v. vs. i.a., tables 2,3 vs. 4,5) and the mode (continuous vs. intermittent, tables 2,4 vs. 3,5) of administration. The data for PGI2 (table 6) and iloprost (table 7) are much less broad documented. Thus, the enormous differences in design of the study, dose of the prostaglandin, duration of therapy, stage of the disease and last but not least the

TABLE 3. Intermittent i.a. PGE1-infusion

Author	design	n	dosis PGE1	duration	stage of PVD	results s/ns
Pilger et al. (1983)	n.c.	20	5,85ng/kg/min	5 d	III/IV	AP,UH 75% (s)
Hach et al. (1986)	n.c.	55	10 µg/90min	19-28 d	IIb	433% painfree walking (s)
Bertuch et al. (1986)	n.c.	64	5ng/kg/min	7 d	III/IV	change IIb 42/64 (s)
Bruch et al. (1986)	n.c.	25	0,1-4ng/kg/min	10 d	III/IV	UH 78% (s)
Blume (1987)	con.	50	10-20µg/90min	21 d	IIb	109% painfree walking (s)
Creutzig et al. (1987)	con.	30	2x5 µg/50min	17 d	IIb	471% painfree walking (s)
Zanke et al. (1987)	n.c.	55	2ng/kg/min	18 - 27d	IIb	433% painfree walking (s)
Rudofsky et al. (1987)	con.	50	20 µg/120min	21 d	IIb	170% painfree walking (s)
Trübestein et al. (1987)	con.	57	20 µg/60min	21 d	III/IV	52% analgetics reduction (s) 90% UH (s)
Creutzig et al. (1988)	con.	40	2x5 µg/50min	21 d	IIb	255% painfree walking (ns) pos. long-term
Balzer et al. (1989)	n.c.	218	10-20µg/120min	28 d	III/IV	84% pain reduction (s) 58% UH (s)
Böhme et al. (1989)	con.	34	10-20µg/60min	23 d	III/IV	39% of III/IV>IIb (ns) 78% UH (ns) pos. long-term

s ... significant; ns ... not significant; UH ... ulcer healing; con ... controlled; n.c. ... not controlled

TABLE 4. Continuous i.v. PGE1-infusion

Author	design	n	dosis PGE1	duration	stage of PVD	results
Carlson et al. (1976)	n.c.	8	2-4ng/kg/min 10min/h	3 d	III/IV	UH: 5/7
Pardy et al. (1980)	n.c.	12	10ng/kg/min	3 d	III/IV	RP: 3/21 UH:11/21
Feldman et al. (1982)	n.c.	14	21ng/kg/min	2 h	III/IV	UH
Martin et al. (1982)	n.c.	12	6-10ng/kg/min	3 d	III/IV	RS:10/12 UH: 2/8
Ambrus et al. (1983)	n.c.	11	0.6-1ng/kg/min	70 h	III/IV	UH:9/11
Rhodes et al. (1983)	con.	8	20ng/kg/min	3 d	IV	RP UH
Schuler et al. (1984)	con.	123	20ng/kg/min	3 d	IV	RP UH
Telles et al. (1984)	con.	30	10ng/kg/min	3 d	IV	RP UH
Clifford et al. (1984)	n.c.	26	6-10 ng/kg/min	3 d	III/IV	UH: 5/8
Joggestrand et al. (1985)	con.	18	3ng/kg/min	3 d	IV	RP UH
Kyle et al. (1985)	n.c.	12	6-10ng/kg/min	3 d	III/IV	RS: 9/12
Heidrich et al. (1986)	n.c.	15	40µg	1 h	II/IV	tcPO2
Hirai et al. (1986)	n.c.	42	40µg	60-90 min	II/IV	ST; PBF
Ehrly et al. (1987)	n.c.	10	40µg	2 h	II/IV	tcPO2

n.c. ... not controlled; con ... controlled;
UH ... ulcer healing; RP ... rest pain; RS ...
ST ... ; PBF ...

TABLE 5. Intermittent i.v. PGE1-infusion

Author	design	n	dosis PGE1	duration	stage of PVD	results s/ns
Eklund et al. (1982)	con.	22	7x20 µg/d	3 d	IV	UH (s) neg. long-term
Diehm et al. (1988)	con.	46	1x60 µg/d	21 d	III	67% pain reduction (s) 36% v. III>IIb (s) pos. follow-up
Rudofsky (1988)	con.	50	1x60 µg/d	28 d	IIb	73% painfree walking (s)
Trübestein et al. (1989)	con.	70	2x40 µg/d	28 d	IV	61% pain reduction (ns) 73 % analg. reduction (s) 59% UH (s) pos. long-term (s)
Balzer et al. (1989)	n.c.	211	1x60 µg/d 2x40 µg/d	28 d	III/IV	85% pain reduction (ns) 62% UH (s)
Diehm et al. (1989)	con.	48	1x60 µg/d	21 d	IIb	97% painfree walking (ns) pos. long-term (s)
Heidrich et al. (1991)	n.c.	203	2x40 µg/d	27 d	III/IV	68% pain reduction 59% UH pos. long-term

s ... significant; ns ... not significant
con ... controlled; n.c. ... not controlled;
UH ... ulcer healing

TABLE 6. PGI2-therapy in patients with PVD

Author	design	n	dosis ng/kg/min	duration	stage	clin. success ulcer	pain relief
Szczeklik et al. (1979)	n.c.	5	5-10	72i.a.	III/IV	+3/5	100%
Szczeklik et al. (1980)	n.c.	30	2-10	72i.a.	III/IV	+17/19	14/16
Pardy et al. (1980)	n.c.	9	8-15	72-96i.v.	III/IV	pos.	n.m.
Hossmann et al. (1981)	co/d	10	5	72i.v.	III/IV	+7/10	n.m.
Olsson et al. (1981)	n.c.	8	1-5 12h/day	72i.v. 72i.v.	III/IV	+6/8	6/8
Belch et al. (1983)	d	28	2.5-10	96i.a.	III	+13/15	100%
Hossmann et al. (1984)	co/d	12	5	168i.v.	III/IV	+8/11	75%
Negus et al. (1985)	con.	33	8	72i.a.	III/IV	*	*
Nizankowski et al. (1985)	d	30	5	72i.a.	III/IV	+7/21	n.m.
Fitscha et al. (1985)	d	108	6 8h/day	120i.v.	II	pos.	

* ... no difference to Praxilen; n.m. ... not mentioned; con. ... controlled; n.c. ... uncontrolled; d ... double-blind; co ... cross-over

clinical endpoint limit the validity of conclusions to be drawn. For taprostene only anecdotal positive findings were communicated, while no well controlled study is available so far for this stable synthetic analog. Nevertheless, beside the significant clinical benefit for PGE1 there are at least 2 well controlled studies for PGI2 and iloprost each providing a similar outcome. Summarizing, only the well controlled studies (double blind, controlled vs. placebo or other substances) in stages III and IV according to Fontaine (table 6) offers a proof for the clinical benefit.

Discussion

No useful parameter providing a reliable predictive value for clinical efficacy of any of the compounds has been discovered so far. The treatment schemes are varying considerably. While some clinical pharmacological studies showed something like a minimal effective dose, no different efficacy was monitored at doses above. Clinical data comparing different doses of one certain compound are not available. Stimulating aspects have been communicated recently by Rudofsky (personal communication) claiming a daily, individual dosing considering circadian aspects, pains, Doppler flow, capillaroscopy and others. Although the platelet rebound (Sinzinger et al., 1981) and desensitisation at the receptor level known to occur after continuous administration of all the PGs and analogs does not seem to be of clinical relevance, the intermittent way of application is the one used in the overwhelming majority of cases today. During the last years the duration of therapy was more and more extended. Intra-arterial and intravenous route of application do not show apparent differences in clinical outcome. This is not surprising for PGI2 and its synthetic analogs, while it is, however, for PGE1. In view of earlier findings, especially by Sir John R. Vane (1964), PGE1 is metabolized during first lung passage to 60-85%. Recent data by Peskar et al. (1991) discovered 13,14-dihydro(DH)-PGE1 as a biologically active metabolite of the parent compound. The listing of biological capacities in table 1 shows, that concerning the mechanisms of action 13,14-DH-PGE1 is very well documented in the meanhile. The fact, that the bilogical profile of the two compounds is almost identical seems to provide the rationale for this longly discussed discrepancy. As the optimal regimen for administration has not been elucidated so far, this could result in a further improvement of the overall benefit induced by the various prostaglandins and their stable analogs.

Conclusion

Prostaglandins seem to represent a group of compounds with potential clinical benefit. This is documented by the

TABLE 7. i.v. Iloprost-infusion versus placebo

Author	n	dosage PGE1	follow	endpoints	results	s -up
Hossmann et al. (1984)	10	0.8-2.5ng/kg/min x12hx7d discont.inf. crossover	end	pain calf blood	red neg	s. 70%
Brock et al. (1986)	101	up to 2ng/kg/min x6hx28d discont.inf.	end	us	red	s. 100%
Balzer et al. (1987)	112	0.5-2ng/kg/min x6hx14d discont.inf.	end	analgesic cons.	red	n.s. 34%
Diehm et al. (1989)	99	up to 2ng/kg/min x6hx28d discont.inf.	end	us	red	s.
Norgren et al. (1990)	103	0.5-2ng/kg/min x6hx14d discont.inf.	end	us	red	n.s. 32%
Brock et al. (1990)	109	0.5-2ng/kg/min x6hx28d discont.inf.	end	us	red	n.s. 100%

s ... statistical significant; end ... end of infusion; neg ... negative; red ... reduced; us ... ulcer size

positive trials done so far for the different compounds and -analogs. The antiatherosclerotic actions suggest that a long-term treatment (by means of more stable orally effective substances) might be of even greater benefit.

Acknowledgements:
The author is gratefully acknowledging the valuable help of Drs P. Fitscha, J. Kaliman, F. Rauscha, K. Silberbauer, Irene Virgolini and the technicians Helga Fischer, Christa Köck and Susanne Granegger for their valuable contribution. The substances used have been kindly provided by Dr. Salvador Moncada, Wellcome Research Labs, Beckenham, Kent, UK, Dr. Waltraud Rogatti, Schwarz Pharma AG, Monheim, Germany, Dr. Theodor Krais, Schering AG, Berlin, Germany, and PD. DDr. Helmut Barth, Grünenthal, Aachen, Germany. The valuable help of Eva Unger in preparing and typing the manuscript is kindly acknowledged.

References

Ambrus, J.L., Taheri, P., Killion, D., and Donaldson, G. (1983) 'Clinical experience with prostaglandin E1 in the treatment of arteriosclerosis obliterans', J. Med. 14, 1-7.

Anitschkow, N. (1913) 'Über die Veränderung der Kaninchenaorta bei experimenteller Cholesterinsteatose', Beitr. Path. Anat. 56, 379-384.

Balzer, K., Rogatti, W. and Rüttgerodt, K. (1989) 'Therapeutische Wirksamkeit von Prostaglandin E1 -intraarterielle und intravenöse PGE1-Therapie bei AVK im Stadium III/IV', Therapiewoche 39, 2736-2742.

Belch, J.J.F., McKay, A., McArdle, B., Leiberman, P., Pollock, J.G., Lowe, G.D.O., Forbes, C.D. and Prentice, C.R.M. (1983) 'Epoprostenol (prostacyclin) and severe arterial disease. A double blind trial', Lancet i, 315-317.

Bergström, S., Ryhage, R., Samuelsson, B. and Sjövall, J. (1963) 'Prostaglandins and related factors. The structures of prostaglandin E1, F1α and F1β', J. Biol. Chem. 238, 2355-2564.

Bertuch, H., Pilger, E. and Sailer, S. (1986) 'Die Prostaglandin Therapie bei AMD. VASA 16: 53

Biedermann, H. (1984) 'Results of i.a. long-term infusion therapy with PGE1 for arterial circulatory disturbances in the extremities in stages III and/or IV', Inter Angio 3, 59-62.

Blume, J. (1987) 'Klinische Wirksamkeit der intraarteriellen Infusionstherapie mit Prostaglandin E1 im Stadium IIb der arteriellen Verschlußkrankheit', Therapiewoche 37, 4819-4823.

Böhme, H., Brülisauer, M., Härtel, U. and Bollinger, A. (1989) 'Periphere arterielle Verschlußkrankheit im Stadium III und IV - Kontrollierte Zweizentren-Studie zur Wirksamkeit von intraarteriellen Prostaglandin E1-Infusionen', Med. Welt 40, 1501-1503.

Bruch, H.P., Hörl, M. and Herold, A. (1986) 'Prostaglandin E1 in peripheral vascular disease in stages III and IV according to Fontaine', in H. Sinzinger and W. Rogatti (eds.), Prostaglandin E1 in Atherosclerosis, Springer Verlag, Berlin, pp. 81-96.

Carlson, L.A. and Eriksson, I (1973) 'Femoral-artery infusion of prostaglandin E1 in severe peripheral vascular disease', Lancet i, 155.

Carlson, L.A. and Olsson, A.G. (1976) 'Intravenous prostaglandin E1 in severe peripheral vascular disease', Lancet ii, 810.

Clifford, P.C. and Martin, M.F.R. (1984) 'The Raynaud phenomenon. Its treatment with intravenous prostaglandin E1', Inter Angio (Suppl), 25-27.

Creutzig, A., Caspary, L. and Alexander, K. (1987) 'Intermittent intraarterial prostaglandin E1 therapy of severe claudication', VASA 17, 44-46.

Creutzig, A., Caspary, L., Radeke, U., Specht, S., Ranke, C. and Alexander, K. (1988) 'Prospektive randomisierte Doppelblindstudie zur Wirksamkeit von i.a. Prostaglandin E1 bei der schweren Claudicatio intermittens', in H. Heidrich, H. Böhme and W. Rogatti (eds.), Prostaglandin E1 - Wirkung und therapeutische Wirksamkeit, Springer Verlag, Berlin, pp. 95-102.

Diehm, C., Stammler, F., Hübsch, C., Wilhelm, C., and Eckstein, H.H. (1987) 'Behandlung von Ruheschmerzen bei peripherer Verschlußkrankheit mit i.v.-Prostaglandin-Infusionen', VASA 20, 204-205.

Diehm, C., Hübsch-Müller, C. and Stammler, F. (1988) 'Intravenöse Prostaglandin E1-Therapie bei Patienten mit peripherer arterieller Verschlußkrankheit (AVK) im Stadium III - eine doppelblinde, plazebokontrollierte Studie', in H. Heidrich, H. Böhme and W. Rogatti (eds.), Prostaglandin E1 - Wirkung und therapeutische Wirksamkeit, Springer Verlag, Berlin, pp. 133-143.

Diehm, C., Kühn, A., Strauss, R., Hübsch-Müller, C. and Kübler, W. (1989) 'Effects of regular physical training in a supervised class and additional intravenous prostaglandin E1 and naftidrofuryl infusion therapy in patients with intermittent claudication', VASA 28, 26-30.

Diehm, C. (1989) 'Plazebo-kontrollierte doppelblinde 13-Center-Studie zum Nachweis der therapeutischen Wirksamkeit von Iloprost bei Patienten mit arterieller Verschlußkrankheit (Stadium IV)', in, 93. Tag. Verh. Dtsch. Ges. Inn. Med., Bergmann, München, pp.

Ehrly, A.M., Schenk, J. and Saeger-Lorenz, H. (1987) 'Einfluß einer i.v.-Gabe von PGE1 auf den Muskelgewebesauerstoffdruck, die transkutanen Gasdrucke und die Fließeigenschaften des Bluten von Patienten im Stadium III und IV der peripheren Verschlußkrankheit', VASA 20, 196-198.

Eklund, A.E., Eriksson, G. and Olsson, A.G. (1982) 'A controlled study showing significant short term effects of prostaglandin E1 in healing of ischaemic ulcers of the lower limb in man', Prostagl. Leukotr. Med. 8, 265-271.

Feldman, S.M., Alpert, J., Dick, L.S., Brief, D.K., Goldkranz, R., Brener, B.J. and Parsonnet, V. (1982) 'Clinical observations with intravenous prostaglandin E1 in peripheral vascular disease', J. Med. Soc. New Jersey 79, 985-991.

Fitscha, P., Sinzinger, H., Greenberg, H., Jennifer, H. and Linet, O. (1985) 'Prostacyclin in peripheral vascular disease - a double-blind trial in 108 patients', Thromb. Haemost. 54, 296.

Gruss, J.D., Vargas-Montano, H., Bartels, D., Simmenroth, H.W., Sakurai, T., Schäfer, G. and Fietze-Fischer, B. (1984) 'Use of prostaglandins in arterial occlusive diseases', Inter Angio 3, 7-17.

Hach, W., Zanke, B.W., Sauerwein, G. and Özen, Y. (1986) 'Teatment of stage IIb peripheral occlusive disease with short-term intra-arterial infusion of prostaglandin E1', in H. Sinzinger and W. Rogatti (eds.), Prostaglandin E1 in Atherosclerosis, Springer Verlag, Berlin, pp. 66-74.

Hecker, G., Ney, P. and Schrör, K. (1990) 'Cytotic enzyme release and oxygen centered radical formation in human neutrophils are selectively inhibited by E-type prostaglandins but not by PGI2', Naunyn-Schmiedbergs Arch. Pharmacol. 341, 308-315.

Heidrich, H., Dimroth, H., Gutman, M., Helmis, J., Peters, A. and Ranft, J. (1986) 'Long-term i.v.-infusion of PGE1 in peripheral arterial blood flow disorders: results of an open screening study with patients in Fontaine's stages III and IV', in H. Sinzinger and W. Rogatti (eds.), Prostaglandin E1 in Atherosclerosis, Springer Verlag, Berlin, pp. 92-98.

Heidrich, H., Brodel, C.H., Meuche, C.H., Hellmann, M. and Ranft, J. (1991) 'Kontrollierte Blutdrucklangzeitmessung unter intravenöser Prostaglandin E1-Infusion', VASA 20, 13-16.

Hirai, M. and Nakayama, R. (1986) 'Haemodynamic effects of intraarterial and intravenous administration of prostaglandin E1 in patients with peripheral arterial disease', Brit. J. Surg. 73, 20-23.

Hossmann, V., Heinen, A., Auel, H. and Fitzgerald, G.A. (1981) 'A randomized placebo controlled trial of prostacyclin (PGI2) in peripheral arterial disease', Thromb. Res. 22, 481.

Hossmann, V., Auel, H., Rücker, W., and Schrör, K. (1984) 'Prolonged infusion of prostacyclin in patients with advanced stages of peripheral vascular disease: a placebo-controlled cross-over study', Klin. Wschr. 62, 1108-1112.

Hossmann, V. (1984) 'Effects of iloprost in patients with peripheral arterial occlusive disease', in Scient. Symp. Iloprost (ZK 36374), a Novel Prostacyclin Analogue in Cardiovascular Disease. Schering, Düsseldorf, p. 57.

Joggestrand, T. and Olsson, A.G. (1985) 'The effect of intravenous PGE1 on ischaemic pain and on leg blood-flow in subjects with peripheral vascular disease: a double-blind controlled study', Clin. Physiol. 5, 495-502.

Kyle, V., Parr, G., Salisbury, P., Page, T.P. and Hazleman, D. (1985) 'Prostaglandin E1, vasospastic disease and thermography', Ann. Rheum. Dis. 44, 73-78.

Martin, M.F.R. and Tooke J.S. (1982) 'Effects of PGE1 on microvascular haemodynamics in progressive systemic sclerosis', Brit. Med. J. 85, 1688-1690.

Moncada, S., Gryglewski, R.J., Bunting, S. and Vane, J.R. (1976) 'An enzyme isolated from arteries transforms prostaglandin endoperoxides to an unstable substance that inhibits platelet aggregation', Nature 263, 663-665.

Negus, D., Irving, J.D. and Friedgood, A. (1985) 'Intra-arterial prostacyclin compared to praxilene in the management of advanced atherosclerotic lower limb ischemia', in A. Gryglewski, A. Szczeklik and J.C. McGiff (eds)., Prostacyclin. Clinical Trials, Raven Press, New York, pp 107-119.

Nizankowski, R., Krolikowski, W., Bielatowicz, J., Schaller, J. and Szczeklik, A. (1985) 'Prostacyclin for ischemic ulcers in peripheral arterial disease: a random assignement, placebo-controlled study', in A. Gryglewski, A. Szczeklik and J.C. McGiff (eds)., Prostacyclin. Clinical Trials, Raven Press, New York, pp 15-27.

Olsson, A.G. and Nilsson, E. (1981) 'The effect of intravenous prostacyclin on resting pain and healing of ischaemic ulcers in peripheral artery disease', Prostagl. Med. 6, 329.

Pardy, B.C., Lewis, J.D. and Eastcott, H.H.G. (1980) 'Preliminary experience with prostaglandins E1 and I2 in peripheral vascular disease', Surgery 88, 826.

Peskar, B.A., Hesse, W.H., Rogatti, W., Diehm, C., Rudofsky, G., Schweer, H. and Seyberth, H.W. (1991) 'Formation of 13,14-dihydro-prostaglandin E1 during intravenous infusions of prostaglandin E1 in patients with peripheral arterial occlusive disease', Prostaglandins (in press).

Pilger, E. and Juan, H. (1983) 'Vorläufige Ergebnisse einer Prostaglandin E1-Therapie bei peripherer obliterierender Arteriopathie', Wr. klin. Wschr. 95, 263-266.

Radomski, M.W., Palmer, R.M.J. and Moncada, S. (1987a) 'The antiaggregatory properties of vascular endothelium: Interactions between prostacyclin and nitric oxide', Brit. J. Pharmacol. 92, 639-646.

Radomski, M.W., Palmer, R.M.J. and Moncada, S. (1987b) 'The role of nitric oxide and cGMP in platelet adhesion to vascular endothelium', Biochem. Biophys. Res. Commun. 148, 1482-1489.

Rhodes, R.S. & Heard, S.E. (1983) 'Detrimental effect of high-dose prostaglandin E1 in the treatment of ischemic ulcers', Surgery 93, 839-843.

Rokitansky, C.von (1852) 'Über einige der wichtigsten Krankheiten', K.u.K. Hof- und Staatsdruckerei, Wien.

Rudofsky, G., Altenhoff, B., Meyer, P. and Lohmann, A. (1987) 'Intra-arterial perfusion with prostaglandin E1 in patients with intermittent claudication', VASA 17, 47-51.

Rudofsky, G. (1988) 'Intravenöse PGE1-Infusionsbehandlung bei Patienten mit arterieller Verschlußkrankheit im Stadium IIb', in H. Heidrich, H. Böhme and W. Rogatti (eds.),

Prostaglandin E1 - Wirkung und therapeutische Wirksamkeit, Springer Verlag, Berlin, pp. 103-111.

Sakaguchi, S. (1984) 'Prostaglandin E1 intra-arterial therapy in patients with ischemic ulcer of the extremeties', Inter Angio 3, 39-42.

Schuller, J.J., Flanigan, D.P., Holcroft, J.W., Ursprung, J.J., Mohrland, J.S. and Pyke, E. (1984) 'The efficacy of PGE1 in the treatment of lower extremity ischemic ulcers secondary to peripheral vascular occlusive disease: result of a prospective, randomized, double-blind, multicenter trial', Vasc. Surg. 1, 160-170.

Sinzinger, H., O'Grady, J., Cromwell, M. and Höfer R. (1983) 'Epoprostenol (prostacyclin) decreases platelet deposition on vascular prosthetic grafts', Lancet ii, 1275-1276.

Sinzinger, H., Fitscha, P., Wagner, O., Kaliman, J. and Rogatti, W. (1986a) 'Prostaglandin E1 decreases activation of arterial smooth muscle cells', Lancet i, 156-157.

Sinzinger, H., Bergmann, H., Kaliman, J. and Angelberger, P. (1986b) 'Imaging of human atherosclerotic lesions using 123-I-low-density lipoproteins', Eur. J. Nucl. Med. 12, 291-292.

Sinzinger, H., Fitscha, P., O'Grady, J., Rauscha, F., Rogatti, W. and Vane. J.R. (1990) 'Synergistic effect of prostaglandin E1 and isosorbide dinitrate in peripheral vascular disease', Lancet i, 627-628.

Sinzinger, H., Virgolini, I., Rauscha, F., Fitscha, P. (1991a) 'Antiplatelet action of isosorbide dinitrate in coronary heart disease', Brit. J. Clin. Pharmacol. (in press).

Sinzinger, H., Virgolini, I., Lupattelli, G., Molinari, A., Gerakakis, A. and Angelberger, P. (1991b) 'Prostaglandin E1 decreases the low-density lipoprotein entry into rabbit arterial wall', Brit. J. Pharmacol. (in press).

Szczeklik, A., Nizankowski, R., Skawinski, S., Szczeklik, J., Gluszko, P. and Gryglewski, R.J. (1979) 'Successful therapy of advanced arteriosclerosis obliterans with prostacyclin', Lancet i, 1111.

Szczeklik, A., Gryglewski, R.J., Nizankowski, R., Skawinski, S., Gluszko, P. and Korbut, R. (1980) 'Prostacyclin therapy in peripheral arterial disease', Thromb. Res. 19, 191

Telles, G.S., Campbell, W.B., Wood, R.F.M., Collin, J., Baird, R.N. and Morris, P.J. (1984) 'Prostaglandin E1 in severe lower limb ischaemia: a double-blind controlled trial', Brit. J. Surg. 71, 506-508.

Trübestein, G., Ludwig, M., Diehm, C., Gruss, J.D. and Horsch, S. (1987) 'Prostaglandin E1 bei arterieller Verschlußkrank-heit im Stadium III und IV - Ergebnisse einer multizentri-schen Studie', Dtsch. Med. Wschr. 112, 955-959.

Trübestein, G., v Bary, S., Breddin, K., Diehm, C., Gruß, J.D., Heinrich, H., Horsch, S., Kriessmann, A., Maass, U.

Martin, M., Maurin, N. and Scheffler, P. (1989) 'Intravenous prostaglandin E1 versus pentoxifylline therapy in chronic arterial occlusive disease - a controlled randomised multicenter study', VASA 28, 44-49.

Vane, J.R. (1964) 'The use of isolated organs for detecting substances in the circulating blood', Br. J. Pharmac. Chemother. 23, 360-373.

Virchow, R. (1856) 'Phlogose und Thrombose im Gefäßsystem', Gesammelte Abhandlungen zur wissenschaftlichen Medizin, Hirsch-Verlag, Berlin.

Virgolini, I., Lupattelli, G., Li, S.R., Pidlich, J., Weiss, K. and Sinzinger, H. (1991) 'Effect of prostaglandin E1 on low density lipoprotein apo-B,E-receptor binding in human, rat and swine liver', Prostaglandins (in press).

Willis, A.L. Smith, D.L. and Viago, C. (1986) 'Suppression of principal atherosclerotic mechanisms by prostacyclin and other eicosanoids', Prog. Lipid Res. 48, 1-22.

Zanke, B.W., Hach, W., Özen, Y. and Sauerwein, G. (1987) 'Treatment of peripheral vascular disease in stage IIb with intermittent short-term infusion of PGE1', VASA 17, 36-38.

ADJUVANT AGENTS TO ENHANCE AND SUSTAIN REPERFUSION WITH t-PA: STUDIES IN EXPERIMENTAL DOG MODELS

H.K. GOLD, T. YASUDA, I.K. JANG, L. GUERRERO, J.T. FALLON, R.C. LEINBACH, D. COLLEN

ABSTRACT. Thrombolytic therapy may be hampered by the resistance of thrombi to dissolution with plasminogen activators and by reocclusion following successful thrombolysis. A number of adjuvant treatments are being evaluated to overcome resistance to lysis, to accelerate recanalization, and to prevent reocclusion. These include potent antiplatelet agents such as combinations of thromboxane A_2 and serotonin receptor antagonists, substances with combined thromboxane synthase inhibitor/prostaglandin endoperoxide receptor antagonist action, antiplatelet glycoprotein (GP) IIb/IIIa monoclonal antibodies, or RGD-containing polypeptides. Alternatively, potent specific thrombin inhibitors such as hirudin or argatroban are being explored as superior agents to heparin for the acceleration and persistence of lysis with plasminogen activators. While it is clear that compounds with antithrombin or antiplatelet properties may enhance and sustain the action of thrombolytic agents, their optimal use and potential (hemorrhagic) side effects remain to be further explored. However, optimized thrombolytic therapy will eventually consist of potent specific plasminogen activators in combination with conjunctive anticoagulants and/or antiplatelet agents.

1. Introduction

Thrombolytic therapy in acute myocardial infarction (MI) is an established procedure for reperfusion of occluded coronary arteries, resulting in reduction of infarct size, preservation of left ventricular function and reduction in early and late mortality [1]. The currently available thrombolytic agents, including streptokinase (SK), anisoylated plasminogen streptokinase activator complex (APSAC) and recombinant tissue-type plasminogen activator (t-PA) suffer from a number of significant limitations, such as resistance to reperfusion in up to 25% of patients even with the most potent thrombolytic agents or combinations [2,3], and angiographically-documated reocclusion in approximately 15% of patients [4-6]. Moreover, the time to reperfusion

A. G. Herman (ed.), Antithrombotics, 221–232.
© 1991 *Kluwer Academic Publishers. Printed in the Netherlands.*

is on average 45 minutes after initiation of therapy [7], and significant bleeding may occur, with a frequency of intracerebral bleeding of approximately 0.5%

Various approaches to overcome the present limitations of thrombolytic therapy are currently under investigation in laboratory animal models. We have developed a model of coronary artery thrombosis in the setting of arterial wall injury and superimposed high-grade stenosis, which more closely resembles the combination of factors underlying coronary thrombosis and reocclusion in man [11]. Indeed, abrasion of endothelium exposing subendothelial thrombogenic structures, uniform production of fixed high-grade stenosis (> 90%), and absence of spontaneous reflow constitute a reproducible quantiative model for the investigation of both coronary thrombolysis and approaches to prevent reocclusion. Morever, the mechanism of reocclusion, consisting of platelet-rich thrombus at the site of endothelial injury and stenosis, appears to be similar to that observed at the site of plaque rupture in man. Indeed, postmortem examination of serial sections of coronary thrombi of patients who died with acute MI has consistently revealed areas of platelet-rich thrombus contiguous to the site of plaque rupture [12].

One cause of resistance of coronary occlusive thrombus to dissolution by thrombolytic agents may be a predominance of platelet-rich thrombus. Indeed, a differential sensitivity to dissolution with t-PA of platelet-rich thrombus relative to erythrocyte-rich thrombus was demonstrated in a femoral arterial thrombosis model in the rabbit [13]. Therefore, we have developed a canine model of platelet-rich coronary arterial thrombus, using eversion of a circumflex coronary arterial segment and a superimposed high-grade stenosis [14]. Exposure of the adventitial surface to flowing blood results in platelet adhesion and aggregation in the everted segment, leading to occlusion with material highly enriched in platelets. This model, where the primary occlusive thrombus is platelet-rich, differs fundamentally from the canine left anterior descending (LAD) coronary artery thrombosis model in which the occlusive thrombus is a whole blood clot [11]. In the latter model, it is not possible to investigate the sensitivity of preformed platelet-rich thrombus to reperfusion strategies.

The aim of the present review is to summarize our experience with these animal models in the investigation of adjuvant therapies to increase the rate and extent of thrombolysis with t-PA, to prevent occlusion and reocclusion, and to evaluate the effect of these procedures on bleeding time.

1.1. COMPARATIVE EFFICACY OF THROMBOLYTIC AGENTS IN THE CANINE LEFT ANTERIOR DESCENDING (LAD) CORONARY ARTERY THROMBOSIS MODEL [11]

The relative efficacy of the thrombolytic agents SK, urokinase (UK), and t-PA was evaluated. In the absence of superimposed stenosis, intravenous (IV) infusion of 750,000 U of SK over 1 hour caused reperfusion in 5 of 6 dogs in 34 ± 25 minutes (mean ± SD). Intravenous infusion of UK, 600,000 U over 30 minutes, followed by 600,000 U over 30 minutes by the intracoronary route, induced reperfusion in 3 of 4 dogs in 64 ± 23 minutes. Recombinant 2-chain t-PA, infused intravenously at rate of 15 μg/kg per minute for 30 minutes or until reflow, induced reperfusion in all of 12 dogs, in 28 ± 13 minutes. In the absence of coronary stenosis, spontaneous reocclusion did not occur within 2 hours after the end of the infusion.

In the presence of coronary artery stenosis, which reduced the blood flow to 40 ± 10% of baseline, SK, UK and t-PA caused coronary thrombolysis to proceed at comparable or only slightly slower rates. Cyclic reocclusion during or after the end of the infusion of these thrombolytic agents, caused by platelet-rich thrombus, was almost invariably observed, generally within 30 minutes after the onset of reperfusion.

1.2. EFFECT OF ANTIPLATELET AGENTS ON REOCCLUSION AFTER REPERFUSION WITH t-PA IN THE CANINE LAD MODEL WITH SUPERIMPOSED HIGH-GRADE STENOSIS [15,16]

Intravenous infusion of t-PA at a rate of 15 to 30 μg/kg per minute for 30 or 60 minutes in 8 dogs induced coronary artery reperfusion within 23 ± 7 minutes (mean ± SD), but reocclusion occurred despite heparin anticoagulation in all but 1 of these dogs within 7 ± 5 minutes. Intravenous injection of 0.8 mg/kg of the $F(ab')_2$ fragment of a monoclonal antibody (7E3), directed against the platelet glycoprotein (GP)IIb/IIIa receptor, prevented reocclusion in all of 10 dogs during an observation period of 2 hours ($p < 0.001$ versus t-PA alone). The antibody abolished adenosine diphosphate (ADP)-induced platelet aggregation and markedly prolonged the bleeding time. Intravenous aspirin or dipyridamole prevented reocclusion for 1 hour or more in only 2 of 7 and 1 of 6 dogs, respectively.

Bolus IV injections of t-PA at a dose of 0.45 mg/kg, repeated at 15-minute intervals until reperfusion occurred or up to a maximum of 4 injections, caused reperfusion in 5 of 7 dogs within 100 minutes (33 ± 15 minutes, mean ± SD). Reperfusion was rapidly followed (generally within 10 minutes) by reocclusion and then by periods of cyclical reflow and reocclusion. A single IV injection of 7E3-$F(ab')_2$ alone at 0.8 mg/kg caused reperfusion within 100 minutes in 2 of 6 dogs (19 and 37 minutes) without subsequent reocclusion. Single bolus injections of different amounts (0.1 to 0.8 mg/kg) of 7E3-$F(ab')_2$ were then combined with bolus injections of 0.45 mg/kg of t-PA. Stable reperfusion without reocclusion was accomplished with 0.8 or 0.6 mg/kg 7E3-$F(ab')_2$ and a single injection of 0.45 mg/kg t-PA, within 6 ± 3 minutes ($N= 6$, $p < 0.01$) and 8 ± 5 minutes ($N= 5$, $p < 0.02$), respectively. None of these animals suffered reocclusion of the coronary artery. Lower doses (0.1 to 0.2 mg/kg) of 7E3-$F(ab')_2$ did not significantly shorten the time to reperfuson and did not prevent reocclusion. Combinations of intermediate doses (either 0.45 mg/kg t-PA with 0.4 mg/kg 7E3-$F(ab')_2$ or 0.225 mg/kg t-PA with 0.6 mg/kg 7E3-$F(ab')_2$) had an intermediate effect on the rate of reperfusion and the frequency of reocclusion. Bleeding times remained unchanged after injection of t-PA alone and were moderately (about 2-fold) prolonged after the injection of 7E3-$F(ab')_2$, at a dose of 0.1

to 0.4 mg/kg. With 0.6 mg/kg 7E3-F(ab')$_2$, the bleeding time was prolonged approximately 4 times and was greater than 30 minutes in 4 of 9 dogs. At 0.8 mg/kg the bleeding time was consistently prolonged to more than 30 minutes; this dose blocked 83 ± 5% of the GPIIb/IIIa receptors on the platelet surface.

1.3. EFFECTS OF ASPIRIN, A SYNTHETIC THROMBIN INHIBITOR, AND A MONOCLONAL ANTIPLATELET GPIIb/IIIa ANTIBODY ON REPERFUSION AND REOCCLUSION WITH t-PA IN THE CANINE LAD MODEL WITH STENOSIS [17]

The comparative effects of IV aspirin, of a synthetic thrombin inhibitor, argatroban, and of F(ab')$_2$ fragments of monoclonal antibody 7E3 against platelet GPIIb/IIIa, 7E3-F(ab')$_2$, on thrombolysis, reocclusion, and bleeding associated with 0.45 mg/kg bolus injections of t-PA were studied. In Group I pretreated with 17 mg/kg IV aspirin, reflow occurred in 4 of 6 dogs but did not persist; reflow was induced in Group II treated with 200 μg/kg/minutes of IV argatroban for 60 minutes, in 4 of 5 dogs, persisting in 1 animal; in Group III treated with aspirin and argatroban combined, reflow occurred in all of 5 dogs, persisting in 4 animals; in Group IV treated with 0.8 mg/kg IV 7E3-F(ab')$_2$ reflow was achieved in 4 of 5 dogs, persisting in 2 animals. The frequency of persistent reflow in Group III was significantly higher than in the combined groups I and II ($p = 0.012$), whereas the time to reflow was significantly shorter in the groups receiving argatroban than in the aspirin group (median 25 minutes versus 55 minutes, $p = 0.04$). There were no significant differences between Groups III and IV. Bleeding times prolonged from 4.2 ± 1.2 minutes (mean ± SD) to 5.0 ± 3.0 minutes at 60 minutes in Group I, to 9.4 ± 11 minutes in Group II, to 12 ± 11 minutes in Group III, and to 27 ± 8 minutes in Group IV. One hour after the end of infusion, the bleeding times were 5.0 ± 0.9, 5.2 ± 1.3, 14 ± 9.2, and 26 ± 9 minutes, respectively.

1.4. LYSIS OF rt-PA-RESISTANT PLATELET-RICH CORONARY ARTERIAL THROMBUS WITH COMBINED BOLUS INJECTION OF t-PA AND ANTIPLATELET GPIIb/IIIa ANTIBODY [14]

In the canine model of platelet-rich coronary arterial thrombus, stable occlusion, as monitored with an ultrasonic flow probe and coronary angiography, was maintained during a 2-hour observation period in all of 5 dogs. Bolus IV injections of t-PA at a dose of 0.45 mg/kg at 15-minute intervals, repeated 4 times, did not cause reperfusion in 4 of 5 dogs and produced cyclic reperfusion and reocclusion in 1 dog. A single IV bolus inejction of 0.8 mg/kg of the F(ab')$_2$ fragment of the monoclonal antibody 7E3 produced stable reperfusion in 2 out of 5 dogs, while occlusion persisted in the other animals. Injection of 7E3-F(ab')$_2$ (0.8 mg/kg) followed by t-PA (0.45 mg/kg) caused stable reperfusion without reocclusion in all of 5 dogs ($p < 0.05$ versus t-PA alone and $p < 0.01$ versus control).

2. Discussion

Thrombolytic therapy for acute MI, even with the most potent thrombolytic agents or strategies presently available, fails in 15 to 25% of patients. In addition, large doses are required and the treatment is associated with unpredictable bleeding and recurrent posttreatment ischemic events. Therefore the quest continues for more improved thrombolytic agents or adjunctive therapeutic regimens.

Acute ischemic coronary syndromes occur in association with plaque rupture [12,18], which triggers intraluminal thrombosis [19]. The composition of the intraluminal thrombus is heterogenous, consisting of platelet-rich material contiguous to the area of plaque rupture, and erythrocyte-rich material extending both proximally and distally. This suggests two alternative and protentially complementary targets for coronary thrombolysis: the erythrocyte-rich whole blood clot and the platelet-rich thrombus. While the potential and limitations of the fibrinolytic agents for the dissolution of whole blood clots is well known, the potential for pharmacological dispersion of platelet clumps and platelet-rich thrombus has not been fully explored.

Although the mechanisms of platelet aggregation and pharmacological approaches to interfere with the process are well known [20], no efficient means are available to disperse preformed platelet-rich thrombus. t-PA disaggregates platelet clumps in vitro [21] but only at a very high concentration, in order of magnitude higher than those currently achievable by IV infusion. Thus, platelet-rich regions of coronary clot might be more resistant to lysis than erythrocyte-rich zones and the predominance of platelet-rich zones may limit the efficacy of IV thrombolytic therapy. Consequently, one approach to increased efficacy and speed of coronary artery reperfusion might consist of the pharmacological dispersion of platelet-rich thrombus in combination with fibrin-dissolving therapy. Alternatively, specific interference with platelet deposition during fibrinolysis might accelerate thrombolysis and prevent reocclusion.

2.1. EFFICACY OF THROMBOLYTIC AGENTS IN THE CANINE LAD CORONARY ARTERY THROMBOSIS MODEL WITH SUPERIMPOSED HIGH-GRADE STENOSIS

To study the mechanism of reocclusion and to investigate new strategies to prevent it, we developed an LAD coronary artery thrombosis model in the dog with superimposed endothelial damage and fixed high-grade stenosis, which simulates anatomical features occurring in patients with acute MI. Indeed, abrasion of endothelium exposing subendothelial thrombogenic structues, uniform production of fixed high-grade stenosis (> 90%), and absence of spontaneous reflow constitute a reproducible quantitative model for the investigation of both coronary thrombolysis and approaches to prevent reocclusion.

The results of thrombolysis obtained by IV infusion of SK, UK, and recombinant t-PA in this canine model parallel those obtained in humans. Indeed, SK and UK had a more limited efficacy than t-PA [22,23], and the invariable occurrence of reocclusion after thrombolysis paralleled the observations in patients with high-grade stenosis, in whom a > 80% reduction of the luminal diameter frequently leads to coronary artery reocclusion [5,24]. Pathologic examination of the material responsible for reocclusion in the dog stenosis model revealed that it consists of a platelet-rich thrombus, possibly of similar composition to the thrombolysis-insensitive material responsible for reocclusion in humans. On the basis of these observations, it became possible to investigate several hypotheses for the prevention of coronary reocclusion. Neither full heparinization nor extensive fibrinogen depletion (for example, with UK) prevented reocclusion, a finding in agreement with observations made in patients [25,26]. This model is stable and reproducible over time but, following thrombolysis of the erythrocyte-rich clot, the reoccluding platelet-rich material does not produce uniform persistent occlusion but results in cycling reflow and reocclusion. Therefore, it is not adequate for the investigation of strategies to overcome resistance of platelet-rich thrombus to dissolution with thrombolytic strategies.

2.2. LYSIS OF PLATELET-RICH CORONARY ARTERIAL THROMBUS

A canine model of platelet-rich coronary arterial thrombus was developed using eversion of a circumflex coronary arterial segment. This model, where the primary occlusive thrombus is platelet-rich, differes fundamentally from the canine LAD model in which the occlusive thrombus is a whole blood clot. The canine eversion graft model therefore allows investigation of the sensitivity of preformed platelet-rich thrombus to reperfusion strategies.

Thrombus models consisting primarily of platelet-rich clot have also previously been described. The original model of Folts et al. [27], consisting of a stenosed coronary artery with an external luminal constriction to 70%, is subject to spontaneous cyclic occlusion with platelet-rich material, which can, however, be prevented with aspirin. More extensive constriction (to 90%) requires more intensive antiplatelet agents to prevent cyclic occlusion, but this modification also does not produce stable coronary artery occulsion [28,29]. Alternatively, models of platelet-rich thrombus based on intraluminal electrical stimulation have been used [30,31], and in these models potentiation of thrombolysis with antiplatelet antibodies has been demonstrated [31].

The eversion graft model is characterized by an intense local triggering mechanism for platelet-mediated occlusion, resulting primarily in a persistent platelet-rich or mixed platelet-rich and erythrocyte-rich occlusive thrombus, which develops within approximately 5 minutes in 80% of the animals. In addition, a superimposed external constriction reduces the luminal diameter by at least 90% and decreases the blood flow to 40% of baseline.

From the results obtained in this model, several conclusions were drawn: (1) platelet-rich thrombus is indeed very resistant to dispersion with t-PA; (2) potent antiplatelet agents, such as 7E3-F(ab')$_2$, do not consistently disperse the occlusive platelet-rich thrombus; and (3) the use of 7E3-F(ab′)$_2$ potentiates reperfusion even with a reduced dose of t-PA.

The mechanism of the enhancing effect of t-PA and 7E3-F(ab′)$_2$ on the lysis of platelet-rich thrombus is not clear. If t-PA would disperse the thrombus by dissolution of the fibrin strands that hold the platelet clumps together, one would not expect such great resistance to thrombolysis with t-PA boluses alone at doses which efficiently dissolve erythrocyte-rich clot [15,16]. Possibly inhibition of the accretion of new platelets on the thrombus surface may shift the dynamic balance of thrombosis and thrombolysis towards the latter.

The marked prolongation of the bleeding time at the high dose of 7E3-F(ab′)$_2$ used in the present study will require further dose-response studies before its potential use in man. In addition, further investigation of alternative reversible antiplatelet agents in combination with t-PA is warranted, both with respect to their effects on platelet-rich coronary thrombus and on bleeding. In view of the known variable morphology of coronary thrombi in patients with acute MI, of the evidence that a combination of antiplatelet and thrombolytic agents improves clinical outcome, and of the results of the present experimental study, optimization of combined antiplatelet and thrombolytic strategies may constitute a successful approach for further improvement of thrombolytic therapy in patients with acute coronary syndromes.

2.3. EFFECTS OF THE MONOCLONAL ANTIPLATELET GPIIb/IIIa ANTIBODY 7E3 ON THROMBOLYSIS WITH t-PA IN THE CANINE LAD MODEL WITH STENOSIS

The effect of 7E3-F(ab′)$_2$ on the rate of coronary artery thrombolysis and the frequency of reocclusion after successful reperfusion with bolus injections of t-PA in the canine LAD model was investigated. When 7E3-F(ab′)$_2$ was given alone at a concentration that nearly saturated the platelet surface GPIIb/IIIa receptors, reperfusion occurred in 2 of 6 dogs and neither dog reoccluded. This suggested that coronary thrombi may be in a relatively dynamic state, with ongoing lysis by endogenous t-PA and continual accretion of platelets and fibrin. The relatively low frequency of reperfusion, however, indicated that the antibody alone was inadequate to secure consistent reperfusion. When t-PA was given alone in up to 4 boluses of 0.45 mg/kg at 15-minute intervals, reperfusion occurred within 33 ± 15 minutes in all of these dogs, after which there were unstable periods of cyclical reocclusion and reperfusion.

The combination of 0.8 mg/kg of 7E3-F(ab′)$_2$ and a single bolus injection of 0.45 mg/kg t-PA was, however, highly effective and reocclusion in this group was prevented. The mechanism of the marked accelerating effect of 7E3-F(ab′)$_2$ on the rate of thrombolysis by t-PA is not evident. Direct triggering of a fibrinolytic pathway by the binding of the antibody to the platelet receptor is not likely. Possibly its mechanism of action is via the inhibition of the accretion of platelets on the thrombus surface, where release of fibrinolytic inhibitors from the platelets might delay the fibrinolytic process. Alternatively, incorporation of functionally intact platelets may constitute a significant pathway in the dynamic equilibrium between thrombosis and thrombolysis leading to thrombus stabilization. Inhibition of platelets with 7E3-F(ab′)$_2$ would then displace this equilibrium toward thrombolysis.

In view of the significant clinical value of rapid reperfusion and prevention of reocclusion of coronary arteries in patients with acute MI, 7E3-F(ab′)$_2$ or alternative agents interfering with the GPIIb/IIIa receptor-mediated pathway of platelet activation may constitute useful adjunctive agents to thrombolytic therapy.

2.4. EFFECT OF THROMBIN INHIBITORS ON THROMBOLYSIS WITH t-PA IN THE CANINE LAD MODEL WITH STENOSIS

The effects of argatroban on the speed of thrombolysis with t-PA, on reocclusion, and on the bleeding tendency as revealed by the template bleeding time were studied as compared with the effects of aspirin and of the monoclonal antiplatelet GPIIb/IIIa antibody. Interference of systemic therapeutic heparin anticoagulation was avoided, either by subcutaneous administration of a low dose of heparin which did not prolong the activated partial thromboplastin time or thrombin time (the prolongation towards the end of the infusion in the aspirin group being the result of excessive fibrinogen breakdown in animals that received 4 bolus injections of t-PA). Alternatively, intravenously injected heparin in the 7E3-F(ab′)$_2$ group was reversed with protamine sulfate.

Intravenous bolus injection of aspirin did not markedly potentiate the efficacy of t-PA for coronary arterial thrombolysis. Short-term infusion of argatroban, in a dose that prolonged the activated partial thromboplastin time from approximately 15 to 85 seconds, accelerated thrombolysis as compared to the aspirin alone group, whereas the combination of argatroban and aspirin prevented reocclusion relative to the groups treated with either drug alone.

We have previously shown that combinations of heparin, 7E3-F(ab′)$_2$, and t-PA accelerate lysis and completely prevented reocclusion in this canine model of MI [16]. However, in the present study, the reversal of heparin with protamine sulfate appeared to diminish the effect of 7E3-F(ab′)$_2$ and consistent prevention of reocclusion was not seen. This suggests an important role for thrombin inhibition in the maintenance of vascular patency, which is not completely blocked by saturation of the platelet GPIIb/IIIa receptors.

The persistence of coronary patency despite the return of the bleeding time, thrombin time, and partial thromboplastin time toward normal suggests that the duration of the bleeding time prolongation induced by antiplatelet therapy that is required to permit deactivation of the damaged endothelial surface may be relatively short.

Combination therapy with antiplatelet agents that affect different platelet activation pathways may permit the reduction of toxicity of any single agent by lowering the dose required to inhibit platelet function. Thus, acceleration of lysis and prevention of reocclusion might be accomplished without or with less prolongation of the bleeding time and a consequently reduced risk of bleeding. Provided these concepts can be extrapolated to man, combination therapy with t-PA, antiplatelet agents, and specific thrombin inhibitors might result in better efficacy-to-toxicity ratios for pharmacological recanalization of occluded coronary arteries in patients with acute MI.

3. Conclusions

The beneficial effects of thrombolytic therapy in acute ischemic coronary syndromes, particularly in acute MI, are now well established. The limited efficacy and potentially life-threatening side effects of thrombolytic agents remain a major problem. The present limitations of thrombolytic therapy can be explained on the basis of the heterogeneity of coronary arterial thrombus, consisting of both erythrocyte-rich and platelet-rich zones, and knowledge of the mechanism of fibrin dissolution and platelet disaggregation. This unified concept suggests alternative and complementary pharmacological approaches to coronary artery recanalization that require evaluation with specific, relevant, in vivo animal models. Available evidence suggests that the efficacy of coronary thrombolysis may be augmented either by improvement of the potency and specificity of fibrin-dissolving agents, by dispersion of aggregated platelets, or by a combination of both. Continued investiations along several new research lines, some reviewed above, will provide new insights and promote progress towards development of the ideal thrombolytic therapy, characterized by maximized stable coronary arterial thrombolysis with minimized bleeding.

4. References

1. Collen, D., Stump, D.C., and Gold, H.K. (1988) 'Thrombolytic therapy', Ann. Rev. Med. 39, 405-423.
2. Collen, D. (1990) 'Coronary thrombolysis: streptokinase or recombinant tissue-type plasminogen activator ?', Ann. Int. Med. 112, 529-538.
3. Chesebro, J.H., Knatterud, G., and Braunwald, E. (1988) 'Correspondence section. Thrombolytic therapy', N. Engl. J. Med. 319, 1544-1545.
4. Gold, H.K., Leinbach, R.C., Palacios, I.F., Yasuda, T., Block, P.C., Buckley, M.J., Akins, C.W., Daggett, W.M., and Austen, W.G. (1983) 'Coronary reocclusion after selective administration of streptokinase', Circulation 68, I50-I54.
5. Johns, J.A., Gold, H.K., Leinbach, R.C., Yasuda, T., Gimple, L.W., Werner, W., Finkelstein, D.B., Newell, J.B., Ziskind, A.A., and Collen, D. (1988) 'Prevention of coronary artery reocclusion and reduction in late coronary artery stenosis after thrombolytic therapy in patients with acute myocardial infarction. A randomized study of maintenance infusion of recombinant human tissue-type plasminogen activator', Circulation 78, 546-556.
6. Raynaud, P. and Desveaux, B. (1988) 'Réocclusion après traitement par l'Actilyse', Arch. Mal Coeur 81, 25-32.

7. Chesebro, J.H., Knatterud, G., Roberts, R., Borer, J., Cohen, L.S., Dalen, J., Dodge, H.T., Francis, C.K., Hillis, D., Ludbrook, P., Markis, J.E., Mueller, H., Passamani, E.R., Powers, E.R., Rao, A.K., Robertson, T., Ross, A., Ryan, T.J., Sobel, B.E., Willerson, J., Williams, D.O., Zaret, B.L., and Braunwald, E. (1987) 'Thrombolysis in myocardial infarction (TIMI) trial, Phase I: a comparison between intravenous tissue plasminogen activator and intravenous streptokinase. Clinical findings through hospital discharge', Circulation 76, 142-154.
8. Rovelli, F., De Vita, C., Feruglio, G.A., Lotto, A., Selvini, A., Tognoni, G., and GISSI investigators, (1987) 'GISSI trial: early results and late follow-up', J. Am. Coll. Cardiol. 10, 33B-39B.
9. ISIS-2 (Second International Study of Infarct Survival) and Collaborative Group, (1988) 'Randomised trial of intravenous streptokinase, oral aspirin, both, or neither among 17,187 cases of suspected acute myocardial infarction: ISIS-2', Lancet 2, 349-360.
10. Wilcox, R.G., von der Lippe, G., Olsson, C.G., Jensen, G., Skene, A.M., and Hampton, J.R. (1988) 'Trial of tissue plasminogen activator for mortality reduction in acute myocardial infarction. Anglo-Scandinavian Study of Early Thrombolysis (ASSET)', Lancet 2, 525-530.
11. Yasuda, T., Gold, H.K., Fallon, J.T., Leinbach, R.C., Garabedian, H.D., Guerrero, J.L., and Collen, D. (1989) 'A canine model of coronary artery thrombosis with superimposed high grade stenosis for the investigation of rethrombosis after thrombolysis', J. Am. Coll. Cardiol. 13, 1409-1414.
12. Friedman, M. and Van den Bovenkamp, G.J. (1966) 'The pathogenesis of a coronary thrombus', Am. J. Pathol. 48, 19-44.
13. Jang, I.K., Gold, H.K., Ziskind, A.A., Fallon, J.T., Holt, R.E., Leinbach, R.C., May, J.W., and Collen, D. (1989) 'Differential sensitivity of erythrocyte-rich and platelet-rich arterial thrombi to lysis with recombinant tissue-type plasminogen activator (rt-PA). A possible explanation for resistance to coronary thrombolysis', Circulation 79, 920-928.
14. Yasuda, T., Gold, H.K., Leinbach, R.C., Saito, T., Guerrero, J.L., Jang, I.K., Holt, R., Fallon, J.T., and Collen, D. (1990) 'Lysis of plasminogen activator-resistant platelet-rich coronary artery thrombus with combined bolus injection of recombinant tissue-type plasminogen activator and anti-platelet GPIIb/IIIa antibody', J. Am. Coll. Cardiol. 16, 1728-1735.
15. Yasuda, T., Gold, H.K., Fallon, J.T., Leinbach, R.C., Guerrero, L., Scudder, L.S., Kanke, M., Shealy, D., Ross, M.J., Collen, D., and Coller, B.S. (1988) 'Monoclonal antibody against the platelet glycoprotein (GP) IIb/IIIa receptor prevents coronary artery reocclusion after reperfusion with recombinant tissue-type plasminogen activator in dogs', J. Clin. Invest. 81, 1284-1291.

16. Gold, H.K., Coller, B.S., Yasuda, T., Saito, T., Fallon, J.T., Guerrero, J.L., Leinbach, R.C., Ziskind, A.A., and Collen, D. (1988) 'Rapid and sustained coronary artery recanalization with combined bolus injection of recombinant tissue-type plasminogen activator and monoclonal antiplatelet GPIIb/IIIa antibody in a canine preparation', Circulation 77, 670-677.
17. Yasuda, T., Gold, H.K., Yaoita, H., Leinbach, R.C., Guerrero, J.L., Jang, I.K., Holt, R., Fallon, J.T., and Collen, D. (1990) 'Comparative effects of aspirin, a synthetic thrombin inhibitor and a monoclonal antiplatelet GPIIb/IIIa antibody on coronary artery reperfusion, reocclusion and bleeding with recombinant tissue-type plasminogen activator in a canine preparation', J. Am. Coll. Cardiol. 16, 714-722.
18. Davies, M.J. and Thomas, A.C. (1985) 'Plaque fissuring - the cause of acute myocardial infarction, sudden ischaemic death, and crescendo angina', Br. Heart J. 53, 363-373.
19. De Wood, M.A., Spores, J., Notske, R., Lowell, T., Mouser, T., Burroughs, R., Golden, M.S., and Lang, H.T. (1980) 'Prevalence of total coronary occlusion during the early hours of transmural myocardial infarction', N. Engl. J. Med. 303, 897-902.
20. Fuster, V., Badimon, L., Badimon, J. Adams, P.C., Turitto, V., and Chesebro, J.H. (1987) 'Drugs interfering with platelet functions: mechanisms and clinical relevance', in M. Verstraete, J. Vermylen, R. Lijnen and J. Arnout (eds.), Trombosis and Haemostasis, Leuven University Press, Leuven, Belgium, pp. 349-418.
21. Loscalzo, J. and Vaughan, D.E. (1987) 'Tissue plasminogen activator promotes platelet disaggregation in plasma', J. Clin. Invest. 79, 1749-1755.
22. The TIMI Study Group, (1985) 'Special Report. The thrombolysis in Myocardial Infarction (TIMI) Trial', N. Engl. J. Med. 312, 932-936.
23. Verstraete, M., Bernard, R., Bory, M., Brower, R.W., Collen, D., de Bono, D.P., Erbel, R., Huhamnn, W., Lennane, R.J., Lubsen, J., Mathey, D., Meyer, J., Michels, H.R., Rutsch, W., Schartl, M., Schmidt, W., Uebis, R., and von Essen, R. (1985) 'Randomised trial of intravenous recombinant tissue-type plasminogen activator versus intravenous streptokinase in acute myocardial infarction', Lancet 1, 842-847.
24. Gold, H.K., Leinbach, R.C., Garabedian, H.D., Yasuda, T., Johns, J.A., Grossbard, E.B., Palacios, I., and Collen, D. (1986) 'Acute coronary reocclusion after thrombolysis with recombinant human tissue-type plasminogen activator: prevention by a maintenance infusion', Circulation 73, 347-352.
25. Harrison, D.G., Ferguson, D.W., Collins, S.M., Skorton, D.J., Ericksen, E.E., Kioschos, J.M., Marcus, M.L., and White, C.W. (1984) 'Rethrombosis after reperfusion with streptokinase: importance of geometry of residual lesions', Circulation 69, 991-999.
26. Gold, H.K., Cowley, M.J., Palacios, I.F., Vetrovec, G.W., Akins, C.W., Block, P.C., and Leinbach, R.C. (1984) 'Combined intracoronary streptokinase and coronary angioplasty during acute myocardial infarction', Am. J. Cardiol. 53, 122C-125C.

27. Folts, J.D., Crowell Jr., E.B., and Rowe, G.G. (1976) 'Platelet aggregation in partially obstructed vessels and its elimination with aspirin', Circulation 54, 365-370.
28. Gallagher, K.P., Folts, J.D., and Rowe, G.G. (1978) 'Comparison of coronary arteriograms with direct measurements of stenosed coronary arteries in dogs', Am. Heart J. 95, 338-347.
29. Aiken, J.W., Shebuski, R.J., Miller, O.V., Gorman, R.R. (1981) 'Endogenous prostacyclin constributes to the efficacy of a thromboxane synthetase inhibitor for preventing coronary artery thrombolysis', J. Pharmacol. Exp. Ther. 219, 299-308.
30. Schumacher, W.A., Lee, E.C., and Lucchesi, B.R. (1985) 'Augmentation of streptokinase-induced thrombolysis by heparin and prostacyclin', J. Cardiovasc. Pharmacol. 7, 299-308.
31. Fitzgerald, D.J., Wright, F., and FitzGerald, G.A. (1989) 'Increased thromboxane biosynthesis during coronary thrombolysis. Evidence that platelet activation and thromboxane A2 modulate the response to tissue-type plasminogen activator in vivo', Circ. Res. 65, 83-94.

EFFECT OF DIETARY MARINE LIPIDS ON (ANTI-)THROMBOTIC MECHANISMS

G. HORNSTRA

ABSTRACT

Animal studies clearly indicate that dietary marine oils have antithrombotic effects, especially when they replace saturated fatty acids in the diet. This chapter reviews the results of human intervention studies on processes involved in thrombus formation (platelet aggregation and blood coagulation) and dissolution (fibrinolysis) as well on clinical conditions associated with ischaemic vascular disease in man.

Dietary marine oils slightly lower platelet aggregation by reducing the potential of activated blood platelets to produce prothrombotic thromboxane A_2. Effects of dietary marine oils on blood coagulability are marginal, if existing at all. Evidence is accumulating that fish oils, by increasing the activity of the plasminogen activator inhibitor, may compromize the fibrinolytic process. This may be the reason why the clinical benefit of dietary marine oils is not very convincing. However, promising results have been obtained in some trials to reduce restenosis after coronary angioplasty and in a secondary prevention trial in post-myocardial infarction patients.

1. Introduction

Arterial thrombosis not only is the major lethal complication of atherosclerosis, it also contributes to the process of atherogenesis. Therefore, any attenuation of the arterial thrombotic process is likely to reduce mortality and morbidity of ischaemic heart- and vessel disease.

Dietary lipids have a profound effect on experimental atherosclerosis in animals, and a number of human intervention studies strongly indicate their value in cardiovascular protection. In recent years, interest has specifically focussed on lipids derived from marine animals, which have a relatively high content of the so-called (n-3) fatty acids, timnodonic acid (TA, 20:5(n-3), eicosapentaenoic acid or EPA) and cervonic acid (CA, 22:6(n-3), docosahexaenoic acid or DHA). This chapter, therefore, reviews recent studies which are relevant to asses the potential importance of marine lipids to lower cardiovascular risk either on its own or as a support of drug therapy. Firstly, studies related to thrombotic and antithrombotic processes will be reviewed. Subsequently, a summary will be given of studies aiming at reducing thrombotic risk in human subjects.

A. G. Herman (ed.), Antithrombotics, 233–249.
© 1991 *Kluwer Academic Publishers. Printed in the Netherlands.*

2. Effect of marine lipids on human platelet function in vitro and in vivo

The tendency of blood platelets to become activated in vivo is of great importance in the development of atherosclerosis and its complications. Therefore, many studies investigated the effect of marine oils on platelet function. So far, the results are equivocal. This is partly due to the fact that many studies have been performed without a proper control group. Of the well-controlled studies, only three (1-3) out of twelve (1, 2, 4-13) describe a limited reduction in platelet aggregation in response to ADP. When collagen is used to trigger platelet aggregation, 7 studies (1, 3-5, 12-14) show a diminished platelet reactivity, whereas in 9 studies (2, 6, 8-12, 15, 16), no effect different from the placebo is observed. Adrenaline-induced aggregation has been reported to be decreased in two studies (1, 7), whereas in two other studies (2, 8) no significant influence could be detected. Aggregation induced by thrombin was reduced in one study (14, low dose only), whereas no effect was demonstrated in 3 other studies (2, 5, 14, high dose). When arachidonic acid or the thromboxane-mimicking agent U46619 was used to activate platelets, no significant effect of marine lipids has been observed so far (2, 4, 6, 12, 13, 16). In the non- or poorly controlled studies, the effects of fish(oils) are considerably more favourable but also equivocal, with the exception of platelet aggregation induced by U46619 or ristocetin (no effect).
In these studies, platelet aggregation was measured with an optical method using platelet-rich plasma (PRP) or washed platelets, resuspended in buffer. Using a test for spontaneous aggregation in PRP (17), 2.5 g of (n-3) fatty acids per day for 5 weeks did not cause significant changes in platelet aggregability as compared to a placebo group, receiving the same amount of saturated medium chain triglycerides (18).
Recently, a new technique for the *in-vitro* measurement of platelet aggregation in whole blood has become available. This method is based on changes in the impedance of blood as a result of platelet adhesion to an electrode, and subsequent aggregation (19, 20). We used this method in a controlled human study in which the effects were compared of the daily dietary supplementation with 135 g of mackerel paste (containing 4.7 g of (n-3) PUFAs) or with 135 g of meat paste. A slight reduction was observed when collagen was used to induce aggregation (21); in addition, the collagen-induced aggregation in PRP was significantly reduced in the fish-treated group (14). However, recent data indicate that the inverse relationship between fish consumption and coronary heart disease mortality, as observed in the Dutch town of Zutphen (22), is not simply explained by an effect on the function of blood platelets (23).

Since it is almost impossible to extrapolate *in-vitro* results to *in vivo* conditions, more research is required to obtain a better insight into the effect of dietary fish(oil) on platelet function *in vivo*. It is of particular interest to apply techniques that truly reflect platelet function *in vivo*. Measurement of the cutaneous bleeding time is considered to be such a test (24).
In traditionally-living Greenland Eskimos, bleeding times are significantly prolonged (25, 26), which is in agreement with the reduced *in-vitro* reactivity of the blood platelets. Oral administration of fish, fish oil, or concentrates of fish oil did induce longer bleeding times in 23 studies. In 16 studies no significant effect was observed. However, it has to be noted that only 16 of these 39 studies comprised an adequate control group. In seven of these well-controlled studies an increase of the bleeding time was observed (2, 6, 9, 13, 16, 27, 28) but the other nine (4, 7, 11, 15, 27, 29-32) did not show this effect. Nonetheless it seems likely that marine oils are able to attenuate the platelet-vessel wall interaction.

Bleeding time prolongation is most probably not due to the reduced formation of thromboxane A_2 (TxA_2) only. Juan and Sametz provide evidence that a fish oil preparation prolongs the bleeding time by antagonizing the vasoconstrictor effect of sympathetic transmitters at the site of the injured vessel (33). In contrast to this, however, Butcher and coworkers (34) observed no effect of a diet, enriched with (n-3) fatty acids, on cold-induced vasoconstriction. Interestingly, dietary arachidonic acid enrichment did reduce the cold pressure response.

Another useful method to measure platelet activation *in vivo* seems the determination of the "survival time" of ^{111}Indium labelled platelets (35). Hay and coworkers (36) reported that the platelet survival time, which is frequently decreased in patients with ischaemic vascular disease (37), can be normalized to some extent by the administration of a fish-oil concentrate. This observation has been confirmed in a (non-controlled) study with 7 healthy volunteers (38).
The presence of circulating platelet aggregates, as measured by a technique described by Wu and Hoak (39), was not significantly altered by the administration of 50 ml of fish oil concentrate per day to atherosclerotic patients for a period of 4 weeks (40). Similar results were obtained in post-myocardial infarction patients receiving 8 g of fish oil per day for 2 weeks (41).
Indirect methods to determine platelet activation *in vivo* are based on the measurement of platelet specific proteins (β-thromboglobulin and platelet factor 4) in plasma, and of the intraplatelet cAMP content.
The effects of treatment with dietary fish(oils) are inconsistent again (5, 7, 11, 30, 36, 40, 42, 43) which may, at least partly, be due to sampling artifacts.

Taken all this evidence together, it can be stated that the effect of dietary marine oils on platelet aggregation *in vitro* and *in vivo* is not very pronounced. There may be a slight reduction, especially when collagen is used as a platelet trigger. This is likely to be due to the lower potential of blood platelets to produce TxA_2 upon activation (44, for a review: see 45), caused by the partly replacement in membrane phospholipids of the TxA_2-precursor arachidonic acid (AA) by the 'fish fatty acids' timnodonic- and cervonic acid (for a review: see 45). In addition, timnodonic acid may also reduce the formation of TxA_2 by inhibiting AA-liberation from membrane phospholipids (46, 47) as well as by competitive inhibition of the cyclo-oxygenase enzyme (48, 49). The Tx-receptor occupancy by timnodonic acid has also been proposed as a mechanism (50). Recent evidence indicates, however, that the Tx-sensitivity of platelets increases when their potential to produce TxA_2 diminishes (51, 52), which would partly counteract the possible beneficial effect of a reduced TxA_2 production upon fish oil administration. Cervonic acid has been suggested to lower platelet aggregability by a direct membrane effect (48). In addition, it may interfere with the formation of TxA_2 via competition with AA (53, 54).

3. Effect of marine lipids on blood coagulation

Blood coagulation and fibrinolysis are likely to play an important role in the development and the complications of ischaemic heart and vessel disease. This is indicated by the fact that the atherosclerotic plaque contains fibrin (55), the end product of the coagulation cascade. Moreover, oral anticoagulants appeared to be effective in the secondary prevention of myocardial infarction (56, 57). Activated platelets stimulate blood coagulation (58-60); furthermore, thrombin -the central enzyme in coagulation- is an extremely potent activator of blood platelets (61, 62). Repeatedly, evidence has been obtained supporting the concept that thrombin, formed as a consequence of vascular injury, is essential for the initiation of the local platelet thrombus (63, 64). The fibrinolytic system has also been implicated in the development of atherosclerosis (65, 66) and an impaired fibrinolytic system has been associated with myocardial ischaemia (67-69). Because of these observations, it seems useful to evaluate the influence of dietary factors on blood coagulation and fibrinolysis. With respect to the influence of fish and fish oils, only limited data are available up till now.

Epidemiological data (which reflect long-term dietary habits) suggest only marginal effects of fish-oil enriched diets on blood coagulation. Traditionally-living Eskimos do not differ from a comparable Danish control group as to the coagulability of their blood plasma. These observations are in accordance with most human intervention studies (for a review: see 45). Plasma fibrinogen was shown to be a powerful cardio- and cerebrovascular risk factor (70-72). Therefore, the effect of dietary marine lipids on the plasma fibrinogen content is of interest. In most studies, the plasma fibrinogen content is not significant affected by dietary fish or by marine oils (9-11, 16, 43, 73-80). In one study, however, an increase was seen in the plasma fibrinogen content (15), which is in agreement with epidemiological findings that Greenland Eskimo's, as compared to Eskimos living in Denmark and Danish controls, have higher plasma fibrinogen levels (81). In another intervention study, a daily dose of 14 g of a fish oil concentrate, administered for 6 weeks (ca. 6.5 g (n-3) fatty acids per day), resulted in a significant reduction of the plasma fibrinogen level (82, 83). The effect was maximal after 3 weeks and tended to normalize (but was still significant) after 6 weeks. No significant effect was observed in a control group, receiving olive oil. At a considerably lower dose (2.2 or 1.1 g/day, given for 20 weeks) plasma fibrinogen content has also been reported to be reduced considerably (31). Ten ml. fish oil (1.8 g of (n-3) fatty acids) per day given to angina pectoris patients for a period of 4 years resulted in a consistent reduction of the plasma fibrinogen content by about 23% over a 4 years period (84). Thus, again, the fish oil effect is equivocal.

The activity of clotting factor VII has also been shown to be a powerful risk indicator for ischaemic cardiovascular disease (85). Intervention studies never demonstrated an effect of marine oils on the activity of this clotting factor in man (5, 15, 74, 76, 78, 79). Administration of a fish-oil concentrate, containing a high concentration (67%) of the ethyl ester of timnodonic acid, induced a significant increase of the circulating amount of activated factor VII at the expense of non-activated factor VII (86). This points to an enhanced consumption of factor VII as a result of *in-vivo* activation. No further studies on this issue have been reported.
Most other coagulation factors do not seem to be influenced by a diet rich in marine oils (45). Some more studies are required, however, with respect to Factor X: in 2 studies no effect was observed (15, 87), but two other studies demonstrated a significant increase (15, 74).

Blood coagulation *in vivo* is controlled by a number of natural anticoagulants present in blood plasma and the vessel wall. One of these physiological anticoagulants is antithrombin III (AT-III), the deficiency of which leads to a prothrombotic state (88). The deficiency of another natural anticoagulant, protein C, may lead to venous thrombosis (89). Experimental results with regard to the effect of dietary fish or marine oils on the AT-III activity are not unanimous: a decrease of AT-III activity has been described following the administration of 20 ml cod-liver oil per day for 6 weeks (76), whereas the administration of the fish-oil preparation MaxEPA (10 ml per day for 5 weeks) did not have an effect (77). In another study with the same dose of MaxEPA for 4 weeks, the AT-III content (immunological activity) increased significantly but this did not result in a significant elevation of AT-III activity. On the other hand, the AT-III content and activity did increase upon the daily administration of 10 ml of a vegetable oil mixture, rich in linoleic acid (9). Administration of the ethyl esters of a cod-liver oil concentrate increased the immunoreactive AT-III significantly but did not change AT-III activity (90). A comparable preparation, given to normal volunteers in an amount of 0.9 g per day for 2-4 weeks, did not change plasma AT-III content (43). Comparable results were obtained when insulin dependent diabetics were given 4 g of (n-3) PUFAs per day for 6 weeks (79). No significant effect was seen on the chromogenic AT-III activity and/or the plasmatic AT-III antigen content, upon giving normal volunteers a fish-enriched diet (about 1.9 g timnodonic acid per day) for 4 weeks (91) or supplementing the diet of insulin-diabetics with 15 g of MaxEPA per day for 6 weeks (15). The daily administration of 1-2 g of a fish oil concentrate for 20 weeks did not alter plasmatic AT III activity (31). In addition, protein C antigen remained the same. In another study, however, the daily administration of 900 mg marine (n-3) fatty acids for 30 days resulted in a significant reduction of protein C and AT-III antigen levels (73). Since the study was uncontrolled and comprized only 9 volunteers, its validity is rather limited. In Type II_a hyperlipidaemic subjects, the daily administration of 6 g (n-3) fatty acids for 6 weeks resulted in a significant increase in protein C, whereas in Type IV patients a significant reduction occurred (78). In the same study, no effect on AT III activity was observed.

These studies do not support the suggestion, derived from epidemiological data, that a fish(oil) enriched diet will increase the physiological anti-coagulatory process via an increased AT-III activity (26, 90). As Eskimos, who emigrated to Denmark, maintain their elevated AT-III activity (90), this elevation seems to be determined more by genetic than by environmental (nutritional) factors.

From these studies it does not seem very plausible that diets enriched with fish, fish oil or fish-oil concentrates influence blood coagulation to a significant extent.

4. The effect of dietary marine lipids on fibrinolysis

The fibrinolytic system is ever more considered to be implicated in the development of atherosclerosis (65, 66) and an unpaired fibrinolytic system has been associated with myocardial infarction (67-69). Because of these observations, it seems useful to evaluate the influence of dietary factors on fibrinolysis. For a long period, measurement of the lysis time of a fibrin clot, suspended in plasma, has been the most widely used method to quantify the fibrinolytic potential of an individual. Using this methodology, it was demonstrated that the daily administration of 20 ml cod-liver oil during 6 weeks to healthy men did not influence fibrinolysis in these volunteers (76). Comparable results were obtained using the highly standardized fibrin plate method (13).

In recent years, the knowledge about the fibrinolytic process increased explosively (66, 92, 93). This resulted in the development of sensitive and specific methods to measure the fibrinolytic process and its regulation (94, 95), some of which have now been used to investigate the effect of dietary fish(oil). Barcelli and coworkers (96) administered 5 g of (n-3) PUFAs per day for 2 weeks to normal volunteers and noted a significant increase in the activity of the vascular plasminogen activator. The activities of the plasminogen activator inhibitor and the plasma content of α_2-antiplasmin decreased slightly. These findings indicate an increased fibrinolytic potential after fish oil administration. Unfortunately, no control group was included in this study. Saldeen and coworkers (97) performed a well-controlled study and also noticed a reduction in the plasminogen activator inhibitor after the administration of MaxEPA. Unfortunately, the measurements were

carried out in serum and are, therefore, not reliable. In a later study, using proper methodology, the same group confirmed their findings but, unfortunately, no control group was included this time (98).
Emeis and coworkers (99) recently demonstrated that the daily intake of 100 g of mackerel for 6 weeks by healthy volunteers did not cause changes in the contents and/or activities of plasminogen, α_2-antiplasmin and tissue plasminogen activator, when compared with a control group receiving 100 g of meat instead. In the fish group, however, the total plasma plasminogen activator inhibitor activity increased by almost 50%, which was mainly due to the type-1 inhibitor. This effect was not observed in the control group. These results are in agreement with the recently published data on traditionally-living Greenland Eskimos who appeared to have significantly higher levels of the fast inhibitor of tissue plasminogen activator in their plasma than a control group, living on a Western diet (100). The same group did not observe a significant effect of (n-3) PUFAs on tissue plasminogen activator inhibitor, when stable angina pectoris patients were given 15 MaxEPA capsules per day for a period of 12 weeks, although fibrinolytic activity at rest decreased significantly (101). In Type I diabetics, however, Fröschl et al (102) noted an increase of the tissue plasminogen activator inhibitor in parallel to a prolonged whole blood clot lysis time after the administration of 4.5 g TA and 2.7 g CA per day for 4 weeks. These results were not confirmed by Schmidt and coworkers (79), who were unable to modulate fibrinolysis by giving 4 g of (n-3) fatty acids per day for 6 weeks to insulin-dependent diabetics. Comparable results were observed by Radack and coworkers for hyperlipidaemic patients (31). Six grams of (n-3) fatty acids per day for 6 weeks, however, resulted in a reduced fibrinolytic activity in hyperlipidemic patients as reflected by the reduction in tPA activity and an increase in PAI activity (78). An increased activity of the plasma plasminogen activator inhibitor has been associated with cardiovascular disease (67-69). The results mentioned above are not unanimous with respect to the effect of dietary fish(oil) on fibrinolytic activity and need, therefore, to be extended. In the mean time the use of fish-enriched diets by people with low endogenous fibrinolytic activity should be discouraged.

5. Influence of (n-3) fatty acids on arterial thrombosis

The study of dietary influences on arterial thrombogenesis in man is severel hampered by the fact that a human thrombosis model is not available.
Recently, the effect of (n-3) PUFAs has been investigated on rate and degree of thrombotic restenosis following percutaneous transluminal coronary angioplasty (PTCA) in man. The first study demonstrated a significant improvement by fish oil supplementation (3.2 g TA per day) in addition to the habitual treatment (325 mg aspirin + 225 mg dipyridamole per day): the incidence of early vessel restenosis was 36% in the control group and 16% in the treatment group ($p = 0.026$, ref 124). These results have been confirmed by others with respect to single-vessel PTCA (103-106). No improvement by fish oil was seen in multivessel PTCA (106). In another study (107) MaxEPA, at a dose of 10 capsules per day in addition to the usual medication, did not lower the risk of stenosis after PTCA as compared with the usual treatment alone. In this study, however, pre-treatment lasted for 24 h only. Reis and coworkers (108) also failed to see any beneficial effect of 6 g/day of (n-3) fatty acids beginning 5 days before PTCA and continuing for 6 months, on top of the usual medication.
As reviewed recently, animal studies suggest a beneficial effect of marine lipids on arterial thrombosis (109). Recent studies of our own group, using an arterial thrombosis model in rats, strongly suggest that the antithrombotic potential of (n-3) fatty acids is very actively counteracted

by saturated fatty acids (110). Consequently, the optimum benefit from (n-3) fatty acids can be expected when their administration is 'supported' by a reduction in saturated fat intake. In this respect it is of interest to note that the traditional Eskimo diet is characterized not only by a high content of (n-3) fatty acids, but by a very low saturated fat content as well (58, 111).

6. Effect of dietary marine oils on ischaemic heart disease and peripheral vascular disease in man.

Angina pectoris is caused by an inadequate blood supply of the myocardium due to atherosclerosis of the coronary arteries. Since the aggregation tendency of platelets from patients with angina pectoris is elevated, (8, 112, 113), local platelet aggregation likely contributes to the anginal complaints (114).

In an uncontrolled study with 12 patients suffering from angina pectoris, Saynor and coworkers (115) noted a dramatic reduction in the consumption of glyceryltrinitrate upon the administration of 10 ml of MaxEPA per day for 9 months. This suggests a reduction of anginal attacks, possibly by lowering platelet aggregability. This suggestion could not be confirmed in another uncontrolled study (116) in which 3 g of (n-3) PUFAs (timnodonic, clupadonic, and cervonic acid, see Table 1) per day was administered to 5 patients with stable angina pectoris. Before and after 6 months treatment, a symptom-limited exercise test with 12-lead electrocardiography was performed to obtain an objective measure of exercise-induced myocardial ischaemia. Exercise duration and maximum ST-segment depression remained unchanged. Moreover, none of the patients reported any change in frequency, duration and intensity of anginal attacks during the study period.
In a double-blind, placebo-controlled trial, two groups of 19 stable angina patients received 15 capsules with MaxEPA or placebo (a linoleic acid rich vegetable oil) per day for 12 weeks after a 4 weeks run-in period on placebo capsules. In both groups a 20-30% reduction was observed in anginal attacks and glyceryltrinitrate consumption. Since the difference between both groups was not significant (not even with the one-sided approach chosen by the investigators), it can be concluded that the treatment with (n-3) PUFAs was unsuccessful. The change in anginal intensity observed during the study was most probably due to seasonal variations: the study started during the winter and was concluded in the spring (7). A comparable design was used in a study with 10 patients with stable angina pectoris. Again, no clinical improvement was observed in the MaxEPA as compared to the control (olive oil) group, although there were significant haemorheological improvements and a prolonged bleeding time (16). Mehta and coworkers (8) administered MaxEPA (3.2 g timnodonic + 2.2 g cervonic acid per day) to 8 patients with stable coronary artery disease and positive exercise stress test results, in a randomized, double blind, cross over fashion over a 12 week period. Despite alterations in platelet and neutrophil functions, arachidonic acid metabolism and myocardial oxygen demand, no significant changes were observed in subjective parameters of coronary artery disease during the MaxEPA phase. Similarly, exercise times to ST-segment depression and to onset of angina were not altered by administration of MaxEPA. They conclude that short-term dietary supplementation with (n-3) PUFAs to patients with stable coronary artery disease does not alter subjective or objective parameters of myocardial ischaemia.

Burr and coworkers (117) performed a secondary intervention study with post myocardial infarction patients who were counseled to change their diet by either reducing fat intake and increasing the polyunsaturated/saturated (P/S) ratio (fat advice), and/or by increasing the intake of fatty fish to at least 2 portions per week (fish advice), and/or by increasing fibre intake. There were thus eight possible combinations of these dietary factors, including a group which received no other advice than just to eat a 'sensible diet' (control group). The subjects adviced to eat fatty fish (either or not in combination with any of the other interventions) had a 29% reduction in 2 year all cause mortality as compared to the volunteers whose diet advice did not include fish ($p < 0.05$). This difference in mortality was entirely attributable to a reduction in IHD deaths ($p < 0.01$). Non fatal MI occurred more frequently in th 'fish advice' groups as compared to the 'no fish advice groups'. As a result, the number of total IHD events was not significantly affected by any of the dietary interventions or their combinations. Interestingly, the fish effect was doubled when the diet advice included the 'fat advice'. This underlines the importance of a high P/S ratio for a beneficial fish effect.

Peripheral vascular disease is associated with *in vivo* platelet activation also (118). In a double-blind, randomized trial 15 patients with intermittent claudication were given 10 capsules a day containing either MaxEPA or a mixture of olive oil and corn oil (placebo). After 7 weeks of experimental or placebo treatment, no changes were found in the disease as investigated by Doppler ultrasound techniques. In neither group did the pressure indices of the affected limbs change with supplementation (119). Comparable results were reported by Knapp and coworkers (120), who studied 6 men with angiographically confirmed Grade III peripheral vascular disease with documented platelet activation *in vivo*. The patients were given 50 ml of MaxEPA per day for 4 weeks as a supplement to their normal diet. No changes were observed in their pedal blood flow as reflected by resting skin colour and temperature, capillary-refill time, and time or extent of position-dependent changes in skin colour. Sakurai and coworkers (121) administered the ethyl ester of timnodonic acid to 41 patients with chronic arterial occlusion associated with ischaemic ulcers of the extremities. Striking clinical improvement was noted in almost 60% of the patients, which included ulcer healing and disappearance of pain at rest.

It should be mentioned here that the clinical improvement of angina pectoris and peripheral vascular disease does not necessarily reflect decreased platelet reactivity; changes in haemorheology may also contribute. This latter possibility is of particular interest, since fish(oil) consumption has repeatedly been shown to lower blood or plasma viscosity (16, 38, 119, 122-127), although this is not a general finding (11, 32, 125, 127-129). Moreover, dietary fish oil improves red cell deformability (16, 38, 122, 127, 130, 131), although not in all studies (11, 126). Both factors are likely to be involved in the increase of the microcirculatory blood flow, which was demonstrated in men receiving MaxEPA (0.15 g/kg/day) for a period of 3 weeks (128). It is tempting to attribute the improved red cell deformability to a decreased microviscosity of erythrocyte membranes upon fish(oil) consumption, because the daily administration of 2.7 g of sardine oil to healthy volunteers and type II diabetic patients for 8 weeks, significantly lowered erythrocyte membrane fluidity as measured by electron spin resonance (132). Another study, with non-insulin dependent diabetic volunteers, however, did not reveal a significant effect of the daily intake of 3 g of (n-3) PUFAs for 8 weeks on erythrocyte membrane fluidity as measured by electron spin resonance and fluorescence polarization (133, 134). The same treatment did reduce the viscosity of erythrocyte suspensions of patients on continuous ambulatory peritoneal dialysis (4). Under almost identical conditions platelet membrane fluidity appeared to be reduced in healthy male volunteers (135).

7. References

1. Driss, F., Vericel, E., Lagarde, M., Dechavanne, M. and Darcet, P. (1984) 'Inhibition of platelet aggregation and thromboxane synthesis after intake of small amount of icosapentaenoic acid', Thromb. Res. 36, 389-396.
2. Goodnight, S.H. Jr., Harris, W.S. and Connor, W.E. (1981) 'The effect of dietary ω 3 fatty acids on platelet composition and function in man: a prospective, controlled study', Blood 58, 880-885.
3. Hänninen, O. and Ågren, J.J. (1989) 'Effects of moderate fresh water fish diet on lipid metabolism of Finnish students', J. Int. Med. 225 Suppl. 1, 77-82.
4. Brox, J.H., Killie, J.E., Gunnes, S. and Nordøy, A. (1981) 'The effect of cod-liver oil and corn oil on platelets and vessel wall in man', Thromb. Haemostas. 46, 604-611.
5. Brox, J.H., Killie, J.E., Østerud, B., Holme, S. and Nordøy, A. (1983) 'Effects of cod-liver oil on platelets and coagulation in familial hypercholesterolemia (Type IIa)', Acta Med. Scand. 213, 137-144.
6. Green, D., Barreres, L., Borensztain, J., Kaplan, P., Reddy, N., Rovner, R. and Simon, H. (1985) 'A double-blind, placebo-controlled trial of fish oil concentrate (MaxEPA) in stroke patients', Stroke 16, 706-709.
7. Kristensen, S.D., Berg Schmidt, E., Rud Anderson, H. and Dyerberg, J. (1987) 'Fish oil in angina pectoris', Atherosclerosis 64, 13-19.
8. Mehta, J., Lopez, L.M., Lawson, D., Wargovich, T.J. and Williams, L.L. (1988) 'Dietary supplementation with stable coronary heart disease. Effects on indices of platelet and neutrophil function and exercise performance', Am. J. Med. 84, 45-52.
9. Mortensen, J.Z., Schmidt, E.B., Nielsen, A.H. and Dyerberg, J. (1983) 'The effect of (n-6) and (n-3) polyunsaturated fatty acids on hemostasis, blood lipids and blood pressure', Thromb. Haemostas. 50, 543-546.
10. Norris, P.G., Jones, C.J.H. and Weston, M.J. (1986) 'Effect of dietary supplementation with fish oil on systolic blood pressure in mild essential hypertension', Brit. Med. J. 293, 104-105.
11. Rogers, S., James, K.S., Butland, B.K., Etherington, M.D., O'Brien, J.R. and Jones, J.G. (1987) 'Effects of a fish oil supplement on serum lipids, blood pressure, bleeding time, haemostatic and rheological variables. A double blind randomised controlled trial in healthy volunteers', Atherosclerosis 63, 137-143.
12. Sanders, T.A.B. and Hochland, M.C. (1983) 'A comparison of the influence on plasma lipids and platelet function of supplements of ω-3 and ω-6 polyunsaturated fatty acids', Brit. J. Nutr. 50, 521-529.
13. Zucker, M.L., Bilyeu, D.S., Helmkamp, G.M., Harris, W.S. and Dujoune, C.A. (1988) 'Effects of dietary fish oil on platelet function and plasma lipids in hyperlipoproteinemic and normal subjects', Atherosclerosis 73, 13-22.
14. Houwelingen, A.C. van , Hennissen, A.A.H.M., Verbeek-Schippers, F., Simonsen, T., Kester, A.D.M. and Hornstra, G. (1988) 'Effect of a moderate fish intake on platelet aggregation in human platelet rich plasma', Thromb. Haemost. 59, 507-513.
15. Haines, A.P., Sanders, T.A.B., Imeson, J.D., Mahler, R.F., Martin, J., Mistry, M., Vickers, M. and Wallace, P.G. (1986) 'Effects of a fish oil supplement on platelet function, hemostatic variables and albuminuria in insulin-dependent diabetics', Thromb. Res. 43: 643-655.

16. Solomon, S.A., Cartwright, I., Pockley, G., Greaves, M., Preston, F.E., Ramsay, L.E. and Waller, P.C. (1990) 'A placebo-controlled, double-blind study of eicosapentaenoic acid-rich fish oil in patients with stable angina pectoris', Curr. Med. Res. Opin. 12: 1-11.
17. Breddin, K., Grun, H., Krzywanek, H.J. and Schremmer, M.M. (1975) 'On the measurements of spontaneous platelet aggregation. III Methods and first clinical results', Thromb. Haemost. 48, 261-272.
18. Bach, R., Schmidt, U., Jung, F., Kiesewetter, H., Hennen, B., Wenzel, E., Schieffer, H., Bette, L. and Heyden, S. (1989) 'Effects of fish oil capsules in two dosages on blood pressure, platelet functions, haemorheological and clinical chemistry parameters in apparently healthy subjects', Ann. Nutr. Metab. 33, 359-367.
19. Cardinal, D.C. and Flower, R.J. (1980) 'The electronic aggregometer: a novel device for assessing platelet behaviour in blood', J. Pharmacol. Meth. 3: 135-158.
20. Ingerman-Wojenski, C.M. and Silver, M.J. (1984) 'A quick method for screening platelet dysfunctions using the whole blood lumi- aggregometer', Thromb. Haemostas. 51, 154-156.
21. Houwelingen, A.C. van, Kester, A.D.M. and Hornstra, G. (1989) 'Effect of moderate fish intake on platelet aggregation and ATP release in human blood', Nutr. Res. 9, 1187-1196.
22. Kromhout, D., Bosschieter, E.B. and de Lezenne Coulander, C. (1985) 'The inverse relation between fish consumption and 20-year mortality from coronary heart disease', New Engl. J. Med. 312, 1205-1209.
23. Houwelingen, A.C. van, Hornstra, G., Stegen, J., Katan, M. and Kromhout, D. (1987) 'Habitual fish consumption, serum lipids and platelet function', in W.E.M. Lands (ed), Polyunsaturated fatty acids and eicosanoids, American Oil Chemists' Society, pp. 368-371.
24. Nieuwenhuis, H.K. and Sixma, J.J. (1983) 'Bleeding time measurements', in L.A. Harker and T.S. Zimmerman (eds), Measurements of platelet function, Churchill Livingstone, Edinburgh, 26-45.
25. Dyerberg, J. and Bang, H.O. (1979) 'Haemostatic function and platelet polyunsatured fatty acids in Eskimos', Lancet ii, 433-435.
26. Jørgensen, K.A., Nielsen, A.H. and Dyerberg, J. (1986) 'Hemostatic factors and renin in Greenland Eskimos on a high eicosapentaenoic acid intake', Acta Med. Scand. 219: 473-479.
27. Harris, W.S., Connor, W.E. and Goodnight, S.H. Jr. (1981) 'Dietary fish oils, plasma lipids and platelets in man', Progr. Lip. Res. 20, 75-79.
28. Houwelingen, A.C. van, Nordøy, A., Beek, E. van der, Houtsmuller, U.M.T., Metz, M. de and Hornstra, G. (1987) 'Effect of a moderate fish intake on blood pressure, bleeding time, hematology, and clinical chemistry in healthy males', Am. J. Clin. Nutr. 46, 871-875.
29. Cleland, L.G., French, J.K., Betts, W.H., Murphy, G.A. and Elliott, M.J. (1988) 'Clinical and biochemical effects of dietary fish oil supplements in rheumatoid arthritis', J. Rheumatol 15, 1471-1475.
30. Demke, D.M., Peters, G.R., Linet, O.I., Metzler, C.M. and Klott, K.A. (1988) 'Effects of a fish oil concentrate in patients with hypercholesterolemia', Atherosclerosis 70, 73-80.
31. Radack, K., Deck, C. and Huster, G. (1989) 'Dietary supplementation with lowdose fish oils lowers fibrinogen levels: a randomized, double-blind controlled study', Am. Int. med. 111, 757-758.
32. Simons, L.A., Hickie, J.B. and Balasubramaniam, S. (1985) 'On the effects of dietary (n-3) fatty acids (Maxepa) on plasma lipids and lipoproteins in patients with hyperlipidaemia', Atherosclerosis 54, 75-88.

33. Juan, H. and Sametz, W. (1989) 'Fish oil diet rich in eicosapentaenoic acid increases bleeding time in the rat by interaction with sympathetic transmitters', Agents and Actions 28, 130-136.
34. Butcher, L.A., O'Dea, K., Sinclair, A.J., Parkin, J.D., Smith, I.L. and Blombery, P. (1990) 'The effects of very low fat diets enriched with fish or kangaroo meat on cold-induced vasoconstriction and platelet function', Prost. Leukotr. and Ess. Fatty Acids 39, 221-226.
35. Hawker, R.J., Hawker, L.M., and Wilkinson, A.R. (1980) 'Indium (^{111}I) labelled human platelets', Optimal method. Clin. Sci. 58, 243-248.
36. Hay, C.R.M., Durber, A.P. and Saynor, R. (1982) 'Effect of fish oil on platelet kinetics in patients with ischaemic heart disease', Lancet i, 1269-1272.
37. Steele, P.P., Weily, H.S., Davies, H. and Genton, E. (1973) 'Platelet function studies in coronary artery disease', Circulation 48, 1194-1200.
38. Terano, T., Hirai, A., Hamazaki, T., Kobayashi, S., Fujita, T., Tamura, Y. and Kumagai, A. (1983) 'Effect of oral administration of highly purified eicosapentaenoic acid on platelet function, blood viscosity and red cell deformability in healthy human subjects', Atherosclerosis 46, 321-331.
39. Wu, K.K. and Hoak, J.C. (1974) 'New method for quantitative detection of platelet aggregates in patients with arterial insufficiency', Lancet ii, 924-926.
40. Knapp, H.R., Rielly, I.A.G., Alessandrini, P. and FitzGerald, G.A. (1986) 'In vivo indexes of platelet and vascular function during fish-oil administration in patients with atherosclerosis', New Engl. J. Med. 314, 937-942.
41. Kahl, P.E., Schimke, E., Hildebrandt, R., Beitz, J., Schimke, I., Beitz, H., Mrochen, H. and Mest, H.-J. (1987) 'The influence of cod-liver oil diet on various lipid metabolism parameters, the thromboxane formation capacity, platelet function and the serum MDA level in patients suffering from myocardial infarction', Cor Vasa 29, 199-208.
42. Rylance, P.B., Gordge, M.P., Parsons, V. and Weston, M.J. (1986) 'Fish oil modifies lipids and reduces platelet aggregability in haemodialysis patients', Nephron 4, 196-202.
43. Yoshimura, T, Matsui, K., Yunohara, T., Kawasaki, N., Nakamura, T. and Okamura, H. (1987) 'Effects of highly purified eicosapentaenoic acid on plasma beta thromboglobulin level and vascular reactivity to angiotension II', Artery 14, 295-303.
44. Hornstra, G., Houwelingen, A.C. van, Kivits, G.A.A., Fischer, S. and Uedelhoven, W. (1990) 'Influence of dietary fish on eicosanoid metabolism in man', Prostaglandins 40, 311-329.
45. Hornstra, G. (1989) 'The significance of fish and fish-oil enriched food for prevention and therapy of ischaemic cardiovascular disease' in A.J. Vergroesen and M. Crawford (eds), The role of fats in human nutrition II, Academic press, London, pp. 151-235.
46. Hirai, A., Terano, T., Hamazaki, T., Sajiki, J., Kondo, S., Ozawa, A., Fujita, T., Miyamoto, T., Tamura, Y. and Kumagai, A. (1982) 'The effects of the oral administration of fish oil concentrate on the release and the metabolism of [^{14}C]arachidonic acid and [^{14}C] eicosapentaenoic acid by human platelets', Thromb. Res. 28, 285-298.
47. Lagarde, M., Drouot, B., Guichardant, M. and Dechavanne, M. (1985) 'In vitro incorporation and metabolism of some icosanoic acids in platelets. Effect on arachidonic acid oxygenation', Biochim. Biophys. Acta 833, 52-58.
48. Crozet, M. and Lagarde, M. (1986) 'In vitro incorporation and metabolism of icosapentaenoic and docosahexaenoic acids in human platelets-effect on aggregation', Thromb. Haemost. 56, 57-62.

49. Needleman, P., Raz, A., Minkes, M.S., Ferrendelli, J.A. and Sprecher, H. (1979) 'Triene prostaglandins: prostacyclin and thromboxane biosynthesis and unique biological properties', Proc. Natl. Acad. Sci. USA 76: 944-948.
50. Gryglewski, R.J., Salmon, J.A. Ubatuba, F.B., Weatherly, B.C., Moncada, S. and Vane, J.R. (1979) 'Effects of all cis-5,8,11,14,17 eicosapentaenoic acid and PGH_3 on platelet aggregation', Prostaglandins 18, 453-478.
51. Heemskerk, J.W.M., Feijge, M.A.H., Kalafusz, R. and Hornstra, G. (1989) 'Influence of dietary fatty acids on membrane fluidity and activation of rat platelets', Biochim. Biophys. Acta 1004, 252-260.
52. Heemskerk, J.W.M., Feijge, M.A.H., Kester, A. and Hornstra, G. (1991) 'Dietary fat modifies thromboxane A_2-induced stimulation of rat platelets', Biochem. J., in press.
53. Corey, E.J., Shih, C. and Cashman, J.R. (1983) 'Docosahexaenoic acid is a strong inhibitor of prostaglandin but not of leukotriene biosynthesis', Proc. Natl. Acad. Sci. USA 80, 3581-3584.
54. Rao, G.H.R. and White, J.G. (1983) 'Effect of docosahexaenoic acid (DHA) on arachidonic acid metabolism and platelet function', Biochem. Biophys. Res. Comm. 117, 549-555.
55. Woolf, N. (1982) 'Pathology of Atherosclerosis', Chapter 10: Thrombosis and atherosclerosis, Butterworth Scientific, pp. 217-259.
56. Loeliger, E.A., Hensen, A., Kroes, F., Dijk, L.M. van, Fekkes, N., de Jonge, H. and Hemker, H.C. (1967) 'A double blind trial of long-term anticoagulant treatment after myocardial infarction', Acta med. Scand. 182, 549-566.
57. Vries, W.A. de, Tijssen, J.P.G., Loeliger, E.A. and Roos, J. (1980) 'A double-blind trial to assess long-term anticoagulant therapy in elderly patients after myocardial infarction', Lancet ii, 989-994.
58. Bevers, E.M., Rosing, J. and Zwaal, R.F.A. (1987) 'Platelets and coagulation', in D.E. MacIntyre and J. Gordon (eds), Platelets in Biology and Pathology III, Elsevier Science Publishers, B.V. Biomedical Division, pp. 127-160.
59. Fantl, P. and Ward, H.A. (1958) 'The thromboplastic component of intact blood is present in masked form', Aust. J. Exptl. Biol. Med. Sci. 36, 499-504.
60. Walsh, P.N. and Griffin, J.H. (1981) 'Contribution of human platelets to the proteolytic activation of blood coagulation factor XII and XI', Blood 57, 106-118.
61. Davey, M.G. and Lüscher, E.F. (1967) 'Actions of thrombin and other coagulant and proteolytic enzymes on blood platelets', Nature 216, 857-858.
62. Majerus, P.W., Tollefsen, D.M. and Shuman, M.A. (1976) 'The interaction of platelets with thrombin', in J.L. Gordon (ed.), Platelets in biology and pathology, Volume 1, Elsevier/North Holland Biomedical Press, pp. 241-260.
63. Ardlie, N.G. and Han, P. (1974) 'Enzymatic basis for platelet aggregation and release: the significance of the 'platelet atmosphere' and the relationship between platelet function and blood coagulation', Brit. J. Haematol. 26, 331-356.
64. Hornstra, G. (1981) 'Platelet-vessel wall interaction: role of blood clotting', Phil. Trans. R. Soc. Lond. B. 294, 344-371.
65. Astrup, T. (1978) 'Fibrinolysis: an overview', in J.F. Davidson, R.M. Rowan, M.M. Samanm and P.S. Desnoyers (eds), Progress in chemical fibrinolysis and thrombolysis, Raven Press, New York, pp. 1-57.
66. Bachmann, F. (1987) 'Fibrinolysis', in M. Verstraete, J. Vermylen, R. Lynen and J. Arnout (eds), Thrombosis and Haemostasis 1987, Leuven University Press, pp. 227-265.

67. Hamsten, A., De Faire, U., Walldius, G., Dahlen, G., Szamosi, A., Landou, C., Blombäck, M. and Wiman, B. (1987) 'Plasminogen activator inhibitor in plasma-risk factor for recurrent myocardial infarction', Lancet ii, 3-9.
68. Hamsten, A., Wiman, B., de Faire, U. and Blomback, M. (1985) 'Increased plasma levels of a rapid inhibitor of tissue plasminogen activator in young survivors of myocardial infarction', New Engl. J. Med. 313, 1557-1563.
69. Paramo, J.A., Colucci, M., Collen, D. and Werf, F. van de (1985) 'Plasminogen activator inhibitor in the blood of patients with coronary artery disease', Brit. Med. J. 291, 573-574.
70. Kannel, W.B., Wolf, P.A., Castelli, W.P. and D'Agostino, R.B. (1987) 'Fibrinogen and risk of cardiovascular disease', J. Am. Med. Assoc. 258, 1183-1186.
71. Meade, T.W., Brozovic, M., Chakrabarti, R.R., Haines, A.P., Imeson, J.D., Mellows, S., Miller, G.J., North, W.R.S., Stirling, Y. and Thompson, S.G. (1986) 'Haemostatic function and ischaemic heart disease: principal results of the Northwick Park heart study', Lancet ii, 533-537.
72. Wilhelmsen, L., Svärdsudd, K., Korsan-Bengtsen, K., Larsson, B., Welin, L. and Tibblin, G. (1984) 'Fibrinogen as a risk factor for stroke and myocardial infarction', New. Engl. J. Med. 311, 501-505.
73. Lox, C.D. (1990) 'The effects of dietary marine fish oils (omega-3 fatty acids) on coagulation profiles in men', Gen. Pharmac. 21, 241-246.
74. Muller, A.D., Houwelingen, A.C. van, Dam-Mieras, M.C.E. van, Bas, B.M. and Hornstra, G. (1989) 'Effect of a moderate fish intake on haemostatic parameters in healthy males', Thromb. Haemost. 61, 468-473.
75. Nagakawa, Y., Orimo, H., Harazawa, M., Morita, I., Yashiro, K. and Murota, S. (1983) 'Effect of eicosapentaenoic acid on the platelet aggregation and composition of fatty acid in man', Atherosclerosis 47, 71-75.
76. Sanders, T.A.B., Vickers, M. and Haines, A.P. (1981) 'Effect on blood lipids and haemostasis of a supplement of cod-liver oil, rich in eicosapentaenoic and docosahexaenoic acids, in healthy young men', Clin. Sci. 61, 317-324.
77. Saynor, R. and Verel, D. (1980) 'Effect of a marine oil high in eicosapentaenoic acid on blood lipids and coagulation', IRCS Med. Sci. 8, 378-379.
78. Schmidt, E.B., Ernst, E., Varming, K., Pedersen, J.O. and Dyerberg, J. (1989) 'The effect of n-3 fatty acids on lipids and haemostasis in patients with Type II[a] and Type IV hyperlipidaemia', Thromb. Haemost. 62, 797-801.
79. Schmidt, E.B., Sørensen, P.J., Pedersen, J.O., Jersild, C., Ditzel, J., Grunnet, N. and Dyerberg, J. (1989) 'The effect of (n-3) polyunsaturated fatty acids on lipids, hemostasis, neutrophil and monocyte chemotaxis in insulin dependent diabetes mellitus', J. Int. Med. 225 Suppl. 1, 201-206.
80. Thorngren, M. and Gustafson, A. (1981) 'Effects of 11-week increase in dietary eicospentaenoic acid on bleeding time, lipids and platelet aggregation', Lancet ii, 1190-1193.
81. Schmidt, E.B., Sørensen, P.J., Ernst, E., Kristensen, S.D., Pedersen, J.O. and Dyerberg, J. (1989) 'Studies on coagulation and fibrinolysis in Greenland Eskimos', Thromb. Res. 56, 553-558.
82. Flaten, H., Høstmark, A.T., Kierulf, P., Lystad, E., Trygg, K., Bjerkedal, T. and Osland, A. (1990) 'Fish-oil concentrate : effects on variables related to cardiovascular disease', Am. J. Clin. Nutr. 52, 300-306.
83. Høstmark, A.T., Bjerkedal, T., Kierulf, P., Flaten, H. and Ulshagen, K. (1988) 'Fish oil and plasma fibrinogen', Brit. Med. J. 297, 180-181.

84. Saynor, R. and Gillett, T. (1988) 'Fish oil and plasma fibrinogen', Brit. Med. J. 297, 1196.
85. Meade, T.W., Chakrabarti, R., Haines, A.P., North, W.R.S., Stirling, Y., Thompson, S.G. and Brozovic, M. (1980) 'Haemostatic function and cardiovascular death; early result of a prospective study', Lancet i, 1050-1054.
86. Hornstra, G. (1982) 'Dietary fats, prostanoids and arterial throm-bosis', Chapter 7, 'Effect of fish oil feeding on arterial throm-bosis, platelet function and blood coagulation', Martinus Nijhoff Publishers, The Hague, pp. 106-137.
87. Hamazaki, T., Urakaze, M., Sawazaki, S., Yamazaki, K., Taki, H. and Yano, S. (1988) 'Comparison of pulse wave velocity of the aorta between inhabitants of fishing and farming villages in Japan', Atherosclerosis 73, 157-160.
88. Rosenberg, R.D. and Rosenberg, J.S. (1984) 'Natural anticoagulant mechanisms', J. Clin. Invest. 74, 1-6.
89. Clouse, L.H. and Comp, P.C. (1986) 'The regulation of hemostasis: the protein C system', New. Engl. J. Med. 314, 1298-1304.
90. Stoffersen, E., Jørgensen, K.A. and Dyerberg, J. (1982) 'Antithrombin III and dietary intake of polyunsaturated fatty acids', Scand. J. Clin. Lab. Invest. 42, 83-86.
91. Atkinson, P.M., Wheeler, M.C., Mendelsohn, D., Pienaar, N. and Chetty, N. (1987) 'Effect of a 4-week freshwater fish (trout) diet on platelet aggregation, platelet fatty acids, serum lipids, and coagulation factors', Am. J. Hematol. 24, 143-149.
92. Collen, D. (1987) 'Molecular mechanisms of fibrinolysis and their application to fibrin-specific thrombolytic therapy', J. Cell. Biochem. 33, 77-94.
93. Sprengers, E.D. and Kluft, C. (1987) 'Plasminogen activator inhibitors', Blood 69, 381-387.
94. Verheijen, J.H., Chang, G.T.G. and Kluft, C. (1984) 'Evidence for the occurrence of a fast-acting inhibitor for tissue-type plasminogen activator in human plasma', Thromb. Haemost. 51, 392-395.
95. Verheijen, J.H., Mullaart, E., Chang, G.T.G., Kluft, C. and Wijngaards, G. (1982) 'A simple, sensitive spectrophotometric assay for an extrinsic (tissue type) plasminogen activator applicable to measurements in plasma', Thromb. Haemost. 48, 266-269.
96. Barcelli, U., Glas-Greenwalt, P. and Pollak, V.E. (1985) 'Enhancing effect of dietary supplementation with omega-3 fatty acids on plasma fibrinolysis in normal subjects', Thromb. Res. 39, 307-312.
97. Mehta, J. (1983) 'Platelets and prostaglandins in coronary heart disease. Rationale for use of platelet-suppressive drugs', JAMA 249, 2817-2823.
98. Mehta, J., Lawson, D. and Saldeen, T.J. (1988) 'Reduction in plasminogen activator inhibitor-1 (PAI-1) with omega-3 polyunsaturated fatty acid (PUFA) intake', Am. Heart J. 116 (5 Pt 1), 1201-1206.
99. Emeis, J.J., Houwelingen, A.C. van, Hoogen, C.M. van den and Hornstra, G. (1989) 'A moderate fish intake increases plasminogen activator inhibitor type-1 in human volunteers', Blood 74, 233-237.
100. Schmidt, E.B., Sørensen, P.J., Ernst, E. and Dyerberg, J. (1988) 'PAI is higher in Greenland Eskimos compared to Danish controls', Fibrinolysis 2, Suppl. 1, 132.
101. Schmidt, E.B., Kristensen, S.D. and Dyerberg, J. (1988) 'The effect of fish oil on lipids, coagulation and fibrinolysis in patients with angina pectoris', Artery 15, 316-329.
102. Fröschl, H., Spannagl, M., Drummer, C., Landgraf-Leurs, M.M.C., Landgraf, R. and Schramm, W. (1988) 'Effect of eicosapentaenoic acid diet on humoral clotting and fibrinolysis parameters in Type 1 diabetes mellitus', Haemostasis 18, Suppl. 2, 27-28.

103. Nye, E.R., Ilsley, C.D.J., Ablett, M.B., Sutherland, W.H.F. and Ram, J. (1987) 'Effect of eicosapentaenoic acid (MaxEPA) on blood lipids, clinical course and coronary vasculature in patients after percutaneous transluminal coronary angioplasty: a comparison with aspirin/dipyridamole and a placebo', Abstr. Int. Symp. on Cholesterol control and cardiovascular diseases: prevention and therapy, Milan, July 7-9,1987, p. 153.
104. Renaud S. and Nordøy, A. (1983) 'Small is beautiful: α-linolenic acid and eicosapentaenoic acid in man', Lancet i, 1169.
105. Schmitz, J.M., Berg, E. van den, Prewitt, J.P., Malley, C.R., Willerson, J.T. and Dehmer, G.J. (1987) 'Dietary supplementation with n-3 fatty acids may reduce the rate of restenosis after coronary angioplasty', Clin. Res. 35, 6A.
106. Slack, J.D., Pinkerton, C.A., VanTassel, J., Orr, C.M., Scott, M., Allen, B. and Nasser, W.K. (1987) 'Can oral fish oil supplement minimize re-stenosis after percutaneous transluminal coronary angioplasty?' J.A.C.C. 9(2), 64A.
107. Grigg, L.E., Kay, T., Valentine, P.A., Larkins, R., Flower, D.J., Manolas, E.G., O'Dea, K., Sinclair, A.J., Hopper, J.L. and Hunt, D. (1989) 'Determinants of restenosis and lack of effect of dietary supplementation with eicosapentaenoic acid on the incidence of coronary artery restenosis after angioplasty', J. Am. Coll. Cardiol. 13, 665-672.
108. Reis, G.J., Boucher, T.M., Sipperly, M.E., Silvermann, D.I., McCabe, C.H., Baim, D.S., Sacks, F.M., Grossman, W. and Pasternak, R.C. (1989) 'Randomised trial of fish oil for prevention of restenosis after coronary angioplasty', Lancet ii, 177-181.
109. Hornstra, G. (1989) 'Influence of dietary fish oil on arterial thrombosis and atherosclerosis in animal models and in man', J. Int. Med. 225 Suppl. 1, 53-59.
110. Hornstra, G. (1989) 'Fish and the heart' (letter), Lancet ii: 1451.
111. Bang, H.O., Dyerberg, J. and Sinclair, H.M. (1980) 'The composition of the Eskimo food in north western Greenland', Am. J. Clin. Nutr. 33: 2657-2661.
112. Hornstra. G. (1978) 'The filtragometer in thrombosis research', in H.J. Day, H. Holmsen, and M.B. Zucker (eds.), Platelet function testing, DHEW Publication (no NIH 78-1087), US Department of health, education and wellfare, Public Health Service, National Institute of Health, pp. 416-427.
113. Weiss, H.J. (1982) 'Platelets, pathophysiology and antiplatelet drug therapy', Alan R. Liss. Inc. New York, 82-83.
114. Jørgensen, L., Haerem, F., Chandler, A.B. and Borchgrevink, C.F. (1968) 'The pathology of acute coronary death', Acta. Anaesth.Scand. Suppl. 29, 193-199.
115. Saynor, R., Verel, D. and Gillot, T. (1984) 'The long-term effect of dietary supplementation with fish lipid concentrate on serum lipids, bleeding time, platelets and angina', Atherosclerosis 50, 3-10.
116. Verheugt, F.W.A., Schouten, J.A., Eeltink, J.C. and Roos, J.P. (1986) 'Omega-3 polyunsaturated fatty acids in the treatment of angina pectoris: effect on objective signs of exercise-induced myocardial ischemia', Curr. Therap. Res. 39, 208-213.
117. Burr, M.L., Fehily, A.M., Gilbert, J.F. Rogers, S., Holliday, R.M., Sweetnam, P.M., Elwood, P.C. and Deadman, N.M. (1989) 'Effects of changes in fat, fish and fibre intakes on death and myocardial reinfarction: diet and reinfarction trial (DART)', Lancet ii, 757-761.
118. Reilly, I.A.G., Doran, J., Smith, B. and Fitzgerald, G.A. (1986) 'Increased thromboxane biosynthesis in a human model of platelet activation: biochemical and functional consequences of selective inhibition of thromboxane synthesis', Circulation 73, 1300-1309.

119. Woodcock, B.E., Smith, E., Lambert, W.H., Morris Jones, W., Galloway, J.H., Greaves, M. and Preston, F.E. (1984) 'Beneficial effect of fish oil on blood viscosity in peripheral vascular disease', Brit. Med. J. 288, 592-594.
120. Knapp, H.R., Whittemore, K.L. and FitzGerald, G.A. (1987) 'Dietary unsaturates and human vascular function', in W.E.M. Lands (ed), Polyunsaturated fatty acids and eicosanoids, American Oil Chemists' Society, pp. 41-55.
121. Sakurai, K., Akabe, N., Sano, F., Washio, M., Mishima, Y., Miyazawa, Y., Terashima, M., Kamiya, K., Inada, K., Matsumoto, K., Okada, M. and Katsumura, T. (1987) 'Clinical results of MND-21 on chronic arterial occlusion', Rinsho Iyaku 3, 605-612.
122. Cartwright, I.J., Pockley, A.G., Galloway, J.H., Greaves, M. and Preston, F.E. (1985) 'The effects of dietary ω-3 polyunsaturated fatty acids on erythrocyte membrane phospholipids, erythrocyte deformability and blood viscosity in healthy volunteers', Atherosclerosis 55, 267-281.
123. Hirai, A., Terano, T., Saito, H., Tamura, Y. and Yoshida, S. (1984) 'Eicosapentaenoic acid and platelet function in Japanese', in W. Lovenberg and Y. Yamori (eds.), Nutritional prevention of cardiovascular disease, Academic Press, pp. 231-239.
124. Kobayashi, S., Hirai, A., Terano, T., Hamazaki, T., Tamura, Y. and Kumagai, A. (1981) 'Reduction in blood viscosity by eicosapentaenoic acid', Lancet ii, 197.
125. Miller, M.E., Anagnostou, A., Ley, B., Marshall, P. and Steiner, M. (1987) 'Effect of fish oil concentrate on hemorheological and hemostatic aspects of diabetes mellitus: a preliminary study', Thromb. Res. 47, 201-214.
126. Rillaerts, E.G., Engelmann, G.J., Kamp, K.M. van and Leeuw, I. de (1989) 'Effect of omega-3 fatty acids in diet on type I diabetic subjects on lipid values and hemorheological parameters', Diabetes 38, 1412-1416.
127. Tamura, Y., Hirai, A., Terano, T., Yoshida, S., Takenaga, M. and Kitagawa, H. (1987) 'Anti-thrombotic and anti-atherogenic action of eicosapentaenoic acid', Jap. Circ. J. 51, 471-477.
128. Bruckner, G., Webb, P., Greenwell, L., Chow, C. and Richardson, D. (1987) 'Fish oil increases peripheral capillary blood flow velocity in humans', Atherosclerosis 66, 237-245.
129. Hamazaki, T., Nakazawa, R., Tateno, S., Shihido, H., Isoda, K., Hattori, Y., Yoshida, T., Fujita, T., Yano S. and Kumagai, A. (1984) 'Effects of fish oil rich in eicosapentaenoic acid on serum lipid in hyperlipidemic hemodialysis patients', Kidney International 26, 81-84.
130. Housley, G., Born, G.V., Conroy, D.M., Belin, J. and Smith. A.D. (1986) 'Influence of dietary lipids on the effect of chlorpromazine on membrane properties of rabbit red cells', Proc. R. Soc. London [Biol] 227, 43-51.
131. Popp-Snijders, C., Schouten, J.A., Jong, A.P. de and Veen, E.A. van der (1984) 'Effect of dietary cod-liver oil on the lipid composition of human erythrocyte membranes', Scand. J. Clin. Lab. Invest. 44, 39-46.
132. Kamada, T., Yamashita, T., Baba, Y., Kai, M., Setoyama, S., Chuman, Y. and Otsuji, S. (1986) 'Dietary sardine oil increases erythrocyte membrane fluidity in diabetic patients', Diabetes 35, 604-611.
133. Popp-Snijders, C., Schouten, J.A., Heine, R.J., Meer, J. van der and Veen, E.A. van der (1987) 'Dietary supplementation of omega-3 polyunsaturated fatty acids improves insulin sensitivity in non-insulin-dependent diabetes', Diabetes Res. 4, 141-147.
134. Popp-Snijders, C., Schouten, J.A., Meer, J. van der, and Veen, E.A. van der (1986) 'Fatty fish-induced changes in membrane lipid composition and viscosity of human erythrocytes', Scand. J. Clin. Lab. Invest. 46, 253-258.

135. Hornstra, G. and Rand, M.L. (1986) 'Effect of dietary (n-6) and (n-3) polyunsaturated fatty acids on the fluidity of platelet membranes in rat and man', Progr. Lip. Res. 25, 637-638.

Index

acetylsalicylic acid (aspirin) 4, 55, 144, 224
adenosine diphosphate (ADP) 3, 51, 83
adenylate cyclase 85, 126
adhesion 68
adhesion molecules 168
ADP receptor antagonist 4, 88
adrenaline 55
alpha-granules 3
AMP-dependent protein kinase 121
amplification 187
angina pectoris 236
anti-aggregating agents 3, 121, 162, 223
α_2-antiplasmin 238
anti-platelet serum 51
antithrombin III (AT-III) 236
arachidonic acid 3, 56, 235
Arg-Gly-Asp (RGD) sequences 86
atherosclerosis 38, 63, 233

bleeding diathesis 31
bleeding time 51, 234
blood coagulation 235

c-fos proto-oncogene 67
c-myc 67
Ca^{2+} fluxes 88
Ca^{2+} indicators 100
Ca^{2+} influx 104
Ca^{2+} spiking 111
calcium channels 99, 125, 229
calcium mobilization 121
calmodulin 88
cAMP 85, 121, 169
cardiopulmonary bypass 51
cellular proliferation 206
cervonic acid 233
cGMP 7, 121
chemotactic 66
clinical efficacy of antithrombotic drugs 19
clinical trials 208
collagen 51, 75, 196
combination of antithrombotic drugs 14
combined thromboxane synthase inhibitors and thromboxane antagonists 6, 148
constitutive No synthase 37
coronary artery disease 239
cranial vasculature 198
creatine phosphate/creatine phosphokinase 88
cyclic nucleotide-dependent protein kinases 121
cyclooxygenase 55
cyclooxygenase inhibitors 4
cyclooxygenase metabolites 140
cytoprotective properties 38

11-dehydro-thromboxane B_2 54
dense granules 3
desintegrins 90
DHA 233
diacylglycerol 102
diet 170, 239
dietary marine lipids 233
2,3-dinor-thromboxane B_2 54
dipyridamole 88, 169
docosahexaenoic acid (DHA) 233
dog models 221

eicosapentaenoic acid (EPA) 57, 233
endothelial cells 29, 99, 121
endothelial denudation 64
endothelium-derived relaxing factor (EDRF) 121
endotoxin shock 31
endotoxins 31
epidermal growth factor (EGF) 66
Eskimos 236, 237
eversion graft model 226
excitatory messenger 108
exercise 239

factor VII 236
factor X 236
fat intake 239
fibre 240
fibrinogen 50, 236
fibrinogen receptor 85
fibrinogen-related peptides 90
fibrinolysis 237
fish oil 57, 234
foamy macrophages 75
fura-2 101

G-proteins 86
Glanzmann's thrombasthenia 86
glucocorticoids 32
glycoprotein (GP)IIb-IIIa complex 83, 106
GMP-dependent protein kinase 121
GP IIb-IIIa-related peptides 90

GP IIb-IIIa structure [24, 25] 85
GPIIb/IIIa receptor 2, 12, 85
growth factors 3
guanylate cyclase 28, 126

12-HETE 163
13-HODE 166
human coronary arteries 68
12-hydroxyeicosatetraenoic acid (12-HETE) 163
13-hydroxyoctadecadienoic acid (13-HODE) 166
5-hydroxytryptamine (5-HT, serotonin) 3, 50, 181
5-HT_2 antigonists 4, 186
hypercholesterolaemia 52
hyperlipidaemic 68

iloprost 88, 205
immune thrombocytopenic purpura 52
indo-1 101
inducible NO synthase 32, 37
inositol 1,4,5-trisphosphate, (IP_3) 102
interferon-γ 32
interleukin-1 67
intermittent claudication 240
intimal thickening 64
ischaemic heart disease 63, 239

ketanserin 186

L-arginine 28

LDL-receptors 207
linoleic acid 166
linolenic acid 170
lipid metabolism 206
lipopolysaccharides 31
lypoxygenase pathway 159

macrophages 68
megakaryocytes 49, 51
membrane fluidity 240
Mn^{2+} 105
molsidomine 36
monoclonal antibodies against GP IIb-IIIa 89
myocardial infarction 49, 63, 221, 235
myosin light chain kinase 109

N^G-monomethyl-L-arginine (L-NMMA) 32
N^G-nitro-L-argon arginine methyl ester (L-NAME) 198
N-iminoethyl-L-arginine (L-NIO) 32
nitric oxide 13, 28, 198
nitroprusside (SNP) 36
nitrovasodilators 35
NO-donors 206

oxyhaemoglobin (Hb) 35

PAF 195
PAF antagonists 4, 195
peripheral vascular disease 239
PGE_1 205
PGE_2 86
PGH_2 84
PGI_2 205
phosphodiesterase 126
phosphodiesterase inhibitors 11, 88, 169
phospholipase C 102, 123
phospholipids 235
plaque injury 63, 75
plasma viscosity 240
plasminogen activator 237
plasminogen activator inhibitor 237
platelet aggregation 83, 234
platelet count 51
platelet derived growth factor (PDGF) 50, 66
platelet factor 4, 55
platelet hypertransfusion 51
platelet inhibitors 121
platelet mass 51
platelet-release reaction 57
platelet survival time 235
platelet volume 51
ploidy 50
potentiation 84
prostacyclin (PGI_2) 13, 121, 205
prostaglandins 205
protein C 236
protein kinase C 102
PTCA 238

quin2 100

receptor-mediated calcium entry 112
receptor-operated calcium channel 125, 129
red cell deformability 240
reocclusion 223
reperfusion 223
S-nitroso-N-acetylpenicillamine (SNAP) 36
salicylate 169
saturated fatty acids 239
septicaemia 31
serotonin 3, 50, 181
shear stress 35
SIN-1 36

spontaneous platelet aggregation 57
stable angina 63
streptokinase (SK) 221
sudden death 49, 63
sulphinpyrazone 57
superoxide anions (O_2^-) 35
synergism 31, 206

taprostene 205
thienopyridines 89
thrombin 196
thrombin inhibitors 228
thrombogenesis 50
β-thromboglobulin 51
thrombolytic therapy 221
thromboses 31, 86, 233, 238
thromboxane A_2 (TXA_2) 3, 50, 84, 235
thromboxane A_2/PGH_2-receptor 142
thromboxane receptor antagonists 6, 147
thromboxane synthase inhibitors 5, 146
thrombus formation 189, 206, 224
ticlopidine 89
timnodonic acid 233, 235
tissue-type plasminogen activator (t-PA) 221
transforming growth factor beta 67

unstable angina 49, 55, 63
uraemia 32
urokinase (UK) 222

vascular proliferation 183
vascular tone 123, 141, 184, 235
vessel wall thrombogenecity 165
vincristine 51
vitronectin receptor 167

Developments in Cardiovascular Medicine

1. Ch.T. Lancée (ed.): *Echocardiology*. 1979 ISBN 90-247-2209-8
2. J. Baan, A.C. Arntzenius and E.L. Yellin (eds.): *Cardiac Dynamics*. 1980 ISBN 90-247-2212-8
3. H.J.Th. Thalen and C.C. Meere (eds.): *Fundamentals of Cardiac Pacing*. 1979 ISBN 90-247-2245-4
4. H.E. Kulbertus and H.J.J. Wellens (eds.): *Sudden Death*. 1980 ISBN 90-247-2290-X
5. L.S. Dreifus and A.N. Brest (eds.): *Clinical Applications of Cardiovascular Drugs*. 1980 ISBN 90-247-2295-0
6. M.P. Spencer and J.M. Reid: *Cerebrovascular Evaluation with Doppler Ultrasound*. With contributions by E.C. Brockenbrough, R.S. Reneman, G.I. Thomas and D.L. Davis. 1981 ISBN 90-247-2384-1
7. D.P. Zipes, J.C. Bailey and V. Elharrar (eds.): *The Slow Inward Current and Cardiac Arrhythmias*. 1980 ISBN 90-247-2380-9
8. H. Kesteloot and J.V. Joossens (eds.): *Epidemiology of Arterial Blood Pressure*. 1980 ISBN 90-247-2386-8
9. F.J.Th. Wackers (ed.): *Thallium-201 and Technetium-99m-Pyrophosphate. Myocardial Imaging in the Coronary Care Unit*. 1980 ISBN 90-247-2396-5
10. A. Maseri, C. Marchesi, S. Chierchia and M.G. Trivella (eds.): *Coronary Care Units*. Proceedings of a European Seminar, held in Pisa, Italy (1978). 1981 ISBN 90-247-2456-2
11. J. Morganroth, E.N. Moore, L.S. Dreifus and E.L. Michelson (eds.): *The Evaluation of New Antiarrhythmic Drugs*. Proceedings of the First Symposium on New Drugs and Devices, held in Philadelphia, Pa., U.S.A. (1980). 1981 ISBN 90-247-2474-0
12. P. Alboni: *Intraventricular Conduction Disturbances*. 1981 ISBN 90-247-2483-X
13. H. Rijsterborgh (ed.): *Echocardiology*. 1981 ISBN 90-247-2491-0
14. G.S. Wagner (ed.): *Myocardial Infarction*. Measurement and Intervention. 1982 ISBN 90-247-2513-5
15. R.S. Meltzer and J. Roelandt (eds.): *Contrast Echocardiography*. 1982 ISBN 90-247-2531-3
16. A. Amery, R. Fagard, P. Lijnen and J. Staessen (eds.): *Hypertensive Cardiovascular Disease*. Pathophysiology and Treatment. 1982 IBSN 90-247-2534-8
17. L.N. Bouman and H.J. Jongsma (eds.): *Cardiac Rate and Rhythm*. Physiological, Morphological and Developmental Aspects. 1982 ISBN 90-247-2626-3
18. J. Morganroth and E.N. Moore (eds.): *The Evaluation of Beta Blocker and Calcium Antagonist Drugs*. Proceedings of the 2nd Symposium on New Drugs and Devices, held in Philadelphia, Pa., U.S.A. (1981). 1982 ISBN 90-247-2642-5
19. M.B. Rosenbaum and M.V. Elizari (eds.): *Frontiers of Cardiac Electrophysiology*. 1983 ISBN 90-247-2663-8
20. J. Roelandt and P.G. Hugenholtz (eds.): *Long-term Ambulatory Electrocardiography*. 1982 ISBN 90-247-2664-6
21. A.A.J. Adgey (ed.): *Acute Phase of Ischemic Heart Disease and Myocardial Infarction*. 1982 ISBN 90-247-2675-1
22. P. Hanrath, W. Bleifeld and J. Souquet (eds.): *Cardiovascular Diagnosis by Ultrasound*. Transesophageal, Computerized, Contrast, Doppler Echocardiography. 1982 ISBN 90-247-2692-1

Developments in Cardiovascular Medicine

23. J. Roelandt (ed.): *The Practice of M-Mode and Two-dimensional Echocardiography.* 1983 ISBN 90-247-2745-6
24. J. Meyer, P. Schweizer and R. Erbel (eds.): *Advances in Noninvasive Cardiology.* Ultrasound, Computed Tomography, Radioisotopes, Digital Angiography. 1983 ISBN 0-89838-576-8
25. J. Morganroth and E.N. Moore (eds.): *Sudden Cardiac Death and Congestive Heart Failure.* Diagnosis and Treatment. Proceedings of the 3rd Symposium on New Drugs and Devices, held in Philadelphia, Pa., U.S.A. (1982). 1983 ISBN 0-89838-580-6
26. H.M. Perry Jr. (ed.): *Lifelong Management of Hypertension.* 1983 ISBN 0-89838-582-2
27. E.A. Jaffe (ed.): *Biology of Endothelial Cells.* 1984 ISBN 0-89838-587-3
28. B. Surawicz, C.P. Reddy and E.N. Prystowsky (eds.): *Tachycardias.* 1984 ISBN 0-89838-588-1
29. M.P. Spencer (ed.): *Cardiac Doppler Diagnosis.* Proceedings of a Symposium, held in Clearwater, Fla., U.S.A. (1983). 1983 ISBN 0-89838-591-1
30. H. Villarreal and M.P. Sambhi (eds.): *Topics in Pathophysiology of Hypertension.* 1984 ISBN 0-89838-595-4
31. F.H. Messerli (ed.): *Cardiovascular Disease in the Elderly.* 1984 Revised edition, 1988: see below under Volume 76
32. M.L. Simoons and J.H.C. Reiber (eds.): *Nuclear Imaging in Clinical Cardiology.* 1984 ISBN 0-89838-599-7
33. H.E.D.J. ter Keurs and J.J. Schipperheyn (eds.): *Cardiac Left Ventricular Hypertrophy.* 1983 ISBN 0-89838-612-8
34. N. Sperelakis (ed.): *Physiology and Pathology of the Heart.* 1984 Revised edition, 1988: see below under Volume 90
35. F.H. Messerli (ed.): *Kidney in Essential Hypertension.* Proceedings of a Course, held in New Orleans, La., U.S.A. (1983). 1984 ISBN 0-89838-616-0
36. M.P. Sambhi (ed.): *Fundamental Fault in Hypertension.* 1984 ISBN 0-89838-638-1
37. C. Marchesi (ed.): *Ambulatory Monitoring.* Cardiovascular System and Allied Applications. Proceedings of a Workshop, held in Pisa, Italy (1983). 1984 ISBN 0-89838-642-X
38. W. Kupper, R.N. MacAlpin and W. Bleifeld (eds.): *Coronary Tone in Ischemic Heart Disease.* 1984 ISBN 0-89838-646-2
39. N. Sperelakis and J.B. Caulfield (eds.): *Calcium Antagonists.* Mechanism of Action on Cardiac Muscle and Vascular Smooth Muscle. Proceedings of the 5th Annual Meeting of the American Section of the I.S.H.R., held in Hilton Head, S.C., U.S.A. (1983). 1984 ISBN 0-89838-655-1
40. Th. Godfraind, A.G. Herman and D. Wellens (eds.): *Calcium Entry Blockers in Cardiovascular and Cerebral Dysfunctions.* 1984 ISBN 0-89838-658-6
41. J. Morganroth and E.N. Moore (eds.): *Interventions in the Acute Phase of Myocardial Infarction.* Proceedings of the 4th Symposium on New Drugs and Devices, held in Philadelphia, Pa., U.S.A. (1983). 1984 ISBN 0-89838-659-4
42. F.L. Abel and W.H. Newman (eds.): *Functional Aspects of the Normal, Hypertrophied and Failing Heart.* Proceedings of the 5th Annual Meeting of the American Section of the I.S.H.R., held in Hilton Head, S.C., U.S.A. (1983). 1984 ISBN 0-89838-665-9

Developments in Cardiovascular Medicine

43. S. Sideman and R. Beyar (eds.): [3-D] *Simulation and Imaging of the Cardiac System.* State of the Heart. Proceedings of the International Henry Goldberg Workshop, held in Haifa, Israel (1984). 1985 ISBN 0-89838-687-X
44. E. van der Wall and K.I. Lie (eds.): *Recent Views on Hypertrophic Cardiomyopathy.* Proceedings of a Symposium, held in Groningen, The Netherlands (1984). 1985 ISBN 0-89838-694-2
45. R.E. Beamish, P.K. Singal and N.S. Dhalla (eds.), *Stress and Heart Disease.* Proceedings of a International Symposium, held in Winnipeg, Canada, 1984 (Vol. 1). 1985 ISBN 0-89838-709-4
46. R.E. Beamish, V. Panagia and N.S. Dhalla (eds.): *Pathogenesis of Stress-induced Heart Disease.* Proceedings of a International Symposium, held in Winnipeg, Canada, 1984 (Vol. 2). 1985 ISBN 0-89838-710-8
47. J. Morganroth and E.N. Moore (eds.): *Cardiac Arrhythmias.* New Therapeutic Drugs and Devices. Proceedings of the 5th Symposium on New Drugs and Devices, held in Philadelphia, Pa., U.S.A. (1984). 1985 ISBN 0-89838-716-7
48. P. Mathes (ed.): *Secondary Prevention in Coronary Artery Disease and Myocardial Infarction.* 1985 ISBN 0-89838-736-1
49. H.L. Stone and W.B. Weglicki (eds.): *Pathobiology of Cardiovascular Injury.* Proceedings of the 6th Annual Meeting of the American Section of the I.S.H.R., held in Oklahoma City, Okla., U.S.A. (1984). 1985 ISBN 0-89838-743-4
50. J. Meyer, R. Erbel and H.J. Rupprecht (eds.): *Improvement of Myocardial Perfusion.* Thrombolysis, Angioplasty, Bypass Surgery. Proceedings of a Symposium, held in Mainz, F.R.G. (1984). 1985 ISBN 0-89838-748-5
51. J.H.C. Reiber, P.W. Serruys and C.J. Slager (eds.): *Quantitative Coronary and Left Ventricular Cineangiography.* Methodology and Clinical Applications. 1986 ISBN 0-89838-760-4
52. R.H. Fagard and I.E. Bekaert (eds.): *Sports Cardiology.* Exercise in Health and Cardiovascular Disease. Proceedings from an International Conference, held in Knokke, Belgium (1985). 1986 ISBN 0-89838-782-5
53. J.H.C. Reiber and P.W. Serruys (eds.): *State of the Art in Quantitative Cornary Arteriography.* 1986 ISBN 0-89838-804-X
54. J. Roelandt (ed.): *Color Doppler Flow Imaging and Other Advances in Doppler Echocardiography.* 1986 ISBN 0-89838-806-6
55. E.E. van der Wall (ed.): *Noninvasive Imaging of Cardiac Metabolism.* Single Photon Scintigraphy, Positron Emission Tomography and Nuclear Magnetic Resonance. 1987 ISBN 0-89838-812-0
56. J. Liebman, R. Plonsey and Y. Rudy (eds.): *Pediatric and Fundamental Electrocardiography.* 1987 ISBN 0-89838-815-5
57. H.H. Hilger, V. Hombach and W.J. Rashkind (eds.), *Invasive Cardiovascular Therapy.* Proceedings of an International Symposium, held in Cologne, F.R.G. (1985). 1987 ISBN 0-89838-818-X
58. P.W. Serruys and G.T. Meester (eds.): *Coronary Angioplasty.* A Controlled Model for Ischemia. 1986 ISBN 0-89838-819-8
59. J.E. Tooke and L.H. Smaje (eds.): *Clinical Investigation of the Microcirculation.* Proceedings of an International Meeting, held in London, U.K. (1985). 1987 ISBN 0-89838-833-3

Developments in Cardiovascular Medicine

60. R.Th. van Dam and A. van Oosterom (eds.): *Electrocardiographic Body Surface Mapping*. Proceedings of the 3rd International Symposium on B.S.M., held in Nijmegen, The Netherlands (1985). 1986 ISBN 0-89838-834-1
61. M.P. Spencer (ed.): *Ultrasonic Diagnosis of Cerebrovascular Disease*. Doppler Techniques and Pulse Echo Imaging. 1987 ISBN 0-89838-836-8
62. M.J. Legato (ed.): *The Stressed Heart*. 1987 ISBN 0-89838-849-X
63. M.E. Safar (ed.): *Arterial and Venous Systems in Essential Hypertension*. With Assistance of G.M. London, A.Ch. Simon and Y.A. Weiss. 1987 ISBN 0-89838-857-0
64. J. Roelandt (ed.): *Digital Techniques in Echocardiography*. 1987 ISBN 0-89838-861-9
65. N.S. Dhalla, P.K. Singal and R.E. Beamish (eds.): *Pathology of Heart Disease*. Proceedings of the 8th Annual Meeting of the American Section of the I.S.H.R., held in Winnipeg, Canada, 1986 (Vol. 1). 1987 ISBN 0-89838-864-3
66. N.S. Dhalla, G.N. Pierce and R.E. Beamish (eds.): *Heart Function and Metabolism*. Proceedings of the 8th Annual Meeting of the American Section of the I.S.H.R., held in Winnipeg, Canada, 1986 (Vol. 2). 1987 ISBN 0-89838-865-1
67. N.S. Dhalla, I.R. Innes and R.E. Beamish (eds.): *Myocardial Ischemia*. Proceedings of a Satellite Symposium of the 30th International Physiological Congress, held in Winnipeg, Canada (1986). 1987 ISBN 0-89838-866-X
68. R.E. Beamish, V. Panagia and N.S. Dhalla (eds.): *Pharmacological Aspects of Heart Disease*. Proceedings of an International Symposium, held in Winnipeg, Canada (1986). 1987 ISBN 0-89838-867-8
69. H.E.D.J. ter Keurs and J.V. Tyberg (eds.): *Mechanics of the Circulation*. Proceedings of a Satellite Symposium of the 30th International Physiological Congress, held in Banff, Alberta, Canada (1986). 1987 ISBN 0-89838-870-8
70. S. Sideman and R. Beyar (eds.): *Activation, Metabolism and Perfusion of the Heart*. Simulation and Experimental Models. Proceedings of the 3rd Henry Goldberg Workshop, held in Piscataway, N.J., U.S.A. (1986). 1987 ISBN 0-89838-871-6
71. E. Aliot and R. Lazzara (eds.): *Ventricular Tachycardias*. From Mechanism to Therapy. 1987 ISBN 0-89838-881-3
72. A. Schneeweiss and G. Schettler: *Cardiovascular Drug Therapoy in the Elderly*. 1988 ISBN 0-89838-883-X
73. J.V. Chapman and A. Sgalambro (eds.): *Basic Concepts in Doppler Echocardiography*. Methods of Clinical Applications based on a Multi-modality Doppler Approach. 1987 ISBN 0-89838-888-0
74. S. Chien, J. Dormandy, E. Ernst and A. Matrai (eds.): *Clinical Hemorheology*. Applications in Cardiovascular and Hematological Disease, Diabetes, Surgery and Gynecology. 1987 ISBN 0-89838-807-4
75. J. Morganroth and E.N. Moore (eds.): *Congestive Heart Failure*. Proceedings of the 7th Annual Symposium on New Drugs and Devices, held in Philadelphia, Pa., U.S.A. (1986). 1987 ISBN 0-89838-955-0
76. F.H. Messerli (ed.): *Cardiovascular Disease in the Elderly*. 2nd ed. 1988 ISBN 0-89838-962-3
77. P.H. Heintzen and J.H. Bürsch (eds.): *Progress in Digital Angiocardiography*. 1988 ISBN 0-89838-965-8

Developments in Cardiovascular Medicine

78. M.M. Scheinman (ed.): *Catheter Ablation of Cardiac Arrhythmias.* Basic Bioelectrical Effects and Clinical Indications. 1988 ISBN 0-89838-967-4
79. J.A.E. Spaan, A.V.G. Bruschke and A.C. Gittenberger-De Groot (eds.): *Coronary Circulation.* From Basic Mechanisms to Clinical Implications. 1987 ISBN 0-89838-978-X
80. C. Visser, G. Kan and R.S. Meltzer (eds.): *Echocardiography in Coronary Artery Disease.* 1988 ISBN 0-89838-979-8
81. A. Bayés de Luna, A. Betriu and G. Permanyer (eds.): *Therapeutics in Cardiology.* 1988 ISBN 0-89838-981-X
82. D.M. Mirvis (ed.): *Body Surface Electrocardiographic Mapping.* 1988 ISBN 0-89838-983-6
83. M.A. Konstam and J.M. Isner (eds.): *The Right Ventricle.* 1988 ISBN 0-89838-987-9
84. C.T. Kappagoda and P.V. Greenwood (eds.): *Long-term Management of Patients after Myocardial Infarction.* 1988 ISBN 0-89838-352-8
85. W.H. Gaasch and H.J. Levine (eds.): *Chronic Aortic Regurgitation.* 1988 ISBN 0-89838-364-1
86. P.K. Singal (ed.): *Oxygen Radicals in the Pathophysiology of Heart Disease.* 1988 ISBN 0-89838-375-7
87. J.H.C. Reiber and P.W. Serruys (eds.): *New Developments in Quantitative Coronary Arteriography.* 1988 ISBN 0-89838-377-3
88. J. Morganroth and E.N. Moore (eds.): *Silent Myocardial Ischemia.* Proceedings of the 8th Annual Symposium on New Drugs and Devices (1987). 1988 ISBN 0-89838-380-3
89. H.E.D.J. ter Keurs and M.I.M. Noble (eds.): *Starling's Law of the Heart Revisted.* 1988 ISBN 0-89838-382-X
90. N. Sperelakis (ed.): *Physiology and Pathophysiology of the Heart.* (Rev. ed.) 1988 ISBN 0-89838-388-9
91. J.W. de Jong (ed.): *Myocardial Energy Metabolism.* 1988 ISBN 0-89838-394-3
92. V. Hombach, H.H. Hilger and H.L. Kennedy (eds.): *Electrocardiography and Cardiac Drug Therapy.* Proceedings of an International Symposium, held in Cologne, F.R.G. (1987). 1988 ISBN 0-89838-395-1
93. H. Iwata, J.B. Lombardini and T. Segawa (eds.): *Taurine and the Heart.* 1988 ISBN 0-89838-396-X
94. M.R. Rosen and Y. Palti (eds.): *Lethal Arrhythmias Resulting from Myocardial Ischemia and Infarction.* Proceedings of the 2nd Rappaport Symposium, held in Haifa, Israel (1988). 1988 ISBN 0-89838-401-X
95. M. Iwase and I. Sotobata: *Clinical Echocardiography.* With a Foreword by M.P. Spencer. 1989 ISBN 0-7923-0004-1
96. I. Cikes (ed.): *Echocardiography in Cardiac Interventions.* 1989 ISBN 0-7923-0088-2
97. E. Rapaport (ed.): *Early Interventions in Acute Myocardial Infarction.* 1989 ISBN 0-7923-0175-7
98. M.E. Safar and F. Fouad-Tarazi (eds.): *The Heart in Hypertension.* A Tribute to Robert C. Tarazi (1925-1986). 1989 ISBN 0-7923-0197-8
99. S. Meerbaum and R. Meltzer (eds.): *Myocardial Contrast Two-dimensional Echocardiography.* 1989 ISBN 0-7923-0205-2

Developments in Cardiovascular Medicine

100. J. Morganroth and E.N. Moore (eds.): *Risk/Benefit Analysis for the Use and Approval of Thrombolytic, Antiarrhythmic, and Hypolipidemic Agents.* Proceedings of the 9th Annual Symposium on New Drugs and Devices (1988). 1989 ISBN 0-7923-0294-X
101. P.W. Serruys, R. Simon and K.J. Beatt (eds.): *PTCA - An Investigational Tool and a Non-operative Treatment of Acute Ischemia.* 1990 ISBN 0-7923-0346-6
102. I.S. Anand, P.I. Wahi and N.S. Dhalla (eds.): *Pathophysiology and Pharmacology of Heart Disease.* 1989 ISBN 0-7923-0367-9
103. G.S. Abela (ed.): *Lasers in Cardiovascular Medicine and Surgery.* Fundamentals and Technique. 1990 ISBN 0-7923-0440-3
104. H.M. Piper (ed.): *Pathophysiology of Severe Ischemic Myocardial Injury.* 1990 ISBN 0-7923-0459-4
105. S.M. Teague (ed.): *Stress Doppler Echocardiography.* 1990 ISBN 0-7923-0499-3
106. P.R. Saxena, D.I. Wallis, W. Wouters and P. Bevan (eds.): *Cardiovascular Pharmacology of 5-Hydroxytryptamine.* Prospective Therapeutic Applications. 1990 ISBN 0-7923-0502-7
107. A.P. Shepherd and P.A. Öberg (eds.): *Laser-Doppler Blood Flowmetry.* 1990 ISBN 0-7923-0508-6
108. J. Soler-Soler, G. Permanyer-Miralda and J. Sagristà-Sauleda (eds.): *Pericardial Disease.* New Insights and Old Dilemmas. Preface by Ralph Shabetai. 1990 ISBN 0-7923-0510-8
109. J.P.M. Hamer: *Practical Echocardiography in the Adult.* With Doppler and Color-Doppler Flow Imaging. 1990 ISBN 0-7923-0670-8
110. A. Bayés de Luna, P. Brugada, J. Cosin Aguilar and F. Navarro Lopez (eds.): *Sudden Cardiac Death.* 1991 ISBN 0-7923-0716-X
111. E. Andries and R. Stroobandt (eds.): *Hemodynamics in Daily Practice.* 1991 ISBN 0-7923-0725-9
112. J. Morganroth and E.N. Moore (eds.): *Use and Approval of Antihypertensive Agents and Surrogate Endpoints for the Approval of Drugs affecting Antiarrhythmic Heart Failure and Hypolipidemia.* Proceedings of the 10th Annual Symposium on New Drugs and Devices (1989). 1990 ISBN 0-7923-0756-9
113. S. Iliceto, P. Rizzon and J.R.T.C. Roelandt (eds.): *Ultrasound in Coronary Artery Disease.* Present Role and Future Perspectives. 1990 ISBN 0-7923-0784-4
114. J.V. Chapman and G.R. Sutherland (eds.): *The Noninvasive Evaluation of Hemodynamics in Congenital Heart Disease.* Doppler Ultrasound Applications in the Adult and Pediatric Patient with Congenital Heart Disease. 1990 ISBN 0-7923-0836-0
115. G.T. Meester and F. Pinciroli (eds.): *Databases for Cardiology.* 1991 ISBN 0-7923-0886-7
116. B. Korecky and N.S. Dhalla (eds.): *Subcellular Basis of Contractile Failure.* 1990 ISBN 0-7923-0890-5
117. J.H.C. Reiber and P.W. Serruys (eds.): *Quantitative Coronary Arteriography.* 1991 ISBN 0-7923-0913-8
118. E. van der Wall and A. de Roos (eds.): *Magnetic Resonance Imaging in Coronary Artery Disease.* 1991 ISBN 0-7923-0940-5
119. V. Hombach, M. Kochs and A.J. Camm (eds.): *Interventional Techniques in Cardiovascular Medicine.* 1991 ISBN 0-7923-0956-1

Developments in Cardiovascular Medicine

120. R. Vos: *Drugs Looking for Diseases.* Innovative Drug Research and the Development of the Beta Blockers and the Calcium Antagonists. 1991 ISBN 0-7923-0968-5
121. S. Sideman, R. Beyar and A. G. Kleber (eds.): *Cardiac Electrophysiology, Circulation, and Transport.* Proceedings of the 7th Henry Goldberg Workshop (Berne, Switzerland, 1990). 1991 ISBN 0-7923-1145-0
122. D.M. Bers: *Excitation-Contraction Coupling and Cardiac Contractile Force.* 1991 ISBN 0-7923-1186-8
123. A.-M. Salmasi and A.N. Nicolaides (eds.): *Diagnosis, Assessment and Management.* 1991 ISBN 0-7923-1188-4
124. J.A.E. Spaan: *Coronary Blood Flow.* Mechanics, Distribution, and Control. 1991 ISBN 0-7923-1210-4
125. R.W. Stout (ed.): *Diabetes and Atherosclerosis.* 1991 ISBN 0-7923-1310-0

Previous volumes are still available

KLUWER ACADEMIC PUBLISHERS – DORDRECHT / BOSTON / LONDON